UROLOGY

A CORE TEXTBOOK

UROLOGY
A CORE TEXTBOOK

Stephen N. Rous, A.B., M.D., M.S. (Urology), F.A.C.S., F.A.A.P.
Professor and Chairman, Department of Urology
Medical University of South Carolina, Charleston, South Carolina
Urologist-in-Chief, Medical University Hospital;
Consultant in Urology, Veterans Administration Hospital,
Charleston, South Carolina
Colonel, United States Air Force Reserve, Medical Corps
and Military Consultant for Urology to the Surgeon General,
United States Air Force

 APPLETON-CENTURY-CROFTS/Norwalk, Connecticut

0-8385-9317-8

Notice: Our knowledge in clinical sciences is constantly changing. As new information becomes available, changes in treatment and in the use of drugs become necessary. The author(s) and the publisher of this volume have taken care to make certain that the doses of drugs and schedules of treatment are correct and compatible with the standards generally accepted at the time of publication. The reader is advised to consult carefully the instruction and information material included in the package insert of each drug or therapeutic agent before administration. This advice is especially important when using new or infrequently used drugs.

85 86 87 88 89/10 9 8 7 6 5 4 3 2 1

Prentice-Hall of Australia, Pty. Ltd., Sydney
Prentice-Hall Canada, Inc.
Prentice-Hall Hispanoamericana, S.A., Mexico
Prentice-Hall of India Private Limited, New Delhi
Prentice-Hall International (UK) Limited, London
Prentice-Hall of Japan, Inc., Tokyo
Prentice-Hall of Southeast Asia (Pte.) Ltd., Singapore
Whitehall Books Ltd., Wellington, New Zealand
Editora Prentice-Hall do Brasil Ltda., Rio de Janeiro

Library of Congress Cataloging in Publication Data

Rous, Stephen N. (Stephen Norman), 1931-
  Urology : a core textbook.

  Rev. ed of: Urology in primary care. 1976.
  Includes bibliographies and index.
  1. Genito-urinary organs—Diseases. 2. Urology.
I. Rous, Stephen N. (Stephen Norman), 1931-
Urology in primary care. II. Title. [DNLM: 1. Urologic
Diseases.   WJ 100 R863u]
RC871.R687 1985   616.6   85-3894
ISBN 0-8385-9317-8

Design: Jean M. Sabato-Morley

PRINTED IN THE UNITED STATES OF AMERICA

*This book is lovingly dedicated to
my darling wife, Margot—still and always the
World's Greatest Woman*

Contents

Preface

It is fitting and proper that this textbook should have a different title and a different publisher than the one I wrote in 1976, which was called "Urology in Primary Care." The present book has been rewritten extensively, many new sections have been added, most of the illustrations are new, and the remarkable advances of the last seveal years in urologic diagnosis and management have been incorporated into the text. Notwithstanding the foregoing, however, the purpose of this book remains the same as it was for its predecessor—that is to address and to cover that body of urologic knowlege worthy of assimilation and mastery by both the medical student and primary care physician. Moreover, this book remains faithful to the basic concept of learning by specific educational objectives rather than by immersion or total inundation in the subject. This book is *not* intended to cover the entire field of urology *nor* is it intended to serve as a text or guide for the practicing urologist or urology resident.

Many medical textbook authors seek to put *all* of their knowledge into a literary effort and make no attempt at all to transmit information selectively based upon the audience for whom the book is intended. They may be motivated by a desire to be honored by their peers for having written a comprehensive text; it should not be forgotten, however, that it is generally easier to be all inclusive in a textbook than it is to discriminate selectively between items that are germane for the intended audience and those that are not. Certainly, there is no disagreement among *any* authors about the fact that the expected level of learning in urology (or any other academic discipline) is quite different for a medical student than it is for a urology resident or a practicing urologist. The problem, then, would appear to be in defining the body of knowledge (see Introduction) necessary for the medical student and then incorporating it in a text while making a conscious effort to *omit* those things that may be vitally important to the urologist but are simply not germane to the needs of the medical student.

This text, therefore, remains faithful to the earlier text in its commitment to selective learning by educational objectives while including the most recent changes and advances in urology, as well as the revisions, and the cumulative suggestions that have arisen in the 9 years of continuous use by hundreds of third-year medical students that the author has been priviledged to teach. Some objectives have been reworded, others have been better combined, and still others have been brought abreast of the progress of medical science as regards diagnosis and management. Totally new in this book, since they were not inlcuded in the earlier book, are sections on the genitourinary history and physical exam and the section on diagnostic procedures has been greatly expanded to include the newer modalities that were not in use just a few short years ago. Studies such as computed tomography (CT) scanning, ultrasonography, nuclear magnetic resonance, urodynamic examinations, and some of the newer forms of renal scanning are all noted in this section. Newer forms of diagnosis and therapy for urolithiasis and advances in chemotherapy for certain cancers are also noted.

I am most appreciative of the understanding, the patience, and the help of Dr. Robert Nelson, Dr. Lee Nyberg, and Dr. William Turner, my colleagues in the urology department at the Medical University of South Carolina. I am particularly indebted to Dr. Turner for his invaluable assistance and his suggestions in preparing the chapter in this book on Pediatric Urology.

Dr. Nancy Curry of our radiology department has been tremendously helpful in sharing her expertise in diagnostic imaging with me. I would like to thank her, as well as her radiology department colleagues, Dr. Leone Gordon and Dr. John Stanley, for their help in locating certain x-rays that were so necessary for this book. Dr. Newton C. Brackett, a member of the nephrology division and an expert in the field of hypertension, was of invaluable assistance in reading over the material in the book relating to renal and adrenal hypertension and in suggesting appropriate changes, and I would also like to thank Dr. Edmund Farrar, Dr. Joseph John, and Dr. Victor DelBene of the infectious diseases division for their gracious assistance in helping me with the material on antimicrobials and mico-organisms. Dr. C. T. Fitts, Dr. P. R. Rajagopalan, and Ms. Donna Priester of the transplantation division were most gracious and helpful in assembling the material on end-stage renal disease and transplantation. Dr. Edward Bannister of the Department of Laboratory Medicine kindly shared with me some of his slides of the urinary sediment and Dr. Richard Dobson of the Dermatology Department was equally kind in providing needed slides of certain venereal lesions.

I also acknowledge with appreciation the suggestions regarding material to be covered in the field of urodynamics that were made by Dr. David Barrett of the Mayo Clinic and Dr. Frank Hinman of the University of California at San Francisco.

I am particularly indebted to Betty Goodwin, Chief of Illustration and Design in the Division of Audio-Visual Production, for her splendid art work and to the photography section of that same division for their excellent cooperation.

Chapter 17 of this book includes an evaluation and self-assessment protocol that has been taken, almost unchanged, from the 1976 textbook for which it was originally prepared. This protocol was assembled by Ms. Donna Edison and Dr. Sara A. Sprafka, who at that time were with the Office of Medical Education, Research, and Development at Michigan State University. Donna Edison is no longer at Michigan State and is now Dr. Donna Edison, a resident in psychiatry, and Dr. Sara Sprafka, still at Michigan State University, is now in the Department of Biomechanics.

Last, but far from least I wish to express my enormous gratitude to my secretary, Mrs. Susan Pullen, whose capacity for work is remarkable and whose cheerfulness and willingness to type, retype, and again retype made the task of putting this book together infinitely more pleasant than it might otherwise have been. I thank her.

Introduction

The objective of this book is to assist the medical student and perhaps the primary care physician in the recognition, assimilation, and mastery of those aspects of urology that are necessary for good patient care. These goals are as applicable to the primary care physician as they are to the graduating medical student since neither are likely to receive any additional instruction in urology.

A comprehensive text on a given subject is often far easier to write than a book for the primary care physician or the medical student. When writing for the specialist, an author can present every bit of available and conceivable knowledge about the subject that is known to him or her. In writing for the medical student, however, using a vast and ever-expanding body of knowledge, how does the author attempt to grasp and to emphasize those items that are essential but not redundant, encompassing but not superfluous? Moreover, once the desired body of knowledge has been defined, how should it best be presented for maximum learning and, most important, for adequate evaluation as to whether it has been learned. For example, if hematuria is considered to be an essential topic, it is not sufficient merely to say that all medical students must *know* about hematuria; this is ambiguous to the learner and difficult to evaluate. Know *what* about hematuria? Medical students need to know specifics about hematuria—color, urologic and non-urologic conditions causing it, diagnostic workup, and treatment, and each of these specifics must be clearly stated.

The concepts of deriving, stating, using, and examining by educational objective is not new to the professional educator, but it is new to physicians involved in medical education and to this date there are *still* very few departments in very few medical schools that actually teach by educational objectives. These objectives in the discipline of urology (or in any other discipline) must state precisely what the medical student must be able to *do*, such as list, describe, discuss, palpate, recognize, and identify; for example, the medical student must be able to *list the causes* of hematuria originating in the bladder.

When educational objectives are clearly and thoughtfully drawn up and presented in this manner, learning is greatly enhanced because (1) the learner knows exactly what is expected of him, (2) the faculty knows exactly what it is supposed to teach; (3) if the objective is clear, the best means to reach it are more readily determined (for example, if the objective is for the physician to be able to palpate a carcinoma of the prostate gland and identify it as such, then clearly the physician should practice using patient mannequins), (4) the likelihood of redundancy and duplication in teaching efforts among departments of a medical school is decreased if each has clearly stated educational objectives, and (5) the process of evaluation is made more precise and specific—individuals are evaluated precisely on those things deemed important enough to be educational objectives. For example, if an educational objective is to list the causes of hematuria originating in the bladder, then the evaluation of that objective simply involves taking that objective and making a question out of it. I feel that it is totally unfair to evaluate medical students on material that they have not been specifically told is subject to evaluation and it is even more unfair to evaluate medical students on material that has not been specifically covered.

Those educational objectives deemed "absolutely necessary" for every graduating medical student are clearly listed in this book at the beginning of each chapter in which those objectives are discussed and also at the very end of the book, in Chapter 17, where they will precede a self-assessment protocol that the student may study at his or her leisure. By perusing the educational objectives as each chapter is studied, the student will be aware of what he or she is expected to learn from the reading. Moreover, the material related to each educational objective is presented in such a manner that, hopefully, the learner will be able to understand the pathophysiology involved and thereby derive the answer to a given objective rather than learn it by rote.

Finally, one arrives at the key question: What material should be included in the educational objectives that have already been defined as "absolutely necessary" for every graduating medical student? Traditionally, the teaching content of medical disciplines has been developed by the professor, acting alone or in consulation with members of the full-time faculty. Commendable as these efforts have been, I feel that it is unrealistic to expect any one individual or group of individuals whose involvement with urology (or any other discipline) is exclusively academic to draw up a set of educational objectives that are applicable to every graduating medical student and will also have relevance to the real world of clinical urology as practiced by nonurologists. Academic urologists are not in an advantageous position to identify the urologic knowledge that will be necessary for the majority of medical school graduates who do not specialize in urology but who are involved in the delivery of primary health care, whether as family physicians, internists, obstetricians and gynecologists, or pediatricians.

Assuming that we train physicians for the purpose of caring for the sick, it should be the practicing primary care physician who tells us what material we should be teaching; that is, what material they have already found to be "absolutely necessary" for the successful outcome of their practice and what material they would like to know in order to better carry out their function.

Establishment of urologic objectives that are fundamental to all physicians regardless of their field of practice is a large endeavor. The starting point for determining which to present in this book was a comprehensive list of edcuational objectives that would cover virtually every aspect of urology up to and including material that a chief resident in urology would be happy to consider knowledge already mastered! Not included in this master list were objectives pertinent to actual surgical procedures because these are usually and properly carried out by specialists only. Also not included were objectives that could be considered as pure, basic science. A list of approximately 500 objectives was developed in this manner and then expanded upon by numerous academic urologists in an attempt to make it as comprehensive as possible. This was to be, then, the "master list" that presumably covers virtually all facets of urology (except as just noted) and from which the educational objectives necessary for the primary care physician would be derived. With the assistance of a team of computer experts and statisticians, this master list was then randomized as follows to 2200 practicing physicians across the United States: 500 members of the American Academy of Family Physicians in private practice, 500 board-certified pediatricians in private practice, 500 board-certified internists in private practice, 500 board-certified urologists in private practice, and the entire membership (200) of the Society of University Urologists. Those objectives deemed "necessary" for every graduating medical student by 70 percent or more of all respondents, plus those objectives felt to be necessary by 70 percent or more of the family physicians (the group identifying the largest number of "necessary" objectives) made up the final list of objectives, which numbered about 160. These constituted the required urologic educational objectives for medical students and formed the basis for the earlier textbook.

Although the original list of educational objectives was derived in the mid-1970s, I am certain that they are as germane today as they were then and as they will be 10 years from now. The objectives themselves are timeless: it is only the responses to these objectives that, in many cases, have changed and will continue to change. For example, "list the symptoms of acute cystitis," or "list the preferred antimicrobials in the treatment of acute cystitis" are objectives that do not change with time. The proper responses, however, obviously *do* change and will continue to do so, and one of the main reasons for writing the present book is to make the proper "responses" to the educational objectives current. In putting the present book together, I have felt it practical to combine some of these objectives and to add some as they applied to newer and changing methods of diagnosis and treatment in urology. For example, "list the indications for a CT scan of the kidneys" is an objective that obviously could not have been derived 10 years ago, but that is most important at this time.

It is my intention to discuss these objectives in sufficient detail in this book to allow the medical student to obtain a full and genuine comprehension of their meanings. I intend also to present these objectives, either visually or in a cognitive manner, in sufficient depth that they may be mastered by the student. This mastery may then be evaluated by means of the assessment test included in this book or, alternatively, the student can convert the educational objectives into questions and test his or her understanding by attempting to answer them.

I would point out that undoubtedly there are certain subjects discussed in this book that are not listed in the master list of educational objectives because, in my opinion, these subjects are so closely related to the objectives that failure to include them would have resulted in an inadequate presentation of the subject. It is of interest to note that in the intervening years since this list of "necessary" educational objectives was derived, it has been endorsed by the Education Council of the American Urological Association as recommended core material for medical students.

1
The Diagnostic Approach to the Urologic Patient

EDUCATIONAL OBJECTIVES

1. List the various symptoms that a patient might have in connection with the following kidney diseases: infection/inflammation, stones, kidney cancer.
2. Explain specifically why each of the symptoms just listed occurs.
3. List the symptoms that a patient might have in connection with infection/inflammation of the bladder.
4. Explain why each of the symptoms just listed occurs.
5. Examine a penis and scrotum (and contents) for normalcy.
6. List the symptoms that a patient might have in connection with the following diseases of the prostate: benign enlargement, acute infection, chronic infection.
7. Explain why each of the symptoms just listed occurs.
8. Discuss the procedure to be used in attempting to palpate the kidney.
9. Explain the procedure to be followed in doing a digital rectal examination of the prostate.
10. List the specific things to be looked for in doing a digital rectal examination of the prostate.
11. Explain the significance of the bulbocavernosus reflex.
12. List the indications for an excretory urogram.
13. Recognize and identify a normal excretory urogram.
14. Explain the significance of a unilateral delay in visualization on the nephrogram phase of the excretory urogram.
15. List the indications for cystoscopy.
16. List the indications for bladder catheterization.
17. Pass a catheter into a bladder atraumatically.
18. List the indications for radioisotope studies of the kidneys (renal scanning).
19. List the indications for CT scanning of the kidneys.
20. List the indications for ultrasonography in urology.
21. List the indications for renal angiography.
22. Describe the two basic functions of the detrusor (bladder).
23. List, in broad terms, the innervation of the detrusor.
24. Discuss the location and the specific type of muscle found in each of the two urinary sphincters.
25. List the available tests that are used to quantitate voiding (urodynamics).
26. Explain and give an example to illustrate the statement that voiding dysfunction may be a result of disease processes originating outside of the urinary tract.
27. Estimate the level of anxiety of a patient over procedures involving manipulation of the genitalia.

INTRODUCTION

Urology, as much as or perhaps even more than any other discipline, consists of disease processes that produce signs and symptoms that, if accurately and properly elicited, will go far towards helping the knowledgeable physician to make an accurate diagnosis. It has often been said that one will never make a correct diagnosis unless one first thinks of it, and this truism applies to urologic disease as well as to any other. The purpose of this chapter is to familiarize the student, in the very broadest sense, with the panoply of urologic signs, symptoms, physical findings, and diagnostic procedures so that he or she will be able to sift through these in order to arrive at an appropriate differential diagnosis. The contents of this chapter and, indeed, of the rest of this book are so structured that hopefully the student will ultimately be able to take an accurate urologic history, perform a urologic physical exam, and then transmit to his or her own brain (the best computer of all) the data accumulated in order to arrive at an appropriate differential diagnosis. After this, those diagnostic studies, be they laboratory, radiographic, or other, can be utilized in the most economical manner possible to reinforce the initial differential diagnosis and, ultimately, lead to a single diagnosis. It is rare indeed in urology that one must resort to an "exploratory" operation in order to reach a diagnosis!

The broad categories of disease that can affect the genitourinary tract are no different than those diseases that can affect any other organ system or any other structure within the body. These categories are neoplasia (which includes benign as well as malignant growths), infection/inflammation (it is convenient, even if not absolutely correct etiologically to include immunologic disease in this category), tuberculosis (this category could alternatively be listed under infection/inflammation), foreign body, such as calculi, or the like, congenital, and traumatic.

The structures involved in the genitourinary tract are the kidneys, the ureters, the bladder, and the urethra in females, and all of the above structures in males, in addition to the prostate gland, the scrotum and intrascrotal contents, the ejaculatory mechanism, and the penis. If the reader becomes familiar enough with the signs and symptoms produced by the more common examples of diseases found in each of the above major disease categories in relation to the specific structure involved, then he or she will be well on the way to a logical thought process by which a given sign or symptom or a group of signs or symptoms elicited from a patient will trigger a logical, and hopefully accurate, differential diagnosis.

HISTORY

The Kidney

Signs and symptoms of the various forms of kidney disease are highly variable and may be localized to the kidney (flank pain or flank mass); they may be quite distant from the kidney (skin or subcutaneous nodules, particularly about the head and neck, which may represent metastatic renal cell cancer); or they may be suggestive of urinary tract disease in general but not specifically kidney disease (microscopic or gross hematuria).

When a patient experiences pain that is referable to the kidney it is because of a stretching of the renal capsule with its sympathetic innervation. Pain may be produced if there is parenchymal edema stretching the renal capsule (as in acute pyelonephritis) or may result from distension of the renal collecting system bringing increased pressure to bear on the renal capsule (as in a sudden hydronephrosis that might be caused by a stone). Disease processes within the kidney that do not bring about any stretching of the renal capsule do not, generally speaking, produce any discomfort or pain referable to the kidney. If a palpable flank mass is noted by the patient, it is likely to be firm in consistency and should bring to mind the possibility of a kidney tumor. A large hydronephrosis could also conceivably be noticed by the patient and it is important to note that either of these conditions may be accompanied by flank pain or by no pain at all depending upon whether the renal capsule was stretched acutely (pain present) or chronically over a long period of time (pain absent). Most often, the flank mass is not accompanied by any particular pain although the patient may claim to be aware of a certain degree of discomfort. Generalized and systemic symptoms may be the first manifestation of renal cell cancer in that it is not unusual for this "great imitator" to present with a fever of unknown origin, metastatic skin nodules, weight loss, anorexia, anemia, or a generalized malaise. Acute glomerulonephritis may present with little else than a periorbital edema noted in the morning upon arising or an ankle edema later on in the day, although this condition will almost always additionally cause micro or gross hematuria.

Hematuria arising in the kidney may produce absolutely none of the signs or symptoms already mentioned or may be accompanied by one or more of the above findings. If blood clots pass down the ureter, these may be accompanied by moderate to severe renal colic simulating the passage of a kidney stone.

Fever, of course, is a totally nonspecific sign, although it is usually present with acute infectious processes involving the kidney such as pyelonephritis.

The foregoing is certainly not a complete listing of the signs and symptoms that can accompany any and all kidney diseases, but it does represent the most common ones and should offer students guidelines regarding those signs and symptoms about which they must ask if they are to learn as much as possible during the course of taking a good urologic history.

The Ureter

Ureteral disease produces relatively few signs and symptoms that are specific for this structure. The most important symptom is probably a colicky pain which may be caused by a calculus moving from the kidney down to the bladder. The pain will be high up in the anterior abdomen or in the flank when the calculus is in the upper ureter, it may be localized in the mid anterior abdomen when the calculus is in the middle portion of the ureter, and it will be in the lower quadrant of the abdomen when the calculus is in the lower ureter. Urgency and frequency may also be present when the stone is in the intramural portion of the ureter (just prior to passing into the bladder) and these symptoms are the ones usually produced whenever there is trigonal inflammation or irritation. If gross or microscopic hematuria originates from a lesion in the ureter, it is usually not possible to discern this from the history of hematuria alone. Obstruction to the ureter caused by an extrinsic lesion (enlarged lymph nodes) or an intrinsic lesion (a ureteral tumor) will usually produce the symptoms of kidney pain if a hydronephrosis has developed rapidly or it may produce no symptoms at all if the obstruction to the kidney has been insidious.

The Bladder

Disease processes involving the bladder generally produce symptoms that are localized to the area of the bladder and that are commonly associated with bladder disease. Suprapubic pain, for example, may be present, as may urgency, frequency, dysuria, stranguria, or hematuria. Urgency, frequency, and dysuria usually suggest an infectious or inflammatory process within the bladder, but it may also be present in the face of bladder cancer. Suprapubic pain may be associated with infection or inflammation within the bladder or with an overdistention of the bladder because of incomplete bladder emptying. A suprapubic mass must, first of all, be considered as a distended bladder until proven otherwise. Stranguria refers to extreme pain on voiding and most often is caused by the presence of a stone in the bladder. Dysuria is pain or discomfort on voiding and is usually caused by infection/inflammation of the bladder mucosa. Gross or microscopic hematuria originating from the bladder may be accompanied by absolutely no other symptoms, in which case bladder cancer is always a major concern, or it may accompany symptoms of infection or inflammation, such as urgency, frequency, and dysuria. Incontinence of urine in an adult man is most often due to bladder outlet obstruction and a "paradoxical" or overflow incontinence. It may also be secondary to extreme urgency, as with infection and inflammation, or (in women) it may be due to a weakening of the support in the region of the bladder neck such that a "stress" incontinence results. Far less frequently is the incontinence due to any sort of neurologic problem.

The Prostate Gland

The prostate gland, the primary function of which is to produce about 90 percent of the fluid that is found in the ejaculate, can become the site of acute or chronic infection/inflammation, benign or malignant neoplasia, foreign bodies (calculi) and even traumatic injuries that may sever it, partially or completely, from the urethra at its distal margin. Perineal pain or discomfort, rectal pain or discomfort, suprapubic pain, inguinal pain, and scanty, but abnormal, urethral discharge can all be caused by chronic infection in the prostate gland or a nonbacterial engorgement of the gland. All of these symptoms plus high fever, malaise, and even acute urinary retention can be caused by an acute prostatic infection.

Hesitancy, intermittency, nocturia, frequency, incontinence, terminal dribbling, hematuria, and urgency and frequency are all symptoms associated with benign prostatic hyperplasia.

The Testes

Patients are generally not able to differentiate signs and symptoms caused by disease processes in the testis from those caused by diseases of the epididymis or the other cord structures and so these are discussed together. Although there are many different forms of intrascrotal pathology, the only ones that would present as signs or symptoms would be conditions that produce pain or enlargement. Intrascrotal pain may be acute in onset, as with torsion of the spermatic cord, or it may be more vague, with gradually increasing severity over a period of hours or even days, as with an epididymitis or an orchitis. The pain of epididymitis and of orchitis both result when the affected structures become edematous secondary to infection and the edematous tissue in turn presses against a fairly rigid capsule with its sympathetic innervation. Far more serious is the case of a patient who has detected (often by serendipity, as when showering) a mass or a swelling within the scrotal sac that is totally nontender. It is very rare that he is able to tell you if this mass or swelling is testicular or belonging to an adjacent structure, but this sign alone should alert the clinician to the absolute necessity of a careful physical examination (see below).

The Penis

The more common penile lesions are readily visible since they are on the skin of the penis although they may be completely concealed under the foreskin in uncircumcised men. A thorough urologic history usually consists simply of ascertaining whether or not the patient has ever noted any lesions on the penis; it is also prudent to inquire about any penile curvature during erection, as well as the adequacy of erections and the patient's sexual life in general. Sexual difficulties, such as erectile dysfunction, are very often the underlying reason for the patient's visit to the urologist but the patient is loathe to volunteer this information and it will only be forthcoming under direct questioning.

The Urethra

Any sort of an abnormal discharge from the urethra, be it mucoid or purulent, suggests inflammation within the urethra. Additional signs of urethral infection/inflammation can be burning, pain, and itching which the patient localizes to the urethra.

PHYSICAL EXAMINATION OF THE GENITOURINARY TRACT

The physical examination is conducted in four parts: (1) the examination of the abdomen and suprapubic area; (2) the examination of the penis and intrascrotal contents; (3) percussion of the kidneys; and (4) palpation of the prostate via digital rectal examination and repeat examination of the intrascrotal contents and inguinal canals. Note that the first and second parts of the examination are best done with the patient lying on his back, and the third part with the patient sitting up on the examining table, leaning forward. The final part of the examination (the fourth part) is best done with the patient in the standing position. It is always a good idea to wash one's hands in front of the patient before beginning the physical exam, as many patients may wonder where the physician's hands may have been just prior to his own examination. Not only will a thorough washing make the patient feel psychologically a little more comfortable but if warm water is used for this purpose the patient's physical comfort will be increased, for the physician will be placing warm (and not cold) hands on the patient during the examination.

The patient should be made comfortable lying on his back, and this may be best done by having him bring his knees up. This position relaxes the rectus abdominus muscles and softens the abdomen. It is also helpful to have the patient cross his hands on his chest: this serves the purpose of preventing him from raising his head by putting his hands behind his neck in order to see what you are doing, a maneuver that tightens the rectus abdominus muscles and makes the examination more difficult. Throughout the procedure, remember to expose only that area of the body that you are examining; this, of course, applies both to men and to women. No one likes to feel completely naked in front of a stranger.

The examination is begun with a visual inspection of the abdomen. Since the human is basically symmetrical, it is important to look for any asymmetry—any lumps, bulges, or unusual findings on one side that are not present on the other.

Palpate the abdomen with whichever hand you prefer, placing your other hand on top of the palpating hand, and use a rolling motion. This makes it possible to feel over a relatively large area with minimal changing of the position of your hand and it is also more comfortable for the patient. Feel for any abdominal masses or signs of guarding or tenderness. Guarding refers to involuntary tenseness of the rectus abdominus muscles and will be present if there is any peritoneal inflammation (peritonitis) such as would result from appendicitis or other pathologic conditions within the peritoneal cavity. Peritonitis, if present, will usually cause the rectus abdominus muscle to go into spasm when it is palpated. Voluntary guarding or rigidity of the rectus abdominus muscles may also result if the patient is ticklish but it is not difficult to differentiate voluntary from involuntary guarding. If the situation is a voluntary one, it is helpful to talk to the patient in order to distract his attention as you palpate more deeply through the rectus muscle. Gradually the muscle will become softer as the patient relaxes. In contrast, the muscles that are made rigid by a true pathologic process resulting in peritonitis will not relax as you talk to the patient in an attempt to distract his attention.

Next, palpate the midline of the lower abdomen for signs of bladder distention. A distended bladder may reach all the way to the umbilicus and is often mistaken for a midline abdominal tumor. It is not unusual to obtain 1 to 2 liters of urine from a bladder in the patient who is suffering from acute urinary retention due to an enlarged and obstructing prostate. An empty bladder that is normally in a collapsed state will lie behind the symphysis pubis and will not be palpable. In a normal individual who perceives that his bladder is "full," the bladder might reach half way to the umbilicus and yield approximately 500 ml of urine should the patient's voided volume be measured. Percussion of the lower abdomen over a distended bladder will result in a dull sound, but percussion of the abdomen over a nondistended bladder will result in a more tympanitic sound because you are really percussing over loops of bowel with air in them. In other words, percussion can serve as another means of demonstrating whether or not the bladder is distended by recognizing the difference between the dull sound of percussion over fluid and the tympanitic sound of percussing over loops of bowel that are filled with air and realizing that when the bladder is empty loops of bowel will most likely be under the percussing fingers in the midline of the lower abdomen.

Next, an attempt should be made to palpate the kidneys, recognizing that in most normal individuals, neither kidney is palpable. It is extremely difficult and unusual to be able to palpate the left kidney, which lies slightly higher than the right kidney (Fig. 1–1). The left kidney is generally only palpable in an extremely thin individual or in pathologic states where there is abnormal enlargement of the kidney, particularly of the lower pole. The right kidney is palpable more often than the left one, but it is still most unusual to be able to feel it unless it is abnormally enlarged. Before beginning to palpate the kidneys, ask the patient to take a deep breath and then to slowly exhale. When the patient inhales, the kidney moves down, but the abdominal muscles also become tense, preventing adequate palpation. Therefore the best time to palpate the kidney (if it is at all palpable) is to wait until the patient exhales and then to try to trap the kidney between your hands. To do this, push up from under the 11th rib with your posterior hand and press down just under the rib cage with your anterior hand (Fig. 1–2). Use the balls of your fingers where the sensory fibres are maximal. If you use the tips of your fingers, you will not feel as well and you also run the risk of hurting the patient if your fingernails are too long. The objective is to bring the fingers of each hand as close together as possible, which obviously is more difficult in very muscular men. If you can feel any mass at all between your fingers, it is very likely kidney. The large bowel normally collapses between your fingers and should not be palpable unless the patient has some impacted barium from a recent barium enema or has very firm stools in the ascending or descending colon, which is usually not the case.

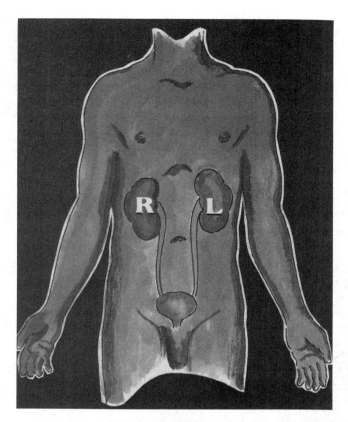

Figure 1–1. A schematic view showing the normal relationship between the two kidneys in which the right is somewhat lower than the left. Note that the terms "right" and "left" refer to the patient's kidneys and *not* to the viewer's right and left. This distinction should be kept in mind when looking at all of the illustrations in this book, particularly the x-ray studies and the CT scans.

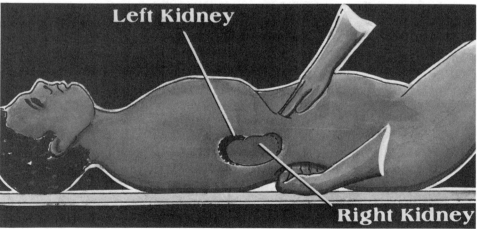

Figure 1–2. The correct maneuver for the attempted palpation of a kidney; in this illustration it is the right kidney which is being palpated. Note that the examiner's left hand is pressing up from underneath the patient in an attempt to move the kidney anteriorly and the right presses downward during expiration in an attempt to "trap" the kidney between the fingers of the two hands.

Next, palpate along the inguinal canals bilaterally: this should be done from the anterior superior iliac spine to the pubic tubercle. The purpose here is to feel for any enlarged and palpable lymph nodes, but do not confuse Poupart's ligament, which will be on the floor of the inguinal canal, with enlarged lymph nodes. An enlarged lymph node will be closer to the surface and fairly easy to feel. If you find any such nodes, they are most likely caused by athlete's foot or some other infectious process on the foot or the leg; however, inflammatory and malignant lesions of the penis will also cause enlarged lymph nodes in this area.

Next, examine the penis and scrotum. First examine the distal urethra by gently everting the meatus. It should be pinkish grey in color if it is normal. By vigorously everting the meatus, it will become a bright, angry red and this is done so as to give the examiner the idea of the bright angry red color to be found in the presence of gonococcal or other acute urethritis when the meatus is gently everted. Also, any urethral discharge present should be noted. Next feel along the dorsum of the penis for induration or hardening. Remember that the penis is a symmetric organ of uniform consistency and any area that feels harder than any other area may represent induration. You are checking for Peyronie's disease, which occurs more frequently in men over 40 years than in younger men. It results from fibrotic plaques forming in the tissues surrounding the corpora cavernosa; these plaques produce deviation of the penis on erection, which is very painful in severe cases and can even make intercourse impossible. Next, feel along the ventral surface of the penis, specifically the corpus spongiosum, in which the urethra lies. Feel the entire length of the urethra all the way down into the perineum; this includes feeling through the scrotal tissue, between the testes. In a normal male the spongiosum will feel soft. If any induration of the spongiosum is present, this may indicate a carcinoma, diverticulum, stricture, or stone in the urethra.

In palpating the scrotum it is important to assure the patient that you will not hurt him. This may be done by gently picking up the scrotal skin and letting it rest on your hand with your fingers closed tightly together. This will give support to the patient's scrotum similar to that offered by an athletic supporter, but even more importantly it gets the patient accustomed to having your hands on this delicate part of his anatomy. Next, bring the fingers of your hands together from above and below along the median raffé between the two testes and gently roll each testis in turn between the fingers. You are feeling for a uniform consistency throughout the testes. A testis of soft or mushy consistency is often a sign of impaired fertility and the examiner can only recognize this from having palpated a sufficiently large number of normal testicles to be able to recognize the difference. Note any signs of testis induration or hardening, which might indicate cancer of the testis, and remember that this disease is most prevalent in 18- to 40-year-old men.

A most important aspect of scrotal palpation is to be able to differentiate testicular hardness from hardness in any other areas within the scrotum, most specifically the epididymis. This hardness of the epididymis is usually caused by epididymitis, which is very common in men in the same age group susceptible to testis cancer, and it is obviously imperative that these conditions be differentiated from one another. Epididymitis will cause the epididymis to swell, initially causing pain; hardness of the epididymis follows, usually with continuing pain. It is extremely important that the examining physician know how to examine the testis and the epididymis so as to be certain as to which of these structures is indurated in cases where one or the other is affected (Fig. 1–3).

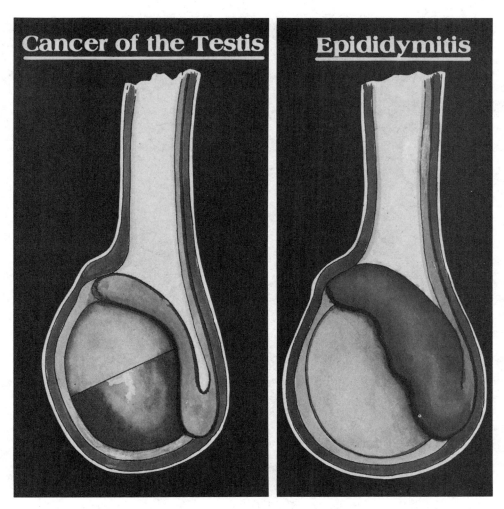

Figure 1-3. This figure illustrates the proximity of the testis to the epididymis, which is the reason for the difficulty in determining the anatomic boundaries of each. On the left (cancer of the testis) the epididymis is totally normal while the testis is indurated; on the right (epididymitis) the epididymis is indurated and enlarged while the testis is perfectly normal.

To palpate the epididymis, pick up the scrotum using the thumb, first finger and middle finger of each hand just beneath the testis. You can bring the fingers of each hand tightly together because you have only scrotal tissue between your fingers since you are *under* the testis. Now move the fingers back a couple of millimeters until you feel the testis. Then, just under or deep to or behind the testis you should feel a tubular structure that collapses when you squeeze it. This is the epididymis. Be sure that you can tell the difference between the testis and the epididymis with regard to where one stops and the other begins. The important point here is to learn the absolute boundaries of the testis (Fig. 1–4) so that if an

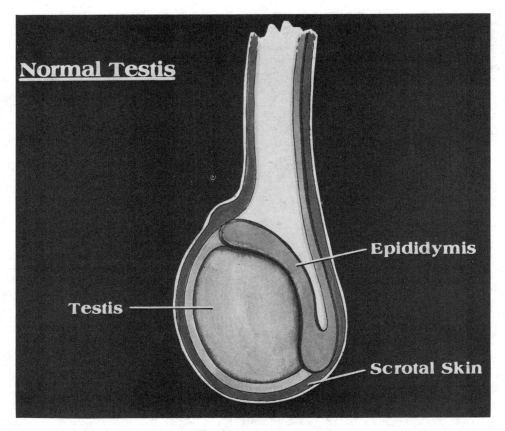

Figure 1-4. The anatomic relationships of the intrascrotal structures. Note the intimate relationship of the epididymis to the testis as well as the distinct boundaries between the two. These must be detected by palpation if the physical examination is to be properly done.

indurated intrascrotal structure is noted, you will be able to clearly determine whether or not this induration is within the testis or adjacent to it (in the epididymis).

Next, with the patient in the sitting position on the examining table and leaning forward, check for any process within the kidney or kidneys such as acute inflammation or hydronephrosis that would bring about tension on the renal capsule and thereby pain when the area over the kidney is percussed. Begin by percussing over the midline area of the spine where you know you will not hurt the patient, and then move into the area of the kidney which is the costovertebral angle. If the patient feels no pain, you can percuss a little harder. Pain in the kidney is caused by swelling of the kidney against the rigid renal capsule that contains the sympathetic pain fibres. The swelling may be caused by inflammation of the renal parenchyma or dilation of the collecting system secondary to obstruction of the urine flow. If the inflammation or obstruction is severe enough, it will usually produce pain without any percussion. Observe the vertebral column while the patient is in this seated position. A curved spine might be congenital, but it might also be caused by a perinephric abscess.

Two intrascrotal conditions not detectable when the patient is lying down are the varicocele and the indirect inguinal hernia and so the patient is next examined in the upright position.

The varicocele consists of dilated veins of the pampiniform plexus (Fig. 1–5) that are collapsed when the patient is lying down and can therefore only be felt with the patient upright. The dilated veins are readily palpable, however, when the patient is standing and these feel like a bag full of worms. Remember that man is symmetric and you need to compare one side with the other. If there is a question of a varicocele on one side, a comparison with the other side will usually give the answer.

To check for an indirect hernia (Fig. 1–6), use your little finger because it will cause the patient least discomfort. Begin by placing the fingernail side of your little finger on the upper part of the testis (use the little finger of your left hand to examine the patient's left inguinal canal, and the little finger of your right hand to examine his right inguinal canal). Gently push the scrotal skin ahead of your finger and avoid sliding the finger against the skin. Follow the cord straight up by moving your finger up along the cord and into the external ring. As you are moving your

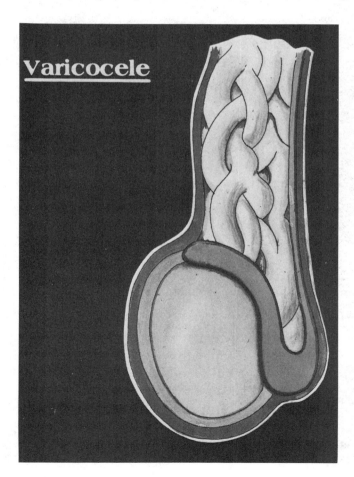

Varicocele

Figure 1–5. A varicocele. Note the numerous and tortuous veins just superior to the testis and the epididymis which have the palpatory feel of "a bag of worms." The patient must be examined in the upright position if this abnormality is to be detected.

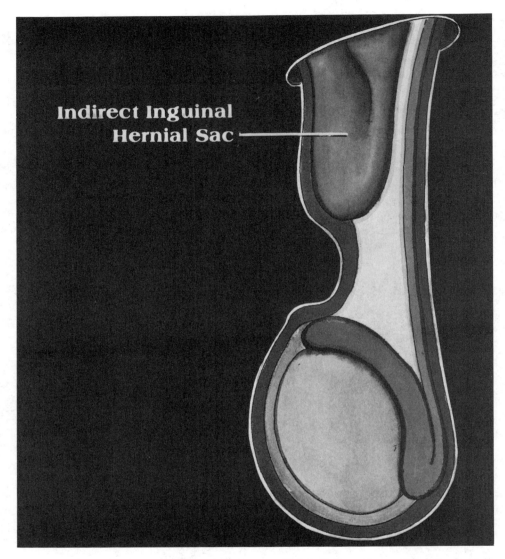

Indirect Inguinal Hernial Sac

Figure 1-6. An indirect inguinal hernia sac that protrudes into the superior portion of the scrotum and comes through the external inguinal ring. Note that this produces a thickening of the cord contents superiorly but the testis and epididymis remain perfectly normal.

finger superiorly in this manner, the back part of your finger will often be in contact with the pubic bone. Once you feel this bone, maintain contact with it, moving your finger in an upward direction until you feel your fingertip caught in the external ring, which has a horseshoelike configuration. At this point, ask the patient to strain and bear down as if moving his bowels, and if an indirect hernial sac is present, you will feel something coming down through the inguinal canal and hitting your finger. It may take a little time to learn to differentiate the feel of a hernial sac against your finger from the gentle bulge behind your fingertip that will be felt from the normal increase in intraabdominal pressure when the patient bears down. Note that if the patient has a *direct* inguinal hernia, this will most readily be palpated as a direct bulge coming right through Hesselbach triangle towards the examiner if the patient is standing upright facing the examiner. This bulge may be seen if the hernia is large or it may be palpated by placing the fingers directly over Hesselbach's triangle and then asking the patient to strain. A large direct inguinal hernia may also go into the scrotum.

To examine the anus, the rectum, and the prostate gland (Fig. 1-7), ask the patient to stand with his feet comfortably far apart, bent at the waist, leaning over an examining table, and with his toes pointed in towards each other. This last maneuver serves to spread the ischial tuberosities and makes it easier to insert the examining finger. Before beginning the examination, it is thoughtful to give the patient some tissues so that he can wipe off excess lubricating jelly after the rectal examination is finished. Ask the patient to spread his own buttocks apart so that you can examine the anus and perianal region for possible hemorrhoids, venereal sores, carcinoma, or other abnormalities. A normal anus has a smooth, accordion-like mucosa all the way around and it literally looks like a pair of well-puckered lips. Using a glove and spreading plenty of lubricating jelly on the distal phalanges of your index and middle finger will minimize the patient's discomfort. After spreading the jelly around the anus, insert your index finger using a pistol grip position, with the thumb pointed straight up and the index finger turned sideways. This facilitates insertion of the examining finger because it is being inserted in its nar-

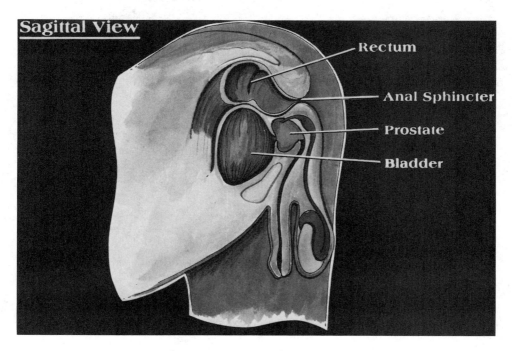

Figure 1-7. A sagittal view of the rectum, prostate, and bladder with the patient bent sharply at the waist in one of the proper positions for performing a digital rectal examination.

rowest dimension from side to side, and keeping the thumb pointed straight up facilitates a deeper entry of the examining finger between the buttocks, which may, at times, be quite large and interfere with proper digital rectal examination. The finger is inserted very slowly, while pressing down slightly, as the anus and rectum are less sensitive anteriorly than posteriorly (Fig. 1–8). After the index finger is fully inserted, wait until the anal sphincter relaxes and then briskly reach around to the front of the patient and squeeze the glans penis with your other hand. This should normally bring about a contraction of the anal sphincter on your fingers, and this is a normal and positive bulbocavernosus reflex. If the anal sphincter does not contract on your finger, it may signify a neurologic deficit that could be related to a neurogenic bladder. The examining finger is then swept around 180 degrees, first to one side and then to the other so that a 360 degree arc is described. This maneuver will ensure that the entire rectal mucosa is examined (within the reach of the examining finger) for any abnormalities, which would, of course, include rectal carcinoma.

The prostate gland is examined next, and to do this satisfactorily, one must be completely familiar with prostate anatomy. Recall the location of the bladder, the external anal sphincter, the posterior lobe, the lateral lobes, and the apex of the prostate and this will facilitate the digital rectal examination of the prostate (Fig. 1–9). In examining the gland, palpate it all the way out laterally to the lateral

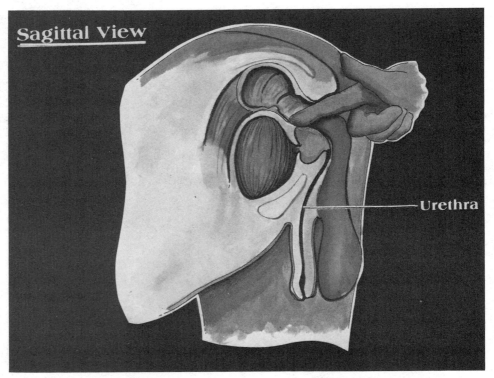

Figure 1–8. The same sagittal view as in Figure 1–7, with the examining finger inserted in the rectum and palpating the prostate gland during the digital-rectal examination.

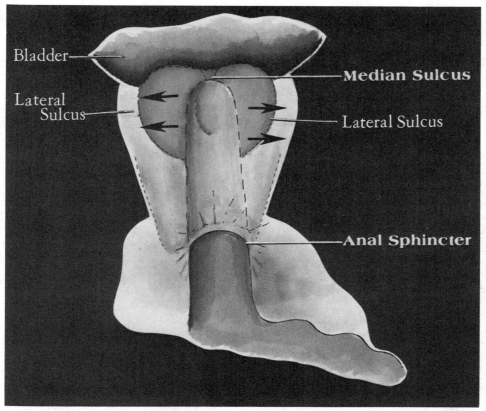

Figure 1-9. A superior view (from above) of the examining finger within the rectum and upon the prostate gland. Note specifically the locations of the median sulcus and the lateral sulci.

sulcus on each side. Next, move your finger across from one side to the other and feel the bumps that are palpable through the floor of the rectum. These are the lateral lobes of the prostate and in between these lobes is a subtle groove called the median sulcus. Feel the entire surface of the prostate for uniform consistency and be aware that when you are actually pressing on the prostate gland while palpating it the patient will often feel as if some fluid is trying to come out of his urethra. This is prostatic fluid, which in fact rarely actually comes out of the urethra during an examination of the prostate. The consistency of the prostate gland, in terms of whether it is soft or firm, varies greatly from person to person, usually depending upon how often it is emptied (during ejaculation). An average adult prostate is the consistency of the thenar eminence with the fist tightly clenched. However, if ejaculation is infrequent, the prostate may be very soft because it is full of prostatic fluid. In addition to noting the consistency of the gland, it is most important to feel whether any areas of the prostate, large or small, are *harder* than the rest of the surrounding gland. Such hardened areas are always suggestive of the possibility of cancer of the prostate, which typically feels like a knuckle with the fist clenched.

The most common mistake made by beginners doing a digital rectal examination of the prostate is to insert the examining finger too far, thereby passing beyond the prostate and poking the finger into the base of the bladder (Fig. 1-10). It is a very frequent occurrence for the beginner to feel the base of the bladder and think that it is an enormous prostate gland that he just cannot quite get his finger around! The trick is to remember to back out with the examining finger until the lateral lobes are readily palpable as bumps on the floor of the rectum poking through the rectal mucosa. It is necessary to do a large number of rectal exams before one is able to recognize a normal prostate gland, and it is necessary to do an even greater number of digital rectal examinations before one is able to recognize gradations in size of the prostate gland. However, even the beginner is frequently able to pick

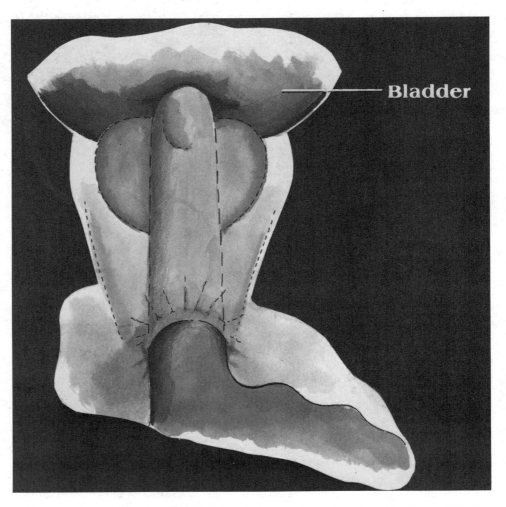

Figure 1-10. The same view as Figure 1-9. Note how easily the examining finger can slide completely over and beyond a normal-sized prostate, thereby poking into the bladder. To the beginner, the bladder is sometimes interpreted as an "enormous" prostate gland.

out a hard area on the prostate from normal surrounding tissue, and I would encourage all medical students to do as many digital rectal examinations as possible in order to become familiar with this key diagnostic exam.

In summary, the physical examination of the genitourinary tract is of paramount importance to evaluate the penis, intrascrotal contents, and prostate in the male as well as the kidney and bladder in both sexes. It is a major part of the physical examination and probably should never be omitted. The genitourinary examination in the female is the same with regard to the abdomen, the suprapubic area, the inguinal area, and the kidneys. Examination of the female genitalia is perhaps better taught in a gynecologic setting, with the exception of the female urethra itself, which is certainly part of the urinary tract. The external urethral meatus should be inspected and periurethral inflammation may sometimes be noted as may urethral caruncles. The latter are most commonly seen in the 6 o'clock position of the urethral meatus and look like very small polypoid growths. Occasionally a prolapse of the urethral mucosa is noted: this is much more common in female children than in adults. Palpation of the anterior vaginal wall in the midline with the index finger is important for detecting a diverticulum of the urethra. The examining finger will feel a midline anterior vaginal mass that may by anywhere from the size of a pea to the size of a golf ball. This is usually soft and an upward pressure will result in an extrusion of the diverticular contents from the urethral meatus.

DIAGNOSTIC PROCEDURES

Excretory Urography

In spite of the remarkable number of recently developed and very excellent diagnostic modalities for the urologic patient, such as CT scanning, nuclear magnetic resonance (NMR), ultrasound, renal scanning, and angiography, the excretory urogram remains the cornerstone of urologic diagnosis and is probably the diagnostic study with which urologists feel the most comfortable.

The Excretory Urogram, sometimes less correctly referred to as the intravenous pyelogram (IVP), is a technique for delineating the entire urinary tract. It was first accomplished in 1929 by the intravenous injection of an aqueous organic iodide compound. Certainly this achievement ranks as one of the major milestones in medical history and much credit is due to the American urologist, Moses Swick, who pioneered the efforts that ultimately led to the excretory urogram as we know it today. Some years earlier, in 1906, the retrograde method of visualizing the urinary tract had been introduced by the German workers Voelcker and Lichtenberg.

As it is commonly performed today, the excretory urogram consists of a preliminary x-ray film of the abdomen prior to injection of contrast medium and, following the injection, a series of x-ray films, usually taken at 1- , 3- , 5- , and 20-minute intervals from the time of the injection, so that the entire urinary tract may be visualized as it is opacified by the contrast medium. The preliminary film is also called the KUB (kidney, ureter, and bladder), scout film, or plain film. It must be emphasized that the clinician should never attempt to interpret an excretory urogram without first viewing a plain film lest he be led to an incomplete and inaccurate diagnosis.

There are many different kinds of contrast medium currently being used in excretory urography. All of these contain a high percentage of radiopaque or organically bound iodine and they are removed from the circulating bloodstream by the kidney and excreted through the urinary tract. In the high doses in which these compounds are injected, contrast medium is both filtered by the glomeruli and secreted by the renal tubules. It is very important for the clinician to realize this because it makes understandable the fact that the patient may have an essentially normal excretory urogram and yet have either severe glomerular or tubular disease. The standard adult dose of injected contrast medium is about 60 ml; in most cases, this will give an excellent and clear delineation of the urinary tract. When the greatest possible clarity in the intravenous roentgenographic visualization is desired, an infusion technique may be used and about 250 ml of a solution that is about half contrast medium and half distilled water is very rapidly infused intravenously. The first film is taken about 2 to 5 minutes after the start of infusion, or when half of the contents of the bottle has been absorbed. This technique is particularly useful in obtaining a so-called hypertension urogram in which the object is to detect subtle and not-so-subtle delays in the contrast medium reaching one or the other kidney because of the narrowing of the affected renal artery.

A particularly important part of the excretory urogram that the author likes very much but that is not commonly performed is to obtain films of the bladder and entire urethra during the act of voiding. This may be done by waiting until the bladder is full of contrast medium and then asking the patient to void under x-ray control. This will allow the physician to obtain a "physiologic voiding cystourethrogram."

KUB Film

Before the physician looks at the excretory urogram and attempts to interpret it, the KUB film must be carefully inspected (Fig. 1–11). It will be noticed that on all excretory urograms (including the preliminary KUB) the usual anatomic position is reversed: the left side of the film as it is seen on the viewing box actually represents the right side of the patient, as shown by the letter R in the left margin of the film. Some radiologists reverse this procedure by placing the letter L along the right margin of the film (the left side of the patient) as it is seen on the view box.

In examining the KUB film, using the labeled x-ray film as a guide (Fig. 1–12), the first thing the clinician should do is look for any evidence of a radiopacity that might be overlying the kidney or bladder areas or the course of the ureters. Observe first the kidney area then the areas through which the ureters will usually travel down into the bony pelvis, and finally the area of the bladder. Radiopacities might represent renal, ureteral, or bladder stones, but the clinician should never make a diagnosis of such stones based on examination of the KUB film alone, as it is two dimensional. The third dimension is not added until the contrast medium has been injected and the appropriate oblique or lateral x-ray films have been taken. On examining the KUB it is sufficient for the clinician to decide whether the possibility of any calculus exists. It is very common to see radiopacities within the bony pelvis, but these usually represent phleboliths, which are calcifications within the pelvic veins. These latter may be provisionally differentiated from true urinary tract calculi by the area of relative radiolucency in the center of the calcification, which is produced by blood within the vein.

The clinician should next carefully examine the renal areas to determine if the renal outlines appear equal in size and of normal contour. It is not at all unusual for the renal outlines to be indistinct on the KUB depending on the weight of the person, the amount of body fat, and particularly on the success that the patient has had in evacuating the bowels prior to the x-ray studies. After looking at the

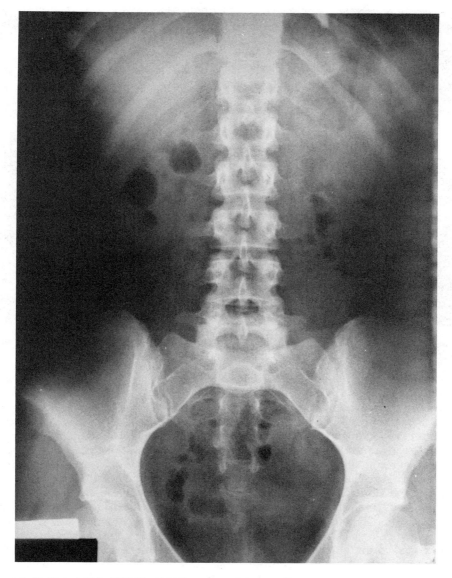

Figure 1-11. Note in this KUB film that there is a minimum of intestinal gas overlying the urinary organs. Small amounts of intestinal gas are, however, within normal limits and usually do not indicate any abnormalities.

renal outlines, the clinician should observe the psoas shadows bilaterally to determine their distinct outlines. The psoas muscles run along the vertebral column, starting at about the level of the first lumbar vertebra, and are frequently visible all the way down to the point where the sacrum and the iliac bones come together. These psoas shadows are normally obscured by overlying gas and feces in the bowels,

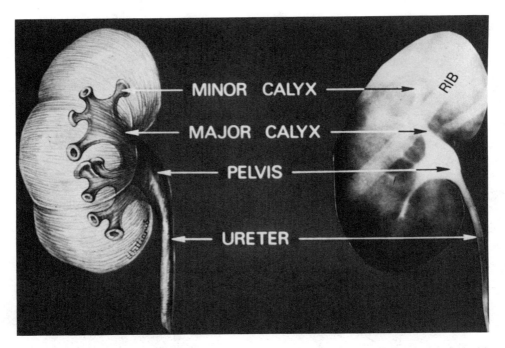

Figure 1-12. Anatomic illustration (left) and x-ray film of kidney (right). Parts are labeled with corresponding ones as seen on the excretory urogram.

but failure to visualize either of them, particularly unilaterally, should alert the clinician to the possibility that some retroperitoneal process such as a hemorrhage or an abscess is causing this nonvisualization. The clinician should next devote attention to the bony structures seen on the KUB films. First the 12th ribs bilaterally should be carefully inspected to see if one is apparently shorter than the other. During renal surgery the 12th rib may be partially amputated to allow for better exposure of the kidney; if such amputation is noticed it may indicate that previous renal surgery has been done. The bony features of all the ribs, the vertebral column, and the pelvis should be carefully inspected for any evidence of abnormal calcification and osteoarthritic changes, the latter being particularly noticeable in the vertebral column. Any diminution of the intervertebral disc spaces and any arthritic changes of the vertebral column or the sacraliliac anastomosis should be noted since these can produce back pain that is often erroreously attributed to disease in the urinary tract. While examining the bony structures, particularly those of the vertebral column and the pelvis, the clinician should look for any increased or decreased bone density since either or both of these findings may represent osteoblastic or osteolytic metastatic lesions from a malignancy somewhere in the body (Fig. 1–13). Carcinoma of the prostate gland is the most common of all malignancies of the genitourinary tract in men and the most likely to produce osteoblastic lesions in the lumbar spine and bony pelvis. These osteoblastic lesions are seen as greatly increased bony densities that can produce an almost pure white appearance of the bone as

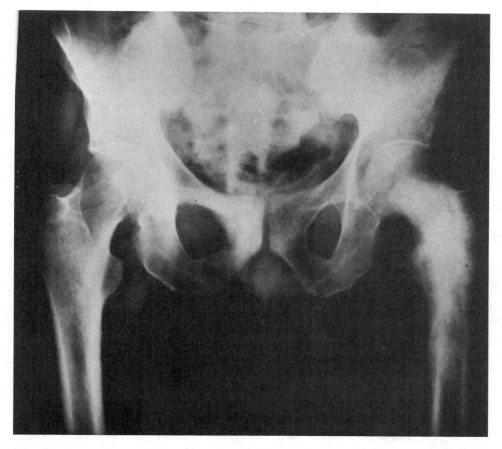

Figure 1–13. This flat plate (without injection of any contrast medium) graphically depicts extensive obsteoblastic metastases involving the upper left femur and virtually the entire bony pelvis in a 63-year-old male with known carcinoma of the prostate gland. Note the greatly increased density in the involved bony areas.

seen on the x-ray film. While still examining the KUB, the clinician should also carefully inspect the vertebral bodies for failure of fusion of the spinous processes posteriorly. Any absence of such fusion will leave an open space between the spinous processes of a given vertebral body. This is referred to as spina bifida occulta. Although this condition is not rare, existing in perhaps 10 percent of normal individuals, it may be associated with a spinal cord lesion or with clinical evidence of a neurogenic bladder.

Within the bony pelvis in the area extending in all directions for a distance of 1 to 2 cm from the superior portion of the symphysis pubis, calcifications that are seen may represent prostatic calculi. Additionally, foreign bodies seen within the bony pelvis in women may represent one of the various intrauterine contraceptive devices that are in common use.

The Excretory Urogram

The timing of the first x-ray film following the injection of contrast medium will depend on the type of urogram that is being done. With conventional urography using about 60 ml of contrast medium injected directly into the veins, the first film is usually exposed 30 to 60 seconds after the injection and a large amount of rapidly absorbed medium will produce an excellent bilateral nephrogram (Fig. 1–14). By definition, the nephrogram refers to the "lighting up" of the entire renal parenchyma so that the renal outlines are very clearly seen. This effect is caused by the contrast medium that is within the renal tubules but that has not as yet entered the actual collecting system of the kidney.

On this 30-second film, it is almost never possible to see contrast medium within any portion of the renal collecting system. However, this very early film serves admirably to compare the two kidneys for size and promptness of visualization. As noted above, delay in visualization on one side is compatible with a renal arterial lesion that may or may not be etiologic in a hypertensive patient (Fig. 1–15). These

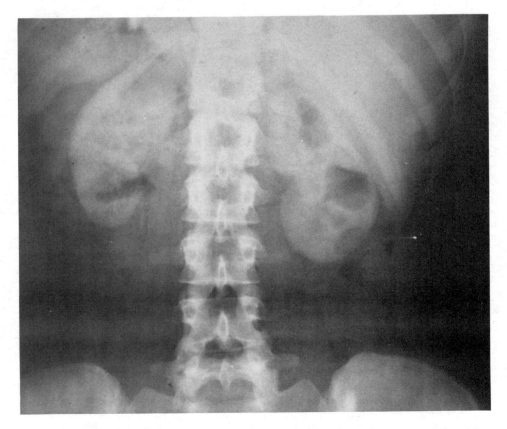

Figure 1-14. Bilateral nephrogram. Both kidneys are very well "lighted up" by the contrast medium within the renal tubules. In this film, exposed 30 to 60 seconds after injection of the contrast medium, the medium has not yet reached the collecting system of the kidney. In this patient, the right kidney is higher than the left, the reverse of the usual situation.

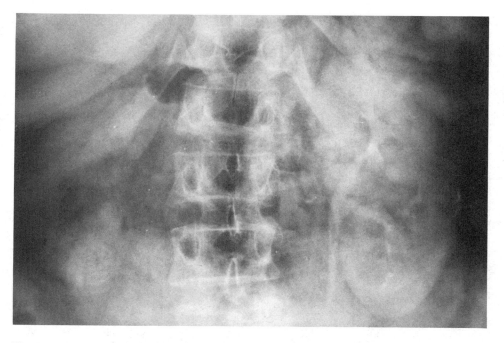

Figure 1–15. An excretory urogram showing a normal collecting system in the left kidney and a marked delay in function of the right kidney. This delay in function was caused by a unilateral renal artery stenosis on the right side.

early nephrograms additionally permit clear visualization of the renal contours for symmetry and for smoothness and accurate comparison of the two renal outlines for size. A disparity of more than 1.5 cm between the kidneys (Fig. 1–16) may be indicative of an atrophy of the smaller kidney, which could be due to a vascular insult, scarring and atrophy secondary to chronic infection, or, uncommonly, simply a normal variance between the kidneys. Films subsequent to the nephrograms are usually taken at 3, 5, 10, and 20 minutes after injection.

When an infusion urogram is being performed, the first film is usually taken 2 to 5 minutes after the infusion is started when half of the contents of the bottle have been absorbed; at this time the renal collecting system is usually well visualized. There may or may not be a residual bilateral nephrogram effect even though it is very apparent that the contrast is present in the collecting system. Whether the excretory urogram is of the conventional or of the infusion type the clinician should carefully examine the structure of the minor calyces, looking for fine cupping and the semicircular elliptical appearance that is normal (Fig. 1–17). This indentation or invagination (cupping) of each calyx is due to the renal papilla that normally invaginates the calyx directly beneath it. When this fine cupping is not present the calyx may appear blunted or clubbed; this is commonly due to the retraction of the renal papilla that results from scarring of the underlying renal parenchyma such as may occur with chronic pyelonephritis. The resulting hydrostatic pressure within the calyx that is unopposed by a renal papilla on the other side will make the calyx appear blunted or clubbed (Fig. 1–18).

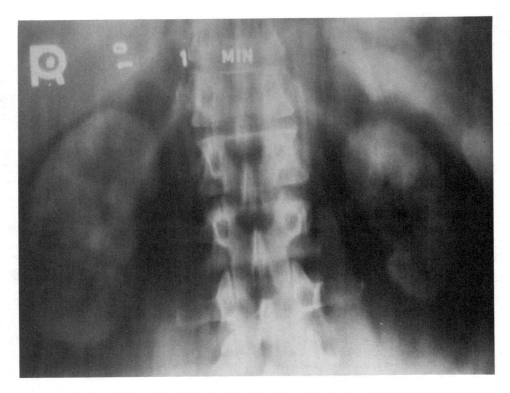

Figure 1-16. An early film taken 1 minute after injection of contrast medium showing a striking disparity in size between the two kidneys, with the left kidney being much smaller. In this case the unilateral atrophy on the left was secondary to severe renal artery stenosis on that side.

It is important for the physician to notice that the architecture of the collecting system of one kidney is not necessarily a mirror image of that of the other kidney, although, more often than not, the kidneys will be similar in appearance. There are many variations; a duplicated renal collecting system is a fairly common one and may be present on both sides or unilaterally (Fig. 1-19). The most important thing a clinician can do to become familiar with the variations of the normal excretory urogram is to view as many as possible.

By far the most frequent error made by the neophyte in looking at urograms is to interpret abnormality where none exists. However, true aberrations from the normal—gross dilatation of the collecting system, inability to visualize the collecting system, or distortion of one or more portions of the collecting system such that the normal intrarenal architecture may no longer be present—should be readily discerned. These distortions may be due to intrarenal masses that impinge on the collecting system, thereby distorting it in one direction or another.

Given that some part or another of the entire urinary tract from the topmost calyx to the lowest portion of the ureter is usually in peristalsis and that this peristalsis propels the contrast medium toward the bladder, the necessity to take more than one x-ray film becomes apparent; any one given film may very well not visualize all of the collecting system of the kidneys and the ureters because those parts that

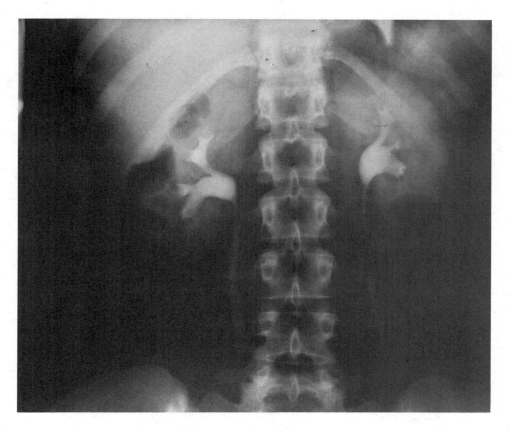

Figure 1–17. Excretory urogram. Five minutes after injection of the contrast medium both renal collecting systems and ureters are very well visualized and the contrast medium has already started to reach the bladder. Note particularly in this film the very sharp detail of the minor calyces, with the normal "cupping" that is characteristic of these calyces in a normal urogram.

are in peristalsis will not be able to fill with contrast media. It is only by viewing *all* of the exposed films that the physician is able to make a rational interpretation of the urograms. The lower ureter, for example, may be seen in only one film and the middle calyx may fill out in only one other film. It is improper to try to interpret each film independently and it may be very misleading to interpret the urogram without seeing *every* film that has been exposed. Correct and successful interpretation of an excretory urogram rests in careful viewing and understanding of each of its component films. At the end of 20 minutes, the patient is usually placed first in the right posterior oblique position and then in the left posterior oblique position for better delineation of the renal outlines that is made possible by changing the angle between the kidneys and the overlying intestines (Fig. 1–20 A and B). Radiopacities seen anywhere along the course of the urinary tract may be ruled outside or inside the tract by using these oblique films as they add a three-dimensional aspect to the study.

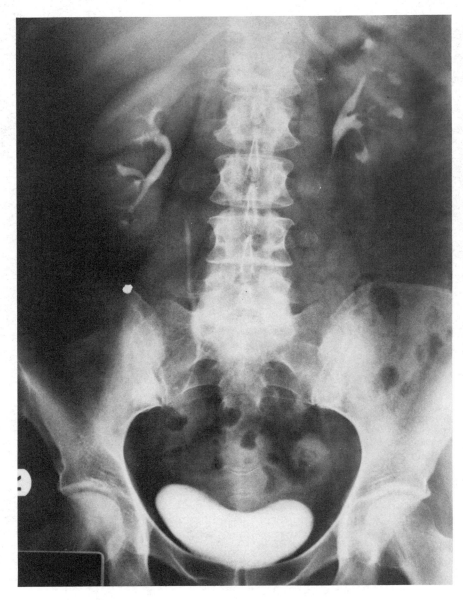

Figure 1-18. An excretory urogram with a normal right kidney and a classical and very characteristic picture of chronic pyelonephritis in the left kidney. Note the clubbing of the calyces on the left side and the marked atrophy of the parenchyma overlying the clubbed calyces.

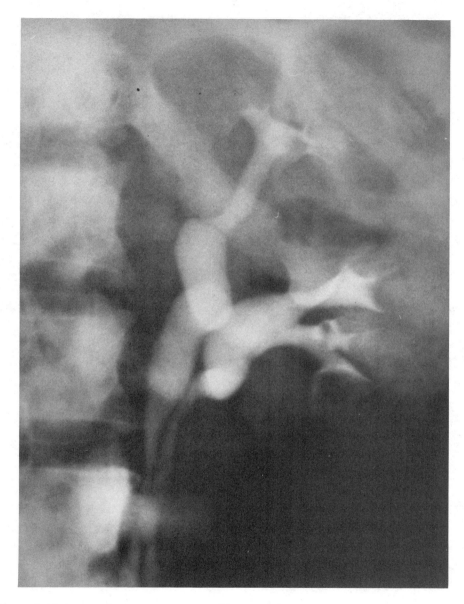

Figure 1-19. A normal excretory urogram with one of the many variations of normal seen on the left side; in this case there is duplication of the left renal and ureteral collecting systems. This is a variant of normal.

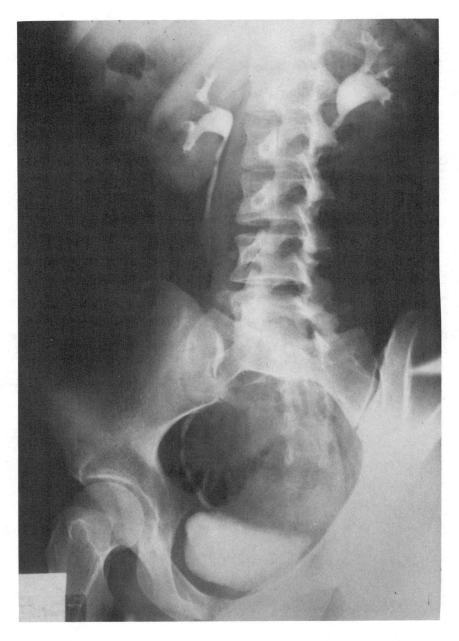

Figure 1-20. A. Excretory urogram. Right posterior oblique view. The patient is positioned with his right hip placed posteriorly against the x-ray cassette and his left hip angled up towards the x-ray camera. The right and left posterior oblique films are particularly advantageous for visualizing the collecting system in another dimension, for seeing the renal outlines more clearly as the intestinal gas is displaced anteriorly, and for localizing calcifications inside or outside of the urinary tract.

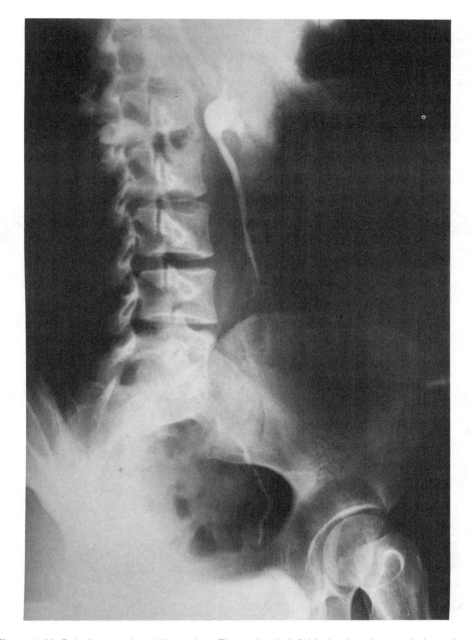

Figure 1-20. B. Left posterior oblique view. The patient's left hip is placed posteriorly against the cassette and the right hip is angled upward toward the x-ray camera. Right and left posterior oblique films are exposed with the patient lying basically in the supine position on the x-ray table.

As time elapses after its injection, more contrast medium reaches the bladder, thereby giving a good roentgenographic depiction of this structure. This phase is called the excretory cystogram, and filling defects within the bladder, such as may be seen with bladder tumors, are often readily identified at this time (Fig. 1–21). Large intravesical filling defects such as may be caused by enlarged lateral or middle prostatic lobes may also be visualized (Fig. 1–22). It is at this point in the sequence of the excretory urogram that the so-called physiologic voiding cystourethrogram can be obtained by having the patient void under fluoroscopic control; when the entire urethra is filled with contrast medium during voiding spot films can be taken. This is obviously more difficult to do in children than in adults, but

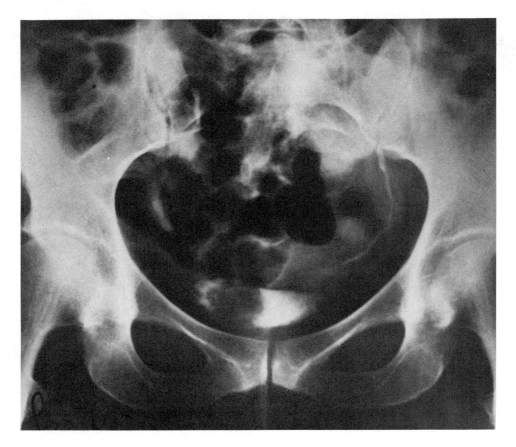

Figure 1–21. The excretory cystogram phase of the excretory urogram can often give a strong suggestion of the presence of a bladder tumor. In this illustration, note the filling defect that is seen on the right side of the bladder. This appears as a negative shadow and is caused by the presence of a bladder tumor keeping the contrast medium from filling the bladder uniformly. This particular film happened to be the postvoiding film but all of the exposures showing the bladder have the same finding.

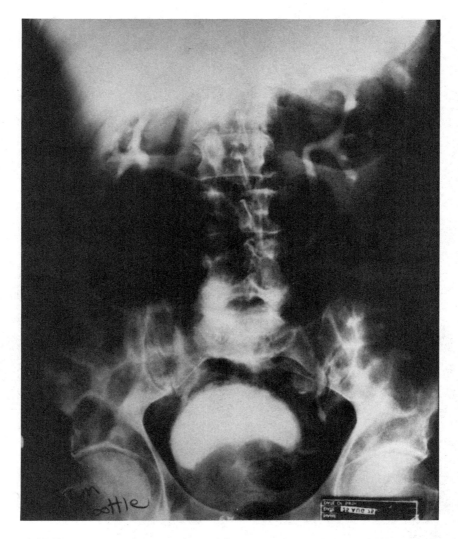

Figure 1-22. The excretory cystogram phase of the excretory urogram in this film shows a marked filling defect on the floor of the bladder caused by massively enlarged prostatic lobes.

it is extremely advantageous to the clinician to have this information and every effort should be made to convince the radiologist to take the time and effort to do this.

Additional films that may be taken during the course of the excretory urography sequence include those with the patient in an upright position for the purpose of documenting renal mobility and in a prone position in which the ureters fall anteriorly, thereby promoting drainage of the contrast medium from the kidneys and ureters (Fig. 1–23). It is also standard procedure in most radiology departments to obtain a postvoiding film which gives a rough estimate of the residual urine based on the amount of contrast medium remaining after voiding (Fig. 1–24). This film

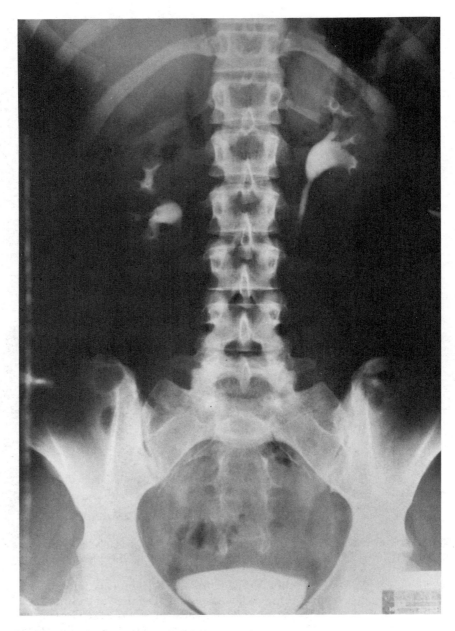

Figure 1-23. Excretory urogram. Sometime toward the end of the x-ray sequence, either before or after the postvoiding film is exposed, the patient is placed on his or her stomach and a prone film is obtained. In this position the ureters fall anteriorly, thereby promoting drainage of the contrast medium from the kidney and ureters and occasionally promoting better visualization of the ureters as they fall anteriorly.

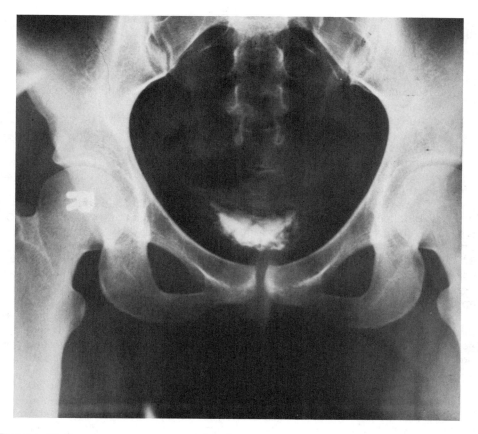

Figure 1-24. Excretory urogram postvoiding film. These films are obtained near the end of the excretory urogram sequence. The patients are instructed to empty their bladders as completely as they can, after which the postvoiding films are exposed. In this manner, a very rough estimate of the postvoiding residual urine can be obtained. In this illustration, there is only a very minimal postvoiding residual urine.

is also helpful if a lower ureteral stone is suspected because the urinary bladder that is distended with contrast medium will usually successfully mask the presence of any lower ureteral stone.

The right kidney is normally lower than the left because of the presence of the liver, but in about five percent of individuals the left kidney is lower than the right. When encountering this relatively uncommon condition, the clinician must consider the possibility of retroperitoneal pathology such as an adrenal or other retroperitoneal mass that is depressing the left kidney, as there is no way of knowing whether or not the patient is in that 5 percent group. In the vast majority of cases, however, it is obvious that no abnormal findings will be present. Of equal importance to this relative position of one kidney to the other is the position of the axis of each kidney, which normally tapers inward toward the vertebral bodies from the lower pole to the upper pole of the kidney. Anything altering this normal axis or causing a lateral displacement of the upper or lower pole away from the vertebral bodies must alert the clinician to the possibility of a retroperitoneal mass as the displacing factor.

The ureters are rarely seen in their entirety on any one film, making it necessary to study several films to visualize the entire ureter. Lateral displacement of the ureters may be due to enlarged retroperitoneal lymph nodes such as may occur from metastatic carcinoma or primary retroperitoneal lymphomas. Medial displacement of the ureters may be simply a variation of normal, a part of the natural history of retroperitoneal fibrosis, or simply a result of earlier retroperitoneal surgery. As a general rule, unless the ureter deviates medially to the medial aspect of the vertebral pedicle on the ipsilateral side, there is no abnormal deviation.

In summary, the excretory urogram, whether of the infusion or conventional variety, is a roentgenographic study intended for the visualization of the intrarenal architecture as well as the ureter, the bladder, and, hopefully, the urethra. The excretory urogram does not necessarily demonstrate all pathologic conditions within the renal parenchyma unless the abnormality is large enough to distort the collecting system or the normal outline of the kidney. Examples of easily visualized abnormal findings are large renal cysts, renal tumors, or tumors of the renal collecting system. The excretory urogram is definitely of no value in documenting so-called medical diseases such as glomerulonephritis and certain of the other less common nephritides. Polycystic renal disease, however, does have a characteristic roentgenographic appearance, as does chronic pyelonephritis.

There are few x-ray studies in all of clinical medicine that can return more information per unit time to the clinician than the correctly ordered and carefully performed excretory urogram. The study, however, is only as valuable as its interpretation and every primary care physician should be able to at least differentiate normal urographic findings from abnormal ones.

A caveat for the clinician is that excretory urography is not without risk and very serious anaphylactic-type reactions, sometimes fatal, will occur in about 1 of 20,000 to 1 of 800,000 excretory urograms. There is no reliable pretest to determine if the patient is likely to be susceptible. Given the catastrophic nature of such reactions, it goes without saying that excretory urograms should only be ordered when the clinician feels that there is a definite indication and that knowledge to be gained can justify the risk.

Cystoscopy

If one were to try to choose the single diagnostic procedure that is unique to urology and that is performed by physicians of no other speciality, it would be the endoscopic examination of the urethra and bladder. It is this extremely precise ability to diagnose pathologic conditions within the bladder and urethra, including the prostatic urethra, that helps to make urology the highly developed specialty that it is.

Cystoscopic examinations in adult men and women can almost always be performed on an outpatient basis using local anesthesia. In children of either sex under the age of 16 or thereabouts, a general anesthetic is often preferable, not necessarily because of any pain inherent in the procedure, but because of the mental trauma and anguish inevitable when procedures are carried out on the external genitalia. At the time of the cystoscopic procedure, men (and women) are placed in the lithotomy position on a cystoscopy table. After suitable draping and cleansing of the external genitalia with soap and water, a generous amount of local anesthesia is introduced into the urethral meatus and allowed to travel through the entire urethra to achieve anesthesia. Agents such as lidocaine jelly (Xylocaine) are ideal for this purpose, with the jelly squeezed out of the tube directly into the urethra. An 18F or 21F cystourethroscope (for adults) is introduced into the urethra using the utmost degree of gentleness; if this is done properly, the patient should experience only minimal discomfort as the instrument is being passed and should have no pain once the cystoscope is within the bladder. Cystoscopy enables the urologist to examine with great accuracy and infinite detail the interior of the bladder, including the ureteral orifices (this is particularly significant in evaluating patients with vesicoureteral reflux), and it additionally facilitates a thorough examination and evaluation of the urethra, including the prostatic urethra, for any objective signs of any disease process and for obstruction as well.

Although a major and very desirable added bonus of cystoscopy is the accurate measurement of the quantity of residual urine present in the bladder (by having the patient void just prior to cystoscopy and then measuring the urine remaining in the bladder when the cystoscope is passed), it is probably not wise to use cystoscopy on patients who are thought to have a *great deal* of residual urine present. Their bladders are obviously not normal and introduction of a foreign body such as a cystoscope can promote severe bladder infection in the presence of residual urine. Cystoscopic evaluation of these patients, with or without determination of residual urine, is best undertaken in a hospital setting to allow close observation following the procedure and prompt treatment if any untoward results occur.

During the course of any cystoscopic exam it is possible to do a very rough sort of urodynamic (see below) evaluation of the bladder by noting the amount of water that has been introduced into the bladder when the patient first reports a voiding urge, by noting the amount of water in the bladder when the patient states that his or her bladder is absolutely full, by poking the four quadrants of the bladder interior with the beak of the cystoscope to see if the patient is able to feel this, by running hot and cold water into the bladder to see if the patient is aware of the difference, and, finally, by noting the expulsive force of the water as it leaves the bladder through the cystoscope when the operating element has been removed from the sheath. All of the foregoing, in the author's opinion, can offer to the clinician, in a very rough manner, much of the knowledge to be gained by using sophisticated urodynamic equipment, although nothing can be determined about intraurethral pressures and the function of the urethral sphincters. Cystoscopy should not really be considered a substitute for sophisticated urodynamic studies in patients in whom bladder sphincter or urethral dysfunction is known or suspected. However, as a simple screening device for the patient felt to have an intact voiding mechanism, the above studies (including the measurement of residual urine) are, in the author's opinion, acceptable.

An additional purpose of cystoscopy is to facilitate the passage of ureteral catheters into the ureters in order to obtain urine from a kidney in an attempt to localize the source of bacteria in certain diagnostically difficult cases. Cystoscopy and ureteral catheterization are also indicated to obtain retrograde ureteropyelograms (Fig. 1–25) when this particular study is indicated; cystoscopy is also necessary to pass long-term indwelling ureteral stents in patients with chronic ureteral obstruction, usually due to extrinsic tumor masses. Finally, the cystoscope may be used in the catheterization of the ureters in those very rare occasions when separated measures of renal function are desired in the diagnostic workup of the patient thought to have renovascular hypertension.

36

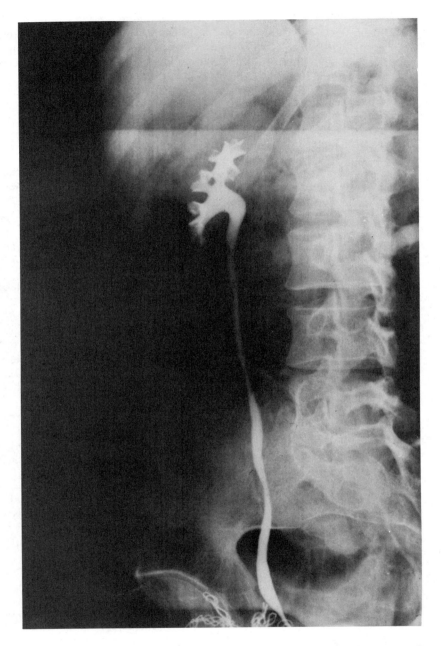

Figure 1-25. A normal right retrograde ureteropyelogram. These studies are most often performed when the excretory urogram discloses a persistent failure to visualize one or another portion of the renal collecting system (or of the ureter) and the retrograde ureteropyelogram is then performed to see if the area in question truly has a filling defect (which may represent a carcinoma) or whether it is merely in spasm, peristalsis, or being compressed externally by a blood vessel.

Bladder Catheterization

Probably the first purpose of a urethral catheter that would come to the mind of the average physician is to provide bladder drainage for the individual unable to void spontaneously. In such circumstances, there is little disagreement among physicians regarding the necessity for catheterization or the fact that the benefits outweigh the inherent risks, and this applies to the one time in-and-out catheterization to relieve acute urinary retention as well as to the use of an indwelling (Foley) urethral catheter for an indefinite period of time to relieve chronic urinary retention. *Intermittent catheterization* is a very excellent technique to facilitate bladder emptying in an individual who is chronically unable to void satisfactorily such that large amounts of residual urine are present following voiding. As a general rule, this problem will be found in individuals with bladder neuropathy due to conditions such as spinal cord injuries, diabetes, multiple sclerosis, and so on. The intermittent catheterization is done every 3 to 6 hours, depending upon fluid intake and may even be done by the patient himself or herself (intermittent self-catheterization) in a most effective manner. This procedure has been a proven one for about the last dozen years, and it is vastly preferable to the long-term chronic use of an indwelling catheter in terms of minimizing bladder infections and their sequelae. When long-term intermittent catheterization is required, it is not necessary and it is almost impossible to follow an absolutely sterile technique.

It is interesting to note, however, that the urethral catheter is probably used much more frequently for diagnosis than for the therapeutic purposes noted above, although such use is not quite as acceptable to the general medical community as is its therapeutic use. The use of the bladder catheter for diagnostic purposes is an inherently safe procedure with little risk to the patient who has an essentially normal bladder. As noted in Chapter 2, there is an intrinsic defense mechanism centered in the bladder mucosa such that small or moderate numbers of bacteria introduced into the bladder are spontaneously shed under usual and normal circumstances without resultant clinical infection. For this reason, it is probably not necessary to follow a sterile technique when performing a diagnostic catheterization but tradition dictates that we *do* follow it. In adults, a well-lubricated catheter of 16F or 18F is probably optimal. For the female child, a significantly smaller size catheter should be used, depending on her age. It is probably wise *not* to catheterize boys under 8 years of age because of the possible risk of traumatizing their very small urethra and thereby producing a stricture; however, if catheterization is absolutely necessary, as small a catheter as possible—certainly one no larger than 8F or 10F in caliber—should be used. Introduction of a catheter into the female meatus may sometimes be a problem because of difficulty in locating the meatus and the catheter may inadvertently be passed into the vagina. With the female in the lithotomy position a bright spotlight focused on the genitalia is absolutely necessary, and when anatomically the meatus is virtually at the anterior vaginal wall, gentle probing with the well-lubricated catheter is sometimes necessary to identify the urethra.

In the male it is particularly important to use sufficient lubricating jelly and to introduce the catheter with extreme care and gentleness. Assuming adequate lubrication and the absence of a urethral stricture, the catheter should pass easily until it meets the external urethral sphincter, which invariably goes into an involuntary spasm when the catheter reaches it. Gentle, inward pressure against the catheter at the level of the urethral meatus while the tip of the catheter rests against the external urethral sphincter (membranous urethra) will shortly result in fatigue and

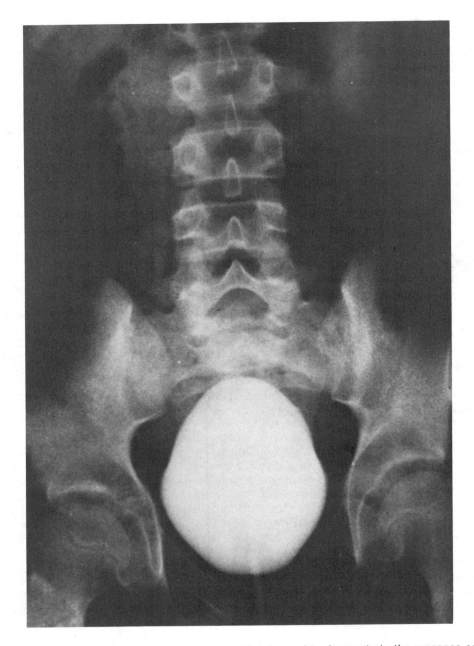

Figure 1-26. A retrograde cystourethrogram, which is used to demonstrate the presence or absence of vesicoureteral reflux. **A.** A normal study showing no reflux at all.

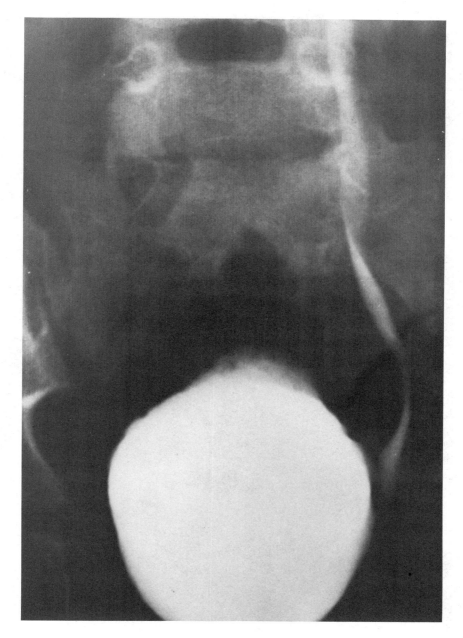

Figure 1-26. B. A different retrograde cystourethrogram showing reflux on the left side, which in this particular patient extended up the entire ureter and into the kidney.

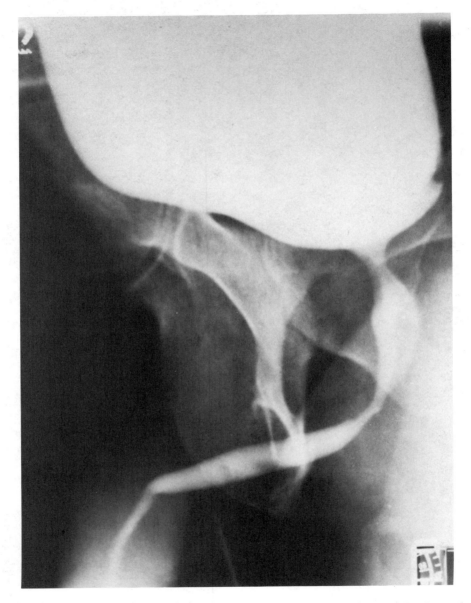

Figure 1–27. A retrograde voiding cystourethrogram that was done in order to visualize the urethra. This is a perfectly normal study showing all of the posterior urethra and a portion of the pendulous urethra.

relaxation of the sphincter and allow the easy passage of the catheter into the bladder. The relaxation of the sphincter can take anywhere from 5 to 20 seconds, and during this time a gentle but steady pressure should be maintained on the catheter but no effort should be made to force it through the sphincter. If it is not possible to pass the catheter into the bladder, as evidenced by urine return through the catheter, attempts should cease and should only be reinstituted by a physician or other individual specially trained and competent in the passage of a catheter (usually a urologist or a urologist's assistant). Persistent efforts to pass a catheter into the bladder by an untrained individual can result in severe trauma to the urethra. The most common reasons for inability to pass a catheter into the bladder are strictures of the urethra and enlargement of the prostate gland, particularly the middle lobe.

The principal reason for diagnostic catheterization of the bladder in men (and sometimes in women) is the accurate measurement of the quantity of residual urine present immediately following voiding (see Chapter 7). Inasmuch as men and older boys can invariably produce midstream urine specimens of an uncontaminated nature for the purpose of obtaining a urine culture, catheterization for this purpose is almost never necessary. Similarly, in the vast majority of females a urine specimen that is satisfactory for culturing can be obtained by means of a midstream collection following thorough cleansing of the urethral meatus and external genitalia. In a small percentage of women and girls, however, it is not possible to obtain an uncontaminated urine specimen, and in these patients bladder catheterization is indicated.

Another reason for bladder catheterization in any individual is to obtain retrograde cystograms and voiding cystourethrograms to verify the presence or absence of vesicoureteral reflux (Fig. 1–26 A and B) and at the same time to visualize the urethra roentgenographically (Fig. 1–27). In such instances contrast medium is instilled by gravity flow up to the capacity of the bladder, after which the catheter is removed and the patient is instructed to void. X-ray films are exposed during the filling of the bladder with contrast medium, after the bladder has been filled, and particularly during the act of voiding. Note that this retrograde manner of bladder filling through a catheter is necessary if the clinician is trying to demonstrate vesicoureteral reflux since the use of a "physiologic" voiding cystourethrogram described above is not satisfactory for this purpose. However, if simple demonstration and delineation of the urethra is all that is desired, then this retrograde approach is most satisfactory and the "physiologic" voiding cystourethrogram is probably just as satisfactory.

Finally, in any patient with known or suspected urethral strictures or diverticula or injury, excellent roentgenographic visualization of such urethral abnormalities is mandatory and may be obtained by inserting a catheter just inside the urethral meatus followed by injection of contrast medium in a retrograde manner through the catheter and into the urethra while x-ray films are exposed.

RADIOISOTOPE STUDIES

Renal Scanning

The principal clinical use of radioisotope scanning of the kidney is to obtain information about various physiologic functions of the kidney. Scanning does not provide any useful information regarding renal morphology and it is not helpful in trying to differentiate renal cysts from renal tumors. However, it can provide very valuable information about plasma clearance, renal accumulation of isotope, acute and chronic renal obstruction, and renal function following transplantation. Perhaps most important of all, it can provide quantitative information about the function of each kidney. For example, coupled with a computer, it can give the percentage of total renal function being provided by each kidney.

Various chemical compounds are handled in various manners by the kidney, that is, some are filtered by the glomerulus, some are secreted by the renal tubules, and so on. Radioactive substances can be used to label these various chemical compounds so that a measurement of the radioactivity at any given point in time serves as an indirect measurement of how the kidney has handled the chemical compound. One commonly performed study is the technetium-99m diethylinetriaminepentacetic acid (Tc-99m-DTPA) scan, which provides information on renal function and perfusion when injected intravenously. The Tc-99m-DTPA is circulated through the vascular system and filtered by the renal glomeruli, in much the same manner as contrast medium is handled. Instead of an x-ray source external to the patient interacting with the tissues to create an image on a film that is underneath the patient, as occurs in radiography, the source of the radiation is internal and the gamma rays emitted from the radioisotope in the body are "captured" by a special camera and recorded on film. Very early, rapid images obtained after injection trace the flow of the Tc-99m-DTPA through the vascular system to the kidneys, providing information on relative renal perfusion (Fig. 1–28).

Another Tc-99m compound that is used in renal scanning is dimercaptosuccinic acid (DMSA), which is retained longer in the cortex than Tc-99m-DTPA. This agent is used primarily to distinguish a pseudotumor of the kidney (a hypertrophied septum of Bertin) from a renal mass such as a neoplasm, cyst, or abscess. The pseudotumor takes up as much Tc-99m-DMSA as the surrounding normal cortical tissue, whereas neoplasms, cysts, or abscesses do not take up the agent and would therefore appear as a "cold" spot within the kidney. It must be noted, however, that this isotope will not serve to differentiate a renal tumor from a renal cyst (Fig. 1–29).

When the Tc-99m-DTPA scan is combined with another radionucleide agent, I-131 orthohippurate, this combination will afford a "triple renal scan." The I-131 orthohippurate is handled differently by the kidney than the Tc-99m-DTPA since it is extracted by the renal tubular cell from the circulation through the kidney and it is excreted into the renal tubular lumina, thereby providing valuable information on renal tubular function. Computer analysis of the data obtained from this study provides a "renogram" consisting of graphs describing plasma clearance, renal accumulation, and clearance and bladder accumulation curves (Fig. 1–30 A and B). As noted above, this triple renal scan has been of use in the evaluation of acute and chronic obstruction and in the status of the grafted kidney in renal transplantation patients.

The advantages of radioisotope renal scans lie in the fact that they can be used in patients with allergy to contrast media in order to provide very gross anatomic details about kidney size, function, and the presence or absence of obstruction. They may also be advantageous when one or both kidneys are not visualized by excretory urography but are still present and functioning minimally. In such a situation a radioisotope scanning *may* demonstrate functioning renal tissue that is present; this is particularly the case in the patient with a high creatinine level. However, a kidney that is nonvisualized by both excretory urography and radioisotope scanning will require ultrasound or CT scanning to detect if any renal tissue is present.

The main disadvantage of radioisotope scans lies in the poor detail of anatomy provided and these scans in no way serve as a substitute for an excretory urogram

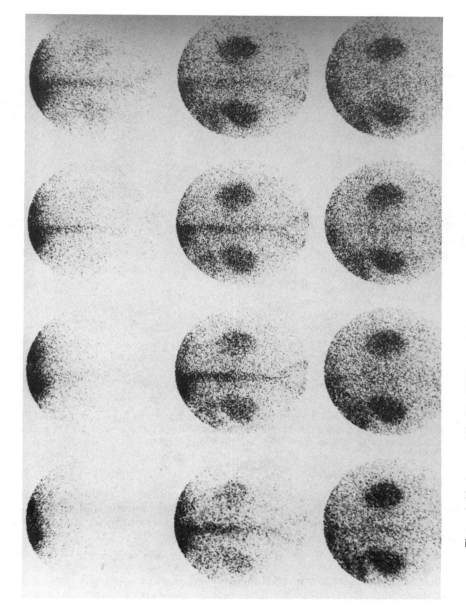

Figure 1-28. A normal Tc-99m-DTPA renal perfusion. This demonstrates a normal and equal bilateral renal blood supply based upon the prompt and symmetric visualization of each kidney.

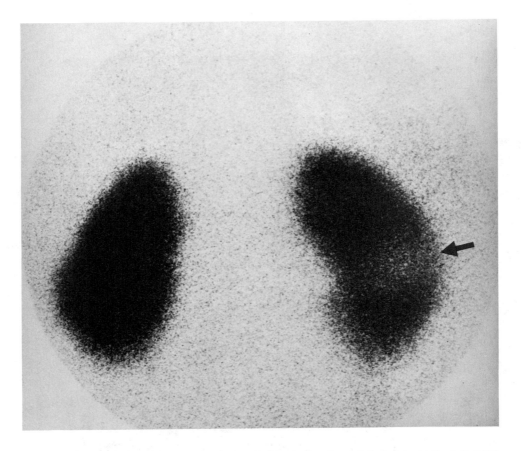

Figure 1-29. A Tc-99m-DMSA renal scan showing lack of radionuclide uptake in the left renal mass (*arrow*). This lack of uptake differentiates this area from a pseudotumor of the kidney, which would have normal uptake, and makes the area identified by the arrow either a tumor, cyst or abscess.

if one is interested in anything but the very roughest outline of renal morphology. Although the radiation dose to the patient is low it can be quite high in cases of obstruction where the radioactive agent remains within the obstructed kidney for long periods of time.

Bladder Scanning

In addition to the bladder accumulation curves alluded to above, in which total renal function can be determined by measuring the radioactivity over the bladder, scanning of the bladder may also be used to measure postvoid residual urine, although in practice it is hardly ever used for this purpose since far more direct, accurate, and less costly methods are available. The isotope used in bladder scanning is Tc-99m-DTPA.

Scrotal Scanning

The differential between torsion of the spermatic cord and epididymoorchitis can

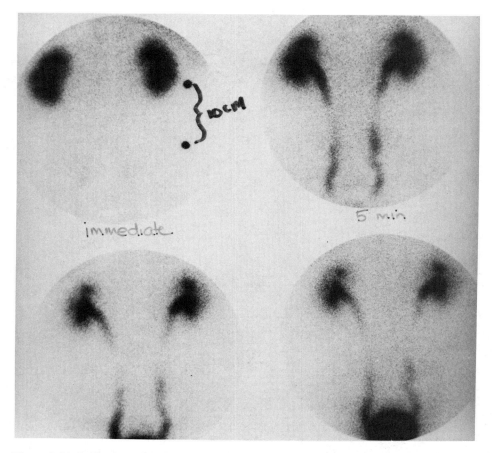

Figure 1-30. A. Tc-99m-DTPA renal scan showing normal renal function. This demonstrates the gross anatomy of the urinary tract and the presence or absence of obstruction.

be an extraordinarily difficult one (see Chapter 11) and, in the final analysis, the decision as to whether or not to explore the scrotum surgically should be a clinical one. However, scrotal scanning may assist the clinician in this diagnosis by demonstrating either an increased blood supply secondary to inflammation on the affected side (epididymoorchitis) or a decreased blood supply secondary to vascular compromise (torsion of the spermatic cord). These findings are determined by comparing the scan on the affected side with the contralateral normal side. Tc-99m-DTPA (pertechnetate) is used as the agent for scrotal scanning.

Bone Scanning

Bone scanning is carried out for the purpose of determining whether or not a given patient has metastatic disease to the bone (most often, in urology, from prostatic carcinoma) and it is used particularly when the bony x-rays are normal. Changes suggestive of metastatic disease will appear in bone scans 3 to 6 months before any changes will be visible on bone x-rays and it therefore is a much more sensitive procedure for the evaluation of metastatic disease. The radioisotope used for this study

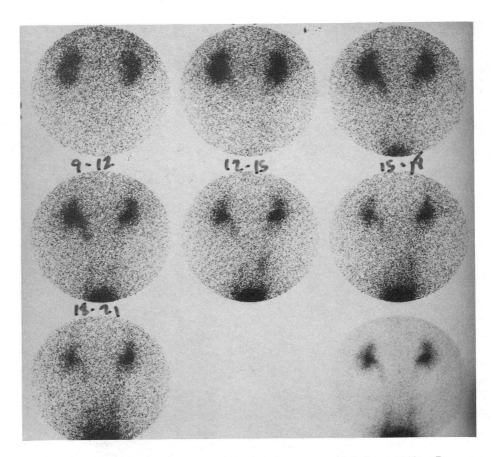

Figure 1–30. B. An I-131 Hippuran scan that demonstrates normal tubular excretion. Renogram curves can be derived by computer from this scan. Combined with that scan shown in Figure 1–28, **A** and **B** form the so-called triple scan.

is Tc-99m-MDP (diphosphonate) and this isotope is taken up by bone in a reparative phase. In other words, whenever there has been any metastatic bone destruction, this is followed by a reparative process and it is this reparative process that is being measured by the bone scan (Fig. 1–31). Unfortunately the reparative process is the same and will appear the same on bone scan whether it is secondary to metastatic disease, trauma, or inflammatory disease such as arthritis. Therefore, a positive bone scan does not constitute firm evidence of metastatic disease, but it is certainly strongly presumptive evidence in the face of a known primary cancer.

Gallium Scanning

Another form of scanning that is not specific for any particular part of the body is done with gallium citrate. This agent is picked up by collections of leukocytes and therefore this type of scanning is helpful in diagnosing abscesses (which are collections of pus cells). Specifically, it is used to confirm or corroborate a suspicion of an intra- or peri-renal abscess, or an abscess in the lower retroperitoneum or pelvis.

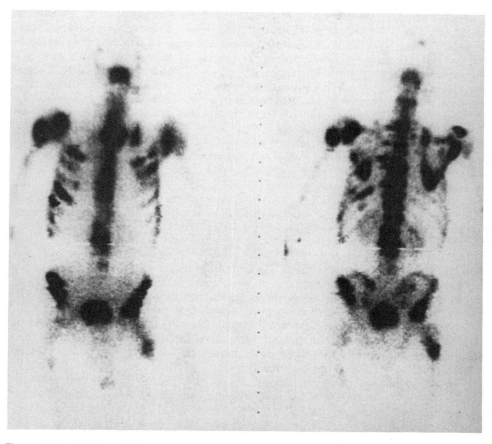

Figure 1–31. A Tc-99m-MDP bone scan showing multiple areas of increased uptake *(black areas)*, suggesting multiple osseous metastases.

Computed Tomography (CT) Scanning

CT scanning, an extraordinary diagnostic methodology, has been in clinical use only since the late 1970s. CT is a cross-sectional imaging modality that represents a combination of x-ray and computer technology. A rotating fan-shaped x-ray beam emanates from a large doughnut-shaped gantry surrounding the patient and penetrates the body in a thin (1 cm) transverse cross section. An array of detectors also located in the gantry records the continuation of the x-ray beam by the tissues of the body and stores the data in digital form in the systems computer. By solving multiple, complex mathematical equations the computer reconstructs a two-dimensional image of the anatomic cross section from the x-ray data. Such multiple scans are obtained through the kidneys at 1-cm intervals. Although in cross section, the resulting images are similar to those of the familiar conventional x-ray: the high density of bone is recorded as white, tissue density as shades of gray, fat as near black, and air as black (Fig. 1–32). The computer can characterize these density differences with a CT number relative to water density, which is arbitrarily designated as 0. Computed tomography is able to detect differences in density far better than conventional radiography, and as such it is highly useful in the evaluation of renal masses. Renal cysts, for example, can usually be easily distinguished from solid neoplasms because of their low density and homogeneous nature, whereas renal malignancies containing calcification or fat are readily identified where they might well be overlooked on plain urography (Fig. 1–33). The indications for CT scanning are many and include the evaluation of a solitary renal mass lesion that is not unequivocally characterized by ultrasound; the evaluation of suspected or known multiple renal mass lesions; the evaluation of suspected or known angiomyolipomas or other vascular malformations; the evaluation of a known renal cell carcinoma as far as its stage (whether or not it is still confined within the renal capsule); the evaluation of suspected recurrent renal cell carcinoma after nephrectomy; the evaluation of a perirenal hematoma or abscess; the evaluation of the kidney with an abnormal axis or an abnormal position of the kidney itself or of the ureter; the evaluation of a filling defect of the renal pelvis or the ureter; the evaluation of possible adrenal lesions, retroperitoneal masses, or pelvic lipomatosis; and to a lesser extent in the staging of known bladder, prostate, kidney, ureteral, or testis cancer.

The CT scan offers several very specific advantages and disadvantages over any other type of roentgenographic study; no special preparation is needed (other than the fact that the patient should be kept NPO as far as recent food intake because contrast material is given); it can detect small lesions that may be missed on the excretory urogram; it will provide additional information about the bones, the liver, the adrenals, the lymph nodes, and vessels beyond the specific purpose for which the study is intended; bone density and gas in the intestines do not interfere with the images, as they do in ultrasound; water, fat, calcium and acute hemorrhage can be confidently identified; and finally, unlike ultrasound, the CT scan offers a standardized and uniform quality.

In the author's opinion, the disadvantages of CT scans are not really significant; misleading numbers (a measure of whether a given lesion is malignant or not) can be obtained from a partial volume effect with small lesions; the fact that one is looking at cross-section anatomy means that one must look at multiple, serial images; even though the density resolution is superior, spatial resolution is poor and excretory urography, for example, is superior for looking at intrarenal collecting structures; the radiation dosage is similar to that received from an excretory urogram and there is the same risk of a severe reaction to the contrast medium; and, finally, the very high cost of the CT scan (about $600.00) is a genuine disadvantage, but as this study may at times obviate the need for an exploratory laporotomy the cost does not seem to be quite so prohibitive.

Ultrasonography

The ultrasound beam may be likened to a beam of light in that it follows the physical laws of optics and can be focused, reflected, or refracted (unlike x-rays). The beam itself, however, is not a light beam but rather a series of high-frequency sound waves that are generated by the vibration of a crystal within an ultrasound transducer. The crystal vibrates in response to an electrical stimulus and the frequency of these vibrations of the crystal are a function of the shape and the thickness of the crystal itself in much the same manner that the sound of a bell will depend upon its shape and size. The ultrasound frequency used for most medical purposes is about 3.5 million cycles per second and the same crystal that transmits the ultrasonic beam also functions as a listening device, which means that a pulse of ultrasound is sent

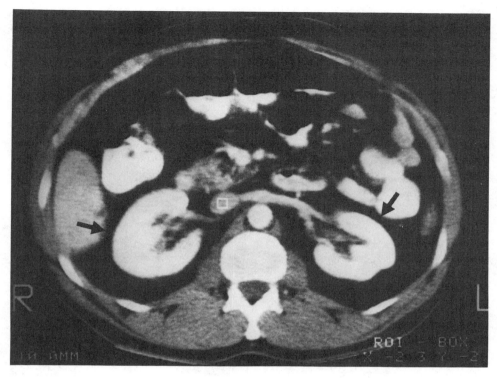

Figure 1–32. A normal CT scan with the body section at the level of the kidneys (*arrows* point to the kidneys).

out for only a fraction of a second and the crystal then "listens" for the echo response. These returning sound waves or echoes produce vibrations that are transmitted as electrical signals to an oscilloscope. These echoes or returning sound waves are produced by what is known as acoustic impedance, which is a fancy term for the fact that the tissues of the body to and through which these sound waves travel differ from each other in their sound-transmission characteristics. When two tissues are of very similar or identical sound-transmission characteristics, it is said that the acoustic impedance is very low and the resulting echoes are very weak. However, when two tissues of very differing acoustic impedance are in apposition to each other, the ultrasonic beam is partially reflected at the interface between them, returning an echo signal to the transducer; the degree of difference in the acoustic impedance determines the strength of the returning echo (the higher the acoustic impedance, the stronger the returning echo). Therefore, strong echoes will be returned if soft tissue, for example, lies next to bone, and weak echoes will be returned if two soft tissues are in apposition to each other, such as one vessel lying against another vessel. The returning echoes may be stored in the digital memory of a scan converter and may then be displayed as dots on a television monitor. This type of ultrasound display is called a B-scan, with the B standing for brightness of the dots on the screen, which vary with the strength of the acoustic impedance. Some ultrasound machines

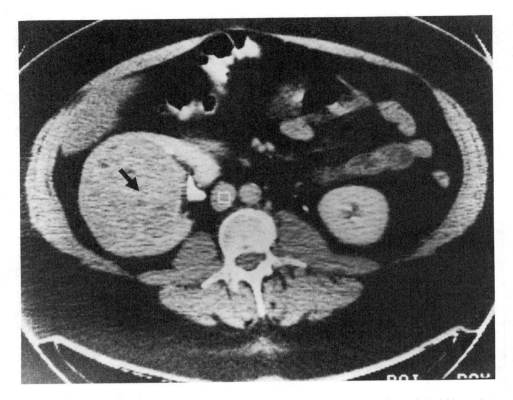

Figure 1-33. A CT scan showing a large mass occupying the middle of the right kidney that is compatible with a hypernephroma (*arrow* in the middle of the tumor mass).

also have "gray scale" capability that allows them to record parenchymal echoes in far greater detail than was previously possible. However, in urologic diagnosis the B-scan displays are the standard that are used when one is scanning the abdomen, retroperitoneum, and pelvis (Fig. 1–34).

A newer and very important form of ultrasound technology has been the development of "real-time" scanning. This may be likened to looking at fluoroscopy whereas standard B-scans are more like static x-rays. One obvious disadvantage of real-time scanning, however, is the resolution, which is much poorer than what is available with static scanning.

The specific indications for ultrasonography in urology include determining whether a mass lesion discovered in the kidney on excretory urography is cystic or solid (Figs. 1–35, 1–36). It cannot determine whether or not a lesion is malignant; it can only tell whether or not a mass lesion is a pure cyst. If it is *not* a pure cyst, then the possibility of a malignancy must be further investigated with angiograms or CT scans. It must be emphasized that ultrasonography is complementary to other studies and should not be used as a screening test except in the presence of serious contrast allergy, profound renal failure, or pregnancy. Other excellent indications for ultrasound in urology are to differentiate medical from surgical causes of acute

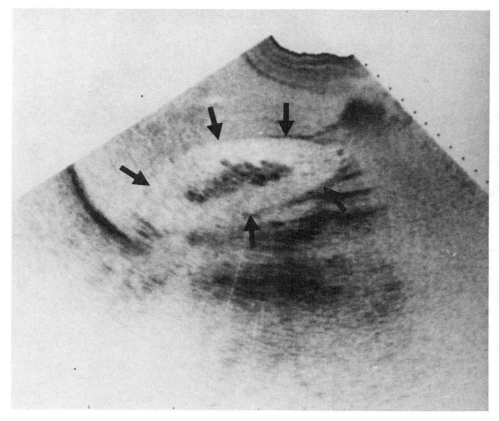

Figure 1-34. An ultrasound exam showing a normal longitudinal section through the kidney (*arrows* point to the kidney).

renal failure by differentiating renal atrophy from the hydronephrosis that is found with renal obstruction. Another good use for renal ultrasound is in evaluating a posttransplantation kidney for obstruction or fluid collection around the kidney.

In addition to the foregoing, there are other far less common and far from universally used applications of ultrasound in urology. Very new endosonic probes can be inserted through a cystoscopy sheath to scan the prostate and bladder from the inside, thereby complementing cystoscopy findings by giving an in-depth picture of tumors and surrounding structures. Also transrectal scanning with the same probe has been shown to be an acceptable method for scanning the prostate and seminal vesicles.

The advantages of ultrasound are significant: it is totally safe, in that there is no radiation present; it is noninvasive and totally painless; it is relatively inexpensive; it is flexible, in that any imaging plane can be selected; it does not require either sedation or preparation; it is independent of any function of a given organ; it tells the consistency of an organ or a mass; and it gives accurate measurements,

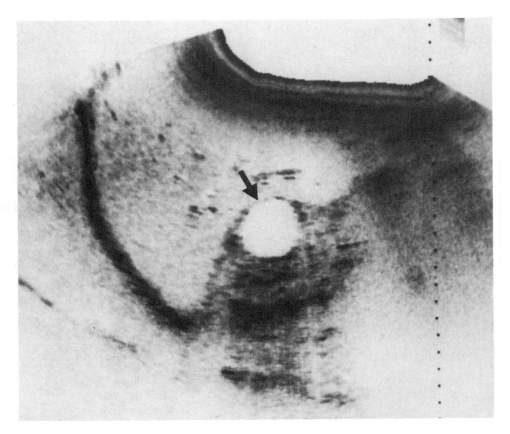

Figure 1-35. An ultrasound exam showing a longitudinal section of the kidney with a mass having no internal echoes and suggesting a cyst of the kidney (*arrows* pointing to cyst).

in that there is no magnification, as there may be with an x-ray. Disadvantages of ultrasound include the fact that bone and gas do not transmit sound well so that structures deep to them cannot be imaged well because they will reflect and disperse sound; also, fat tends to attenuate the sound waves so studies of obese people are usually poor in quality; perhaps the most important disadvantage is that the exam is highly dependent upon the skill of the person performing it and a high degree of technical competence is required.

In summary, the ultrasound wave is partially reflected at an interface between two tissues of differing acoustic impedance. The degree of difference in the acoustic impedance determines the strength of the returning echo, that is, the higher the acoustic impedance, the stronger the echo. Solid organs and masses generally do not show much acoustic enhancement but fluid-filled organs and masses show prominent acoustic enhancement since they have no internal echoes. It is the author's opinion that the principal use of ultrasound in clinical urology is in receiving an initial strong impression as to whether or not a mass lesion within the kidney found

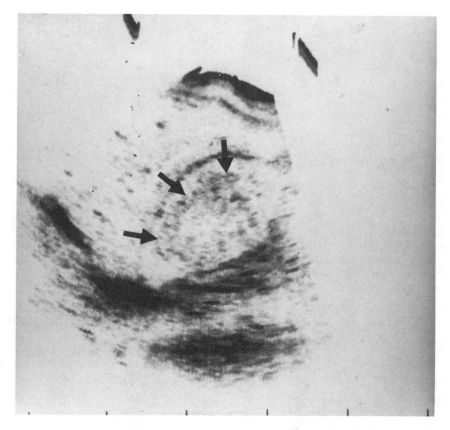

Figure 1-36. An ultrasound exam showing a longitudinal section of the kidney with a large central mass with internal echoes suggesting a solid mass lesion (*arrows* pointing to mass within the kidney).

on excretory urography is cystic. A second important clinical use for ultrasound is in diagnosing the presence or absence of retroperitoneal or pelvic abscesses or other masses.

Renal Angiography

Basically there are two indications for renal angiography (Fig. 1–37 A and B). In the hypertensive patient suspected of having a renal artery narrowing, renal angiography enables a precise visualization of the renal arteries to determine the presence of any abnormalities (Fig. 1–38). Much more commonly, renal angiography is used to determine if a mass lesion seen in the kidney on excretory urography is a malignant tumor or a benign cyst. Although ultrasound and CT scanning have tended to replace the renal angiogram in some patients for this purpose, the author still feels that there is a major role for renal angiography inasmuch as it alone illustrates the vascularity of the involved kidney and will show a characteristic pud-

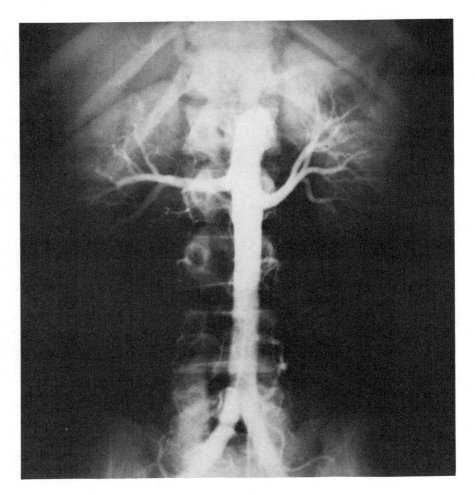

Figure 1–37. A. A normal flush renal angiogram showing the aorta, both renal arteries, and the various branches of each renal artery.

dling of the contrast media within a tumor that may be present (Fig. 1–39). Also, the vessels feeding into a tumor will often have a characteristic "corkscrew" appearance. If the mass lesion is a benign cyst, it will appear to be completely avascular on angiographic study (Fig. 1–40), although it must be noted that a benign cyst and an avascular hypernephroma can have a similar appearance on angiography.

Renal angiography is carried out most commonly under local anesthesia by catheterization of the femoral artery under x-ray control. The roentgenologist (who most often carries out such procedures) gently threads the catheter from the femoral artery into the aorta and then into the appropriate renal artery. A large volume of contrast medium is then injected and the intrarenal vasculature and any mass lesions can be visualized.

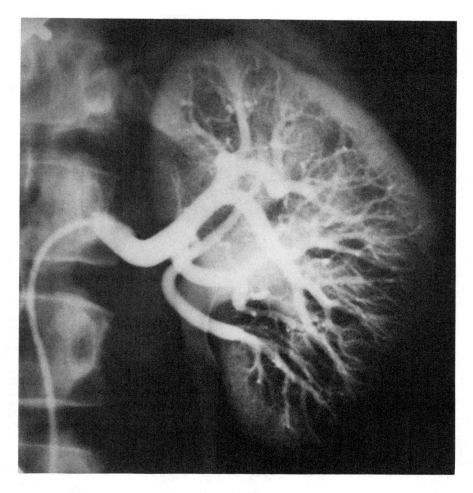

Figure 1-37. B. A normal left selective renal angiogram (not the same patient as in **A**) showing the normal details of the renal vasculature.

Nuclear Magnetic Resonance (NMR)

NMR is somewhat similar to CT scanning in that cross-sectional images are obtained, although the methodology is entirely different. Nuclear magnetic resonance imaging of the kidneys is presently in its very early stages, but it already promises to be a very valuable diagnostic tool. The images obtained are the result of complex interactions that occur whenever hydrogren atoms—abundant in the human body—are exposed to applied radio-frequency waves in a strong magnetic field. Excellent anatomic detail, similar to CT scanning, can be obtained without exposing the patient to any ionizing radiation, and this is probably the principal and major advantage of NMR over CT scanning. There is no known hazard to this study and no contrast material need be introduced into the bowel or kidney, another major

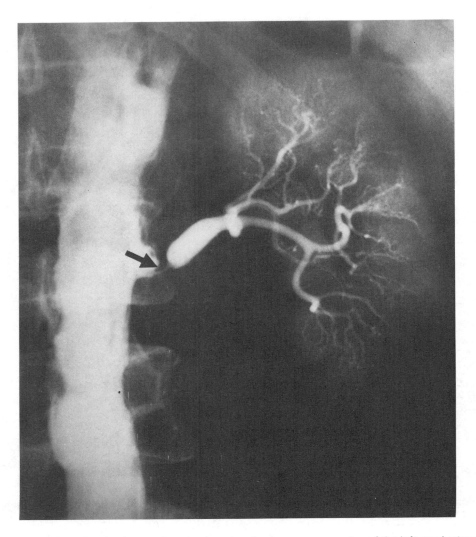

Figure 1–38. A left selective renal angiogram showing a severe narrowing of the left renal artery just distal to the point where it branches from the aorta (*arrow*). This patient was severely hypertensive.

advantage of NMR over CT scanning. Further, there are fewer artifacts generated than with CT scanning and renal cortex and medulla can more readily be distinguished from each other. Fat appears white (high density) whereas fluids appear dark (low density) and bone cannot be visualized at all on NMR. At the present time the drawbacks of NMR include the fact that calcifications cannot be detected and the scan time at present is lengthy in comparison to CT scanning—on the order of minutes versus seconds. Also the study is much more expensive than CT scanning. However, it is likely that vast improvements will be seen in this new age of

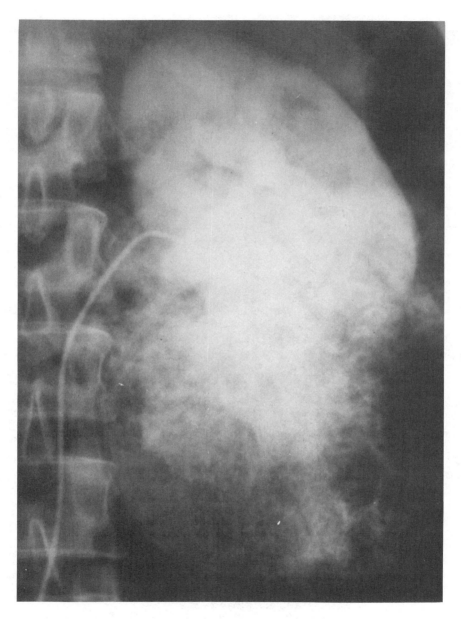

Figure 1-39. A left selective renal angiogram showing the characteristic appearance of renal cell carcinoma of the lower pole of the kidney. Shortly after injection of the contrast medium, a "puddling" of the medium is seen in the region of the tumor; this is very characteristic and diagnostic of renal cell carcinoma.

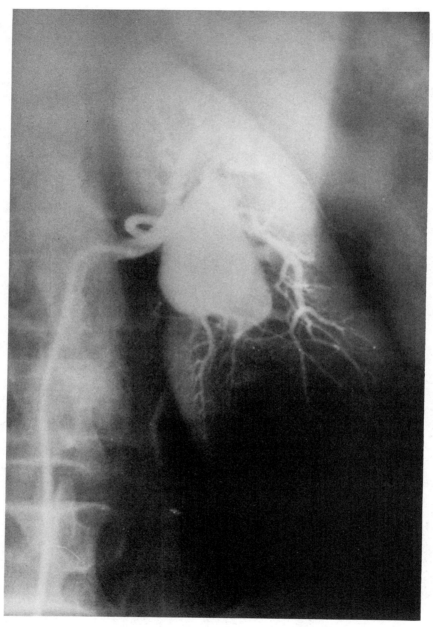

Figure 1-40. A left selective renal angiogram depicting a cyst of the lower pole of the left kidney. A mass lesion had been found on excretory urography and this selective renal angiogram demonstrated that there was no abnormal vascularity within the mass lesion, thereby strongly pointing to the diagnosis of a cyst.

imaging technologies and it may very well replace CT scanning in areas where both are applicable.

Lymphangiography

Lymphangiography has been used to visualize the lymph channels and the lymph nodes in the retroperitoneum and pelvis in an effort to determine if any lymph nodes are abnormal and potentially involved with metastatic carcinoma. This procedure is quite nonspecific, however, because retroperitoneal lymph nodes may appear large and shoddy as a result of either inflammatory or malignant disease and it is not possible to differentiate with certainty between the two on a lymphangiogram.

Lymphangiography is usually carried out by injecting contrast medium, under pressure and over several hours, into the lymphatic channels in the webbed space of the feet. X-ray films of the iliac and retroperitoneal areas are obtained after 24 and 48 hours and show the contrast medium in good concentration within the appropriate lymph channels and nodes and tentative evaluation of these nodes for metastatic disease can then be made. It must be emphasized, however, that lymphangiography is rarely carried out because it is a very difficult and tedious procedure, the pulmonary complications can be significant, the diagnostic accuracy is low, and, most important, CT scans provide the same (or more) information with far less patient morbidity.

Needle Aspiration of Enlarged Lymph Nodes

The procedure of needle aspiration of enlarged lymph nodes for diagnostic purposes started in the 1920s in this country but was not well received at the time. It remained for the Swedes to develop and polish the technique in the 1950s and it has now become a standard diagnostic study. A very small-caliber, hollow needle (less than 1 mm in diameter) is used and is the reason that the procedure is called the "skinny" needle biopsy technique. A needle size of 22 or 23 gauge is fairly standard. Lesions that can be palpated readily, such as inguinal lymph nodes, can be aspirated directly without any roentgenographic studies. However, lesions known to be present or suspected as such can be visualized on CT scans or, very occasionally, on lymphangiograms and needled under CT scan or fluoroscopic control. Obviously, the success of the aspiration biopsy technique will depend largely upon the skill of the individual performing it. However, once a fair amount of experience is gained, better than 80 percent of the nodes can successfully be needled with better than a 95 percent diagnostic accuracy.

Urodynamic Studies

The bladder, also known as the detrusor, is a smooth muscle organ that is innervated by the autonomic nervous system and it has two basic functions: urine storage and urine evacuation. There are two urinary sphincters: the internal sphincter, which is composed of smooth muscle and is actually a part of the detrusor itself; and the external sphincter, which is composed of skeletal muscle. The individual and the collective function of the detrusor and these two sphincters is to control voiding and they are responsible for any abnormalities thereof. *Urodynamics* are simply tests by which the clinician is able to quantitate the functions of the detrusor and the two urinary sphincters as an objective means of evaluating the physiology of voiding and, more specifically, abnormalties of voiding. The urodynamic tests that are available to assist the clinician in these evaluations of a patient's voiding pattern

NORMAL BLADDER

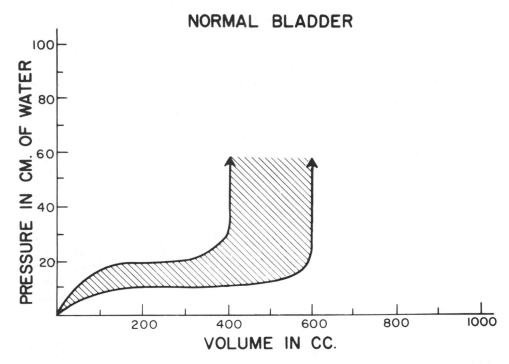

Figure 1-41. Cystometrogram. A schematic drawing of a perfectly normal cystometrogram which demonstrates the relationship of the pressure within the bladder to the volume of water within the bladder. Variations in this pressure–volume relationship, when taken in conjunction with other studies and other clinical findings, are helpful in diagnosing abnormalities of voiding.

are *cystometry, urinary flow, urethral pressure evaluation,* and *electromyography (EMG) of the pelvic floor muscles.*

Cystometry is the method by which the pressure–volume relationship of the bladder is measured, with the pressure recorded in centimeters of water. Normal values for intravesical pressures that will vary with the intravesical volume of water have been derived (Fig. 1–41). These will vary with the techniques used, the rate of bladder filling, and some other parameters, but they all serve the same fundamental purpose, which is to evaluate the bladder capacity, compliance (the change in intravesical pressure that accompanies changes in intravesical volume), and contractility (bladder contractions while filling is occurring but not appropriate to the degree of filling as compared with standards of normal). Cystometry may provide valuable clinical information but it should not be regarded as an absolute measure of physiologic activity, and diagnostic conclusions from it should only be made by combining the results of cystometry with all of the other available clinical information.

Urinary flow is the simplest of the urodynamic investigations and it involves an assessment of the rate of urine flow, in milliliters per second after an individual's maximum urine flow rate has been reached. The validity of the urinary flow measurement ideally requires a voided volume of at least 200 ml and if the total volume voided is less than 100 ml the study is probably not valid. Nevertheless, with these caveats norms have been obtained and it has been found that males under 40 years old should have a urinary flow rate greater than 22 ml/sec; males 40 to 60 years old should have a flow rate greater than 18 ml/sec; and males over 60 years old should have a flow rate greater than 13 ml/sec. For females under 50 years, a flow rate greater than 25 ml/sec and for females over 50 years a flow rate greater than 18 ml/sec is normal. The urinary flow rate is a fundamental urodynamic measurement that is of great value in the clinical evaluation of voiding disorders. However, it must be recognized that flow rates are determined by the relationship between detrusor force and urethral resistance and that therefore abnormalities of the flow rates do not necessarily pinpoint the reason for the decreased flow. Nevertheless, the urine flow rate is a very simple and good means of "screening" those with a normal flow rate from those with less than a normal flow rate, although it must again be emphasized that abnormally low flow rates must then be interpreted in light of other clinical studies because they do not by themselves point to a specific diagnosis. However, they are particularly valuable in evaluating patients with bladder outlet obstruction due to prostatic enlargement where, many clinicians feel, a flow rate of less than 10 to 12 ml/sec should be established before prostatic surgery is undertaken.

Urethral pressure evaluation measures the resistance of the urethral walls to the distension caused by a catheter that is slowly being withdrawn from the bladder neck to just beyond the urethral sphincter and also to the perfusing fluid as it leaves the eyeholes of the catheter. This resistance is expressed in terms of the pressure necessary to maintain a steady flow of perfusant through the catheter system. An 8F catheter with two side holes is commonly used and is generally withdrawn from the bladder at a rate of about 0.05 cm/sec using a machine to ensure a constant rate of withdrawal. The urethral pressure evaluation is of particular use in assessing the degree of prostatic obstruction that may be present and also for assessing postprostatectomy problems such as continuing outflow obstruction or urinary incontinence. With the latter problem, urethral pressure evaluation may be of considerable help in differentiating patients with urgency incontinence from those with true stress incontinence. If the urethral pressure evaluations are performed frequently, they can become highly reproducible diagnostic tests. It must be remembered, however, that this is a static investigation and the intraurethral pressures being measured represent measurements made during the storage phase of bladder function. Nevertheless, some valid observations may still be made regarding the behavior of the urethra during micturition based on these studies. This validity, however, does not apply to the bladder neck and the proximal urethra since the urethral pressure profile cannot reliably identify whether an obstructed bladder neck is competent, incompetent, or obstructed.

Electromyography of the pelvic floor muscles is used to determine the electrical activity within the muscles of the external urethral sphincter and the pelvic floor which normally cease with the onset of detrusor contraction. Direct needle electromyography of the urethral sphincter is the best possible way to assess the activity of this group of muscles but is not always feasible, particularly in children, and the pasting of pediatric electrocardiogram electrodes in the immediate proximity of the anal sphincter may be almost as useful. The anal plug electrode is another method of obtaining the necessary information. This assessment via electrical activity of the pelvic floor muscles and the urethral sphincter is done in conjunction with cystometry and urinary flow studies and enables the clinician to detect the

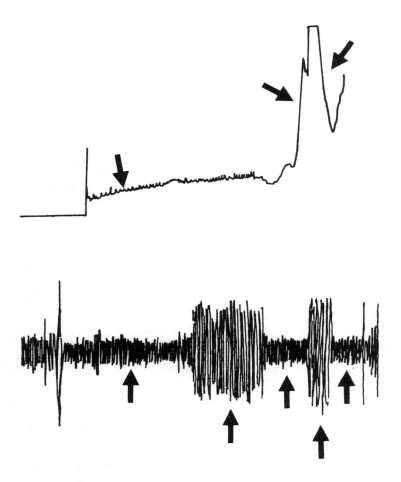

Figure 1-42. A normal cystometrogram (above) performed simultaneously (below) with electromyography of the pelvic floor musculature (the urethral sphincter). Note that as the bladder fills (*first arrow*, top) the external urethral sphincter is relaxed and there is minimal electrical activity (*first arrow*, bottom). As the bladder continues to fill, the patient has an urge to void and voluntarily contracts his external urethral sphincter to counteract the voiding urge (*second arrow*, bottom). The bladder filling continues and the patient is told to relax his external urethral spincter as the bladder is allowed to fill (*third arrow*, bottom). As bladder filling continues, there is a marked spike in the intravesical pressure as the bladder nears its capacity (*second arrow*, top). Finally, with the intravesical pressure high and a very strong voiding urge present, the patient is told to inhibit voiding by contracting his external urethral sphincter (*fourth arrow*, bottom). After this, the patient is told to relax his sphincter and void and the intravesical pressure drops sharply (*third arrow*, top) while the urethral sphincter relaxes to permit voiding (*fifth arrow*, bottom). This particular type of study is particularly useful in detecting abnormalities in the normally reciprocal functions of the detrusor and the external urethral sphincter. Note that the numbers have been omitted from this graph as they would be superfluous to its understanding.

various forms of detrusor sphincter dyssynergia that can occur. Simply stated, the external urethral sphincter should relax completely during detrusor action (Fig. 1–42) and when it does not then various types of voiding dysfunction may occur (see Chapter 5). The use of electromyography of the pelvic floor muscles, as just mentioned, is the best means of assessing the various sorts of dyssynergia of the detrusor and the sphincter.

It should also be realized that various voiding dysfunctions may be a result of disease processes that are outside of the urinary tract but only manifested through the voiding abnormality, and interpretation of the various urodynamic studies must be done with this in mind.

It is the author's feeling that urodynamic studies have provided a major contribution to the knowledge about the physiology of micturition and they are undoubtedly of great assistance in the clinical evaluation of particularly difficult problems, especially in the pediatric age group. Unquestionably, however, as occurs with any new clinical tool, the use of urodynamic studies is probably overemphasized and overdone, providing information that could be gained by less expensive and more common techniques.

REFERENCES

Abrams P: Urodynamic investigations. In Stamey TA (ed), 1982 Monographs in Urology. Princeton, NJ, Custom Publishing Services, 1982

Witten DM, Myers GH Jr, Utz DC (eds): Emmett's Clinical Urography, 4th ed. Philadelphia, Saunders, 1977

Friedland GW: Urography. In Stamey TA (ed), 1984 Monographs in Urology. Princeton, NJ, Custom Publishing Services, 1984

Greene LF, Parsons CL: Urologic diagnosis. In Karafin L, Kendall AR (eds), Urology. Philadelphia, Harper and Row, 1980, vol 1, chap 81

Malmud LS, Lessig HJ, Makler PT: Nuclear medicine in urologic practice. In Karafin L, Kendall AR (eds), Urology. Philadelphia, Harper and Row, 1981, vol 1, chap 10

Pollack HM: Radiologic examination of the urinary tract. In Karafin L, Kendall AR (eds), Urology. Philadelphia, Harper and Row, 1979, vol 1, chap 9N

Rous SN: Urology in Primary Care. St. Louis, Mosby, 1976

Rous SN: Understanding Urology. Basel, Karger, 1973

2

Infection and Inflammation of the Urinary Tract

EDUCATIONAL OBJECTIVES

1. Discuss the significance and the management of asymptomatic bacteriuria.
2. Discuss the management of acute pyelonephritis in a man and in a woman.
3. Discuss the management and therapy of chronic or recurrent pyelonephritis in a man and in a woman.
4. List and discuss the theories of etiology of pyelonephritis.
5. List the symptoms and the physical (including any urine) findings of acute pyelonephritis.
6. List the symptoms and physical (including urine) findings of chronic pyelonephritis.
7. List the diagnostic tests needed to make a diagnosis of renal tuberculosis.
8. List the symptoms of renal tuberculosis.
9. List the symptoms of acute cystitis.
10. Discuss the management of postcoital cystitis in a young woman.
11. Discuss the pathogenesis of acute cystitis in males and females.
12. Describe the management of acute cystitis in males and females.
13. Describe what is meant by "bacterial adherence" in terms of lower urinary tract infections in women.
14. Discuss the rationale of collecting urine from a man sequentially in three glasses to localize the source of infection.
15. List the antimicrobials effective against the most common organisms that cause cystitis.
16. List the symptoms of acute prostatitis.
17. Discuss the management of acute prostatitis.
18. Discuss the use of prostatic massage in the management of chronic bacterial prostatitis and prostatostasis.
19. Discuss the causes of acute prostatitis.
20. List the symptoms of chronic bacterial prostatitis and prostatostasis.
21. List the symptoms of posterior urethritis.
22. Explain, on an anatomic basis, why the symptoms of prostatitis and posterior urethritis may be so similar.
23. Describe how to "strip" a prostate gland to obtain prostatic secretions for microscopic and bacteriologic studies.
24. Describe the differential diagnosis among chronic bacterial prostatitis, chronic nonbacterial prostatitis (prostatostasis), and prostatodynia.
25. List the methods used in the treatment of acute epididymitis.
26. List the symptoms and the causes of epididymitis.
27. List the methods used in the treatment of orchitis.
28. Describe the palpatory findings used to differentiate epididymitis from orchitis.
29. Obtain and examine a smear from a urethral discharge to find pus and bacteria.
30. Explain how the infecting organism in epididymitis varies with the age of the patient.

65

INTRODUCTION

Infection and inflammation of the entire genitourinary tract probably comprise the most important disease processes in clinical urology in terms of numbers of patients. They are the cause of symptomatology or disease in a plurality and quite possibly a majority of all patients seen by urologists and definitely constitute a majority of all patients with urologic disease that are seen by primary care physicians. These statements are based upon data gathered in a nationwide survey of 2200 physicians (see Introduction). A far greater number of educational objectives dealing more with infection and inflammation than with any other topic were deemed "necessary" for every graduating medical student by 70 percent or more of all participants. Since the participants in the survey were themselves predominantly primary care physicians in private practice their responses undoubtedly reflected experiences in the delivery of health care.

DEFINITIONS AND GENERAL COMMENTS

What is meant by infection and inflammation in the genitourinary tract? As with so much in medicine, absolute answers may be confusing and are not always valid. Nevertheless, inflammation may be considered to exist when white blood cells (pus cells), with or without bacteria, are found in the urine. The diagnosis of infection is proper only in instances where the presence of an invading organism has been documented. Inflammation or infection may be suspected when a patient complains of a feeling of irritation or discomfort in any part of his or her urinary tract, or, as often occurs, when the discomfort is located in the male genital tract. The finding of bacteriuria in a properly collected urine specimen or from an examination of prostatic or urethral secretions may also indicate infection whether or not the patient is symptomatic.

The entire concept of infection and inflammation is not always easy to comprehend. The disease process itself may exist in any part of the genitourinary tract, but the history, symptoms, physical and x-ray findings, and laboratory results will vary greatly according to the location of the pathology. For example, infection and inflammation within the renal parenchyma may cause high fever and profound illness whereas infection within the male urethra may produce only minimal symptomatology that is of little or no clinical significance but may well result in a psychologic cripple. Although it is gratifying to relieve the acute distress of a patient with an uncomplicated bladder infection it can also be embarrassing to the physician and harmful to the patient if the signs, symptoms, or laboratory findings indicative of severe underlying genitourinary tract disease are overlooked.

Establishing with certainty a diagnosis of infection or inflammation may be difficult. In the patient who complains of severe burning upon urination, a provisional diagnosis of bladder infection is relatively simple. When a few pus cells (white blood cells) are found on routine urine examination (such as is done as part of a preschool checkup or a regular adult physical examination) in a completely asymptomatic patient, the possibility, however slight, of a urinary tract infection must be considered. Additionally the finding of totally asymptomatic bacteriuria with or without pyuria in a healthy individual whose urine is being examined routinely may be the first and only finding to indicate serious underlying genitourinary tract disease.

GENERAL CONSIDERATIONS IN INTERVIEWING AND EXAMINING THE PATIENT

A carefully taken urologic history is usually able to direct the physician towards an accurate diagnosis, although in certain cases, such as an asymptomatic patient with bacteriuria, the urologic history may be of little or no value.

A very basic and important step that physicians should employ when interviewing patients is to be absolutely certain that the patient understands the anatomic terms used by the physician and it is preferable for the physician to use the correct anatomic terms when speaking to the patient. Unfortunately, however, in our culture anatomic parts of the genitourinary tract are very rarely correctly named when parents talk to and teach their children so that these children grow up and pass onto their children a woefully inadequate knowledge about the correct terms for virtually all of the parts of the genitourinary tract. It is perfectly appropriate and proper for clinicians to interrupt interviews with patients as frequently as it is felt necessary in order to point out that some of the words or terms being used might be unfamiliar and to ask patients if the terminology is in fact being understood.

It is also important for clinicians to keep in mind throughout the history taking and physical examination (and, indeed, during every aspect of working with patients with urologic problems) that the psychologic or emotional input to the disease process is very prominent because of the anatomy and function of the parts of the body dealt with in urology. The intimate and almost sacred connection, particularly in males, between the psyche and the genitalia is well illustrated in treating patients with minimal prostatitis or urethritis, where the most minor symptoms are often accompanied by a tremendous anxiety and concern in the patient.

Just as the signs and symptoms of genitourinary tract disease often cause the patient anxiety that is far out of proportion to the disease process, so too does anticipation of any diagnostic or other manipulative procedures involving the genitalia. Most patients are not even slightly anxious about a physician putting an otoscope into their ear or a tongue depressor into their mouth; the vast majority of patients, however, are extremely concerned about even palpatory examination of the external genitalia. This concern is appreciably heightened if a digital rectal examination of the prostate gland is contemplated and the prospect of a catheterization or cystoscopic examination may be absolutely terrifying to the patient. As a general rule, pelvic examinations cause females the same degree of anxiety and concern as genital or rectal examinations do males. It is incumbent upon the caring physician to be aware of the anxiety present in these situations. It is usually wise to describe the procedure in advance of carrying it out and to ask patients about any concerns they might have. A very objective measurement of fears or concerns may be obtained by direct observation of patients, who may demonstrate a degree of trepidation, or even diaphoresis or hyperventilation that reveals their emotions. By being aware of their patients' fears and concerns regarding examinations and other procedures involving the external genitalia, the physician is better able to gain their confidence and ultimately to effect better patient management.

UPPER TRACT INFECTION AND INFLAMMATION

Acute Pyelonephritis

History and Symptoms. Infection within the kidney may produce a variety of symptoms. Renal pain is generally produced only when the renal capsule is stretched by rapidly induced edema of the parenchyma or sudden obstruction of the collecting system. Such parenchymal edema can be produced by acute pyelonephritis and it is characteristic of this condition that pain in the costovertebral area is present. Parenchymal edema may be mild, moderate, or severe; in mild cases there may be minimal distention of the renal capsule with minimal or no costovertebral angle pain perceived by the patient. It is particularly important when eliciting a history of past or present kidney pain to be certain about the area of the body to which the patient is referring when he or she speaks about the pain. It is not uncommon for patients to equate low back pain either in the midline or more laterally with kidney pain because in the minds of many patients pain anywhere in the back means that the kidney is involved. In point of fact, the pain must be in the region of the 11th or 12th ribs posteriorly for it to be of renal origin unless an abnormally mobile or ptotic kidney exists. The patient with acute pyelonephritis may or may not have concomitant symptoms of lower urinary tract infection.

The patient will usually complain of malaise and will appear to be sick. The temperature will almost always be elevated and is commonly in the range of 102°F but may be as high as 105° or 106°F.

Etiology. By far the majority of cases of acute pyelonephritis are secondary to ascending infection from the bladder. This bacterial ascent to the kidney may be a current or a past phenomenon; in the latter case, the chronic foci of infection have been seeded into the kidney, with the present episode representing an acute exacerbation of a chronic infection. The ascent of urine from the bladder to the kidney, which never occurs as a normal phenomenon, is referred to as *vesicoureteral reflux* (see Chapter 5). Two other etiologies are considered significant, though uncommon, for this condition. One is the hematogenous spread of bacteria to the kidney from a distant focus of infection such as furunculosis, infected teeth or gums, or infections in the ears or the throat. In such cases, the offending organism is usually gram-positive staphylococcus or streptococcus. The other, which is very rare, involves the lymphatic spread of bacteria from the large intestines to the kidney. In these cases, the offending organism is usually one of the gram-negative bacteria that normally inhabit the large intestine.

Physical, Laboratory, and X-Ray Findings. When acute pyelonephritis exists, the patient is usually in moderate to severe distress, with a generalized malaise. The most notable physical finding is exquisite tenderness over the involved costovertebral angle when that area is struck briskly with the hypothenar eminence while the fist is clenched (Murphy's sign). In the absence of this percussion, the patient will usually but not always complain of pain in the affected costovertebral angle. The temperature will usually be elevated to 102°F or higher, and this may or may not be accompanied by chills. Also, such nonspecific findings as nausea, vomiting, malaise, lassitude, and anorexia may be present.

Laboratory work may be helpful but is generally not diagnostic. Urinary sediment will *usually* show pyuria and bacteriuria, but the absence of either or both of these findings does not rule out the diagnosis of acute pyelonephritis. This is because if an individual has an acute infectious process within the parenchyma of the kidney that does *not* communicate with or involve the collecting system, it is possible to have sterile urine without either pyuria or bacteriuria. It should also be noted that in the presence of acute pyelonephritis the urine sediment may show some microscopic hematuria and may on rare occasions even show gross hematuria. Note again that the absence of any or all of these findings in the urine makes a diagnosis of acute pyelonephritis much less likely but certainly does not rule it out. The peripheral hemogram will usually have a leukocytosis with a shift to the left, but this also is a nonspecific finding.

Roentgenographically, there are no findings that could be called pathognomonic of acute pyelonephritis. However, in about one third to one half of patients with this clinical entity edema and inflammation of the parenchyma and the collecting system may produce x-ray findings such as narrowed and incompletely filled infundibulae and fractionally seen calyces, both of which are compatible with acute pyelonephritis.

Diagnostic Methodology. In an adult patient with flank pain, fever, pyuria, bacteriuria, and generalized malaise, all of which should alert the clinician to the diagnosis of acute pyelonephritis, a precise diagnostic approach should be maintained. Should the patient not have all of the above findings, this diagnosis should still be entertained *provided* a bacteriuria is present. In the absence of a bacteriuria it is doubtful whether the thorough urologic workup outlined below is warranted insofar as it is predicated on the presence of bacteriuria and directed towards identifying how the organisms reached the urinary tract in the first place (in the male) as well as how they reached the kidney (in the female).

Acute Pyelonephritis in Adult Males. If a patient is a male adult, it should be understood that an underlying disease process may be causing the acute pyelonephritis. Since most cases of acute pyelonephritis occur from a bladder infection by way of the ascending route, the very presence of a bladder infection in a male should suggest some underlying condition. Although the pyelonephritis may be secondary to a hematogenous or a lymphatic spread of bacteria from a distant source, the odds so heavily favor the ascending route of infection that the author feels an extensive urologic investigation is virtually mandatory in the adult male with documented acute pyelonephritis.

After a complete history, physical examination, microscopy of the urine sediment, and urine culture have been carried out, an excretory urogram is indicated in order to rule out any obvious urinary tract abnormalities that might be causative of acute pyelonephritis. Conditions such as ureteropelvic junction obstruction, chronic pyelonephritis with a clinically superimposed acute process, urinary tract calculus disease, or hydronephrosis of any etiology are examples of fairly common findings related to acute pyelonephritis in the male. Additionally, persistent dilatation of the lower ureters seen on all or most of the films suggests the presence of vesicoureteral reflux. If any significant degree of lower ureteral dilatation is present or if any findings on the excretory urograms suggest that vesicoureteral reflux might exist, a retrograde voiding cystourethrogram should be carried out to determine the presence or absence of reflux. A careful examination of the excretory cystogram and the postvoiding film also should be carried out to discern evidence of bladder trabeculation or diverticulae or a significant postvoiding residual, each or all of which could be etiologic in a lower urinary tract infection, resulting in ascending infection with pyelonephritis. If a "physiologic" voiding film has been obtained (see Chapter 1), the configuration of the entire urethra will also be seen. Cystoscopy in the adult male may also be warranted to evaluate the bladder outlet more definitively and discern any obstructive urologic disease; however, most often a totally normal excretory urogram with an insignificant postvoid residual and a normal-appearing urethra when the physiologic voiding cystourethrogram is done obviate the necessity for cystoscopic exam. If cystoscopy is carried out, however, accurate residual urine measurement should be obtained by having the patient void immediately prior to cystoscopy and then noting the amount of urine still present that flows out of the cystoscope following its introduction into the bladder.

Finally, the possibility of chronic bacterial prostatitis seeding bacteria into the bladder and thence into the kidney must also be considered. In addition to the diagnostic studies already noted, culture of the prostatic fluid or of the postprostatic massage urine may be diagnostic.

Acute Pyelonephritis in Adult Females.   In women, the same diagnostic methodology applies as is outlined for the adult male. However, it must be remembered that the adult female may develop lower urinary tract infections without having any underlying urologic abnormalities and so the thrust of the diagnostic study in women is to determine the presence or absence of vesicoureteral reflux and not, as with men, to find out why the urinary tract infection developed in the first place. Cystoscopy is sometimes indicated so that direct observation of the ureteral orifices may be done in the patient with vesicoureteral reflux that has already been documented. Observation of the ureteral orifices enables the clinician to make a very educated guess as to whether the reflux is a transient phenomenon or is likely to require ultimate surgical correction.

Management.   Patients with acute pyelonephritis, regardless of sex or age, are usually moderately to severely ill and are febrile. Management of the disease is specific, but also includes nonspecific treatment for the symptoms such as bed rest during the acute phase, aspirin for temperature over 102° F, and forced fluids if the patient is able to tolerate them. If the patient is nauseated and unable to hold down sufficient quantities of fluids then intravenous feeding is necessary. Specifically, culture and sensitivity studies should be done on properly collected bladder urine and the appropriate antibiotics chosen. If the patient is able to take oral medication and is not too ill, then a first-generation cephalosporin or cinoxacin or Cefaclor or Macrodantin would be perfectly acceptable therapy. If the patient's clinical condition is such that hospitalization is required and intravenous antibiotics must be administered, then a second- or third-generation cephalosporin or an aminoglycoside would be indicated. In any case, if the antimicrobial agent chosen is found to be incorrect based on the in vitro sensitivity studies or if the clinical response within 2 to 3 days suggests a lack of in vivo sensitivity, then the antibiotic therapy should be switched to a more appropriate one. If it is not possible to isolate any specific organism from the bladder, but the clinical impression is that of acute pyelonephritis, then the empirical use of antimicrobials as outlined above is warranted. Treatment for acute pyelonephritis should continue for approximately 2 weeks, after which time the urine should be recultured. This should be repeated 1 and 3 months posttherapy to be sure that there are no subclinical recurrences. A caveat to be borne in mind is that if the patient does not respond to what is felt to be an appropriate antibiotic, then excretory urograms should be obtained as promptly as possible because of the distinct possibility of a stone obstructing the drainage of an infected kidney.

Chronic Pyelonephritis

History and Symptoms. Chronic pyelonephritis will rarely produce any flank pain or any other symptoms, although an acute exacerbation of the chronic condition may certainly produce any of the symptoms associated with acute pyelonephritis. Individuals with chronic pyelonephritis, particularly women, may have recurring lower urinary tract infections that do not seem to be related to sexual intercourse or to anything at all. In such patients the possibility of showers of bacteria entering the bladder from a focus in the kidney should always be considered. These patients may have a low-grade temperature of perhaps 100°F and they are usually well except when they have symptoms of lower urinary tract infection. Another, perhaps more common, presentation of chronic pyelonephritis involves the totally asymptomatic individual who visits the physician for an unrelated reason and is found to have asymptomatic bacteriuria when the urine is properly collected and cultured. In this case, the possibility of chronic pyelonephritis must be considered since this condition is frequently asymptomatic and may go undiscovered but for the fortuitous finding of the asymptomatic bacteriuria. Bacteriuria in the asymptomatic patient means, by definition, a colony count of over 100,000 organisms per milliliter, almost always gram-negative organisms, in each of more than one properly collected urine specimens. In the truly asymptomatic individual this will usually involve the collection of urine by catheterization or suprapubic needle aspiration in order to document the disease itself (and to rule out contamination of the urine) before submitting the patient to the extensive, expensive, and possibly unpleasant diagnostic and therapeutic regimen that is mandatory in cases of asymptomatic bacteriuria.

Etiology. The etiology of chronic pyelonephritis is not always easy to determine. In some patients a prior history of acute pyelonephritis may be ascertained and it is easy to speculate that insufficient treatment of this acute episode resulted in a failure to eradicate all of the bacteria within the renal parenchyma, thereby rendering the condition subclinical or chronic. In other individuals there have possibly been repeated attacks of subclinical acute pyelonephritis that have become chronic. It is possible that a bacterial conversion to the L form at the time of therapy for acute pyelonephritis might be etiologic in some few individuals. Because these L forms lose their cell walls, they are much less affected by certain types of antimicrobial therapy and can lie dormant within the renal parenchyma. At a future date, under some unknown stimulae, the L forms may regain their cell walls and regain their virulence and cause chronic pyelonephritis.

Physical, Laboratory, and X-Ray Findings. Chronic pyelonephritis is usually distinguished by an absence of physical findings and, as often as not, is diagnosed as a result of an investigation triggered by the serendipitous finding of asymptomatic bacteriuria in a routine general physical examination. In other patients, chronic pyelonephritis does indeed produce symptoms or physical findings. The patient may have an occasional temperature elevation of otherwise unexplained origin that may be accompanied by headache, malaise, and pain over the affected costovertebral angle. Sometimes the patient may have intermittent symptoms of lower urinary tract infection such as dysuria or frequency and urgency of urination.

Laboratory studies, particularly of the urine, are most significant in the diagnosis of chronic pyelonephritis. Pyuria and bacteriuria will almost always be present and there may be microscopic hematuria as well.

Roentgenographic studies are very helpful in establishing the diagnosis of chronic pyelonephritis and films of the affected kidney will often show caliceal blunting, usually limited to part of the renal collecting system but that may uncommonly involve the entire system. Caliceal blunting results from retraction of the renal papilla that is secondary to scarring of the renal parenchyma adjacent to the papilla. Since the renal papilla normally invaginates the minor calyx to produce a characteristic "cupping" of the calyx the retracted renal papilla no longer invaginates the calyx and hydrostatic pressure within the collecting system distends the calyx to produce the characteristic "blunting" or "clubbing" of that calyx. Note that there must also be parenchymal atrophy or scarring directly over the point of the blunted calyx for chronic pyelonephritis to be correctly diagnosed from an excretory urogram (Fig. 2–1). It is extremely dangerous to diagnose chronic pyelonephritis roentgenographically without these twin findings of calyceal blunting and parenchymal atrophy directly over the blunted calyx. Differential diagnosis of roentgenograms showing caliceal blunting without parenchymal atrophy or vice versa or showing both but without the atrophic area noted *directly* over the blunted calyx are many and include the following:

1. Segmental renal infarction, in which the calyx may retain its normal cupping directly under the area of parenchymal atrophy.
2. Total renal infarction, in which the parenchymal atrophy is uniform throughout but the underlying calyces all retain their normal cupping.
3. Hydronephrotic atrophy, in which there is parenchymal loss due to back pressure from the dilated calyces, but this is a diffuse atrophy and chronic pyelonephritis is generally not diffuse. Moreover, the calyces will usually be far larger and more dilated than they would be from chronic pyelonephritis.
4. Localized calyceal obstruction, in which there is dilation secondary to a narrowed infundibulum or a nonopaque calculus may produce enough back pressure locally to bring about parenchymal loss. This condition may be indistinguishable from chronic pyelonephritis.
5. Fetal lobulation, in which the calyces are normal and the lobulations, which may look like parenchymal atrophy, are actually *between* the calyces and *not overlying them.*
6. Chronic glomerulonephritis, in which the kidneys may be uniformly contracted overall but the calyces are usually normal.
7. Congenital renal hypoplasia, in which the calyces will remain normal.

Although one should hesitate to make a roentgenographic diagnosis of chronic pyelonephritis without the caliceal blunting and overlying parenchymal atrophy, it is an accepted fact that chronic pyelonephritis may exist even when the excretory urograms are normal. This occurs if the disease developed *after* the patient reached 7 or 8 years of age. Most kidney growth has been completed by 7 years of age, and the parenchymal atrophy that is classically seen in chronic pyelonephritis occurs as a result of *continued renal growth* around a scarred or a fibrosed area that resulted from infection and not from *retraction* of a scarred area in a fully grown

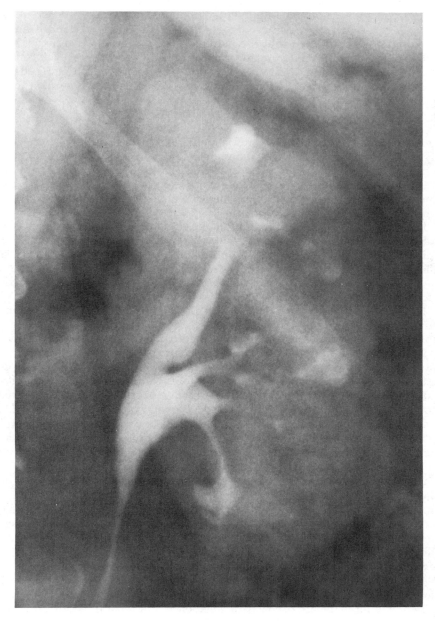

Figure 2-1. Chronic pyelonephritis. An excretory urogram showing the left kidney with the classic findings of pyelonephritis. Note the blunting or clubbing of the calyces with atrophy of the overlying parenchyma. The atrophy is irregular and specifically located directly over the blunted calyces.

kidney. If the scarring or the fibrosis, therefore, occurs *after* renal growth has stopped (or after age 7 or thereabout) then any fibrosis that occurs within the parenchyma of the kidney will *not* produce the roentgenographic appearance of parenchymal atrophy. Thus, when the classic roentgenograms of chronic pyelonephritis are discovered in an adult it is felt that the patient had the disease when he or she was a child and probably suffered from upper urinary tract infection due to vesicoureteral reflux. However, it must constantly be borne in mind that chronic and severe pyelonephritis can be present in the adult in the face of perfectly normal excretory urograms and should one of these kidneys be removed surgically, histologic examination will confirm severe and chronic pyelonephritis.

Diagnostic Methodology. The diagnostic methodology for chronic pyelonephritis is fairly comprehensive and certainly mandates an excretory urogram. Recall that chronic pyelonephritis is often discovered by the chance finding of asymptomatic bacteriuria during the course of a screening examination or a routine physical examination. In view of the paucity of symptoms it is extremely difficult to determine by clinical history the duration or even the existence of a disease process.

Inasmuch as the finding of asymptomatic bacteriuria requires an extensive and not always comfortable patient evaluation and may then result in long-term therapy the physician must be certain that asymptomatic bacteriuria (or bacteriuria accompanied by some symptoms) does in fact exist. The clinician must be certain that urine collection has been carried out with meticulous care (as outlined in Chapter 15) to avoid false-positive results.

If bacteriuria truly is present it must be established that the bacteriuria is originating in the upper urinary tract in one or both kidneys. An x-ray finding compatible with chronic pyelonephritis is not absolute proof that the pyelonephritic kidney is the site of the bacteriuria; it is not uncommon for kidneys that are roentgenographically pyelonephritic to be "burned out" and sterile at least as far as being the source of the bacteriuria. In view of the recent knowledge that chronic pyelonephritis *can* exist in the kidney that is roentgenographically normal it should be equally obvious that the presence of a roentgenographically pyelonephritic kidney does not preclude the possibility of the bacteria arising from the roentgenographically normal contralateral kidney. Finally, it must be remembered that the bacteriuria can arise from a chronic bladder infection without any lower urinary tract symptoms. This is particularly true in older patients.

Probably the most reliable test to document bacterial presence in the upper urinary tract is the bacterial localization test of Stamey, in which infected urine from the bladder is obtained through a cystoscope, after which the bladder is lavaged copiously with several liters of sterile water to mechanically remove bacteria present and then ureteral catheters are placed to each kidney. After the first few milliliters of urine obtained from each kidney are discarded (in case bacteria was inadvertently pushed up to the kidney from an incompletely lavaged bladder), several milliliters of urine are then collected from each kidney for culture. Bacteria present in either kidney (or both kidneys) that match those found in the initially obtained bladder urine are pretty strong evidence of a renal infection and serve to justify long-term antimicrobial therapy. This bacterial localization test is generally carried out under local anesthesia on an inpatient or an outpatient basis.

If the excretory urogram suggests the presence of chronic pyelonephritis (this is only an x-ray diagnosis and does not necessarily imply currently active infection in the kidney), a voiding cystourethrogram is indicated to see if vesicoureteral reflux is present. This can be done before or several days after the Stamey bacterial localization test.

Management. The management of chronic pyelonephritis is considerably more complex than that of acute pyelonephritis both because a disease that has been present for a long time is often more difficult to eradicate than an ailment of short duration and because associated urologic abnormalities are more likely to be present in cases of chronic pyelonephritis.

For purposes of management, patients may be divided into those who are urologically normal (no underlying abnormalities) and those who have urologic abnormalities.

For patients in whom no structural abnormalities can be demonstrated as a result of the excretory urograms or the voiding cystourethrograms (and this will undoubtedly encompass a majority of patients in whom chronic pyelonephritis is diagnosed), long-term therapy is indicated to eradicate any existing foci of bacteria within the kidney. An agent such as trimethoprim/sulfamethoxazole (Bactrim or Septra) is probably as efficacious as any for this therapy because of its relatively few major side effects (although occasional blood dyscrasias may develop with this drug in some individuals on long-term therapy). The usual dosage is one double strength tablet twice daily for 3 to 6 months and it should only be used for patients with normal renal function. During the course of therapy the patient's urine should be cultured monthly to ensure that a drug-resistant strain of organism has not emerged; the patient's urine is then cultured monthly for at least 6 months after therapy has been terminated. A recurrence of the bacteriuria (ascertained from a properly collected specimen) mandates a return to antimicrobial therapy, which may be necessary for as long as 1 to 3 years. If the infection does not recur after therapy has been terminated, the patient's urine should be recultured every 3 to 6 months for at least 1 year and probably yearly thereafter to be certain that the condition does not return.

A problem that invariably arises in the management of individuals with chronic pyelonephritis, particularly if the condition has been diagnosed because of asymptomatic bacteriuria, is convincing these patients of the importance of maintaining long-term therapy with frequent cultures. In particular, patients who do not and never did have any symptomatology can find little justification for taking three or four pills every day for a seemingly endless period of time. The challenge to the physician is great and is best met by carefully going over patients' x-ray films with them and explaining in as much detail as is necessary the existing pathology as well as the natural history of untreated pyelonephritis, which may well result in renal failure in the affected kidney.

Patients with Urologic Abnormalities

Existing abnormalities of the urinary tract that can be demonstrated as the probable reason for present and active chronic pyelonephritis are best corrected, surgically or otherwise. Examples of such urologically correctable lesions include primary vesicoureteral reflux (most commonly seen in children but still an occurrence in adults), bladder outlet obstruction such as might be caused by a congenitally contracted vesical neck or a benign prostatic hyperplasia and ureteropelvic junction obstruction. It is axiomatic in urology that where obstruction and infection coexist it is fruitless to attempt to cure the infection without relieving the obstruction. Although not primarily obstructive, vesicoureteral reflux allows bladder bacteria a ready portal of entrance to the kidney and could be the cause of unending attacks of pyelonephritis unless corrected. Finding an underlying urologic abnormality contributing to chronic pyelonephritis is more likely in males in whom uncomplicated pyelonephritis is rare unless of hematogenous origin. On the other hand, few women afflicted with chronic pyelonephritis show a demonstrable urologic abnormality as an etiologic factor. This may well be because most of them developed chronic pyelonephritis secondary to vesicoureteral reflux in childhood, which in many cases ceases spontaneously during the years of puberty and adolescence.

Following the surgical correction of any associated urologic abnormalities, long-term therapy is still necessary to eradicate existing foci of bacteria remaining within the renal parenchyma. Achieving high intrarenal tissue levels of antibiotics is difficult, which helps to explain why chronic pyelonephritis tends to recur despite long-term therapy. Appropriate therapy is administration of an antimicrobial of choice (based on sensitivity studies) for 3 to 6 months; an agent such as trimethoprim/sulfamethoxazole (Bactrim or Septra) is often very excellent for this purpose. While the patient is having antimicrobial therapy, monthly cultures (for at least 6 months) are necessary to be certain that the treatment has been efficacious and to assure that there is no bacterial breakthrough and recurrence of infection. If reinfection should occur, additional therapy is necessary, in some cases for 1, 2, or even 3 years. If the patient's urine remains sterile after the first course of therapy (3 to 6 months) and for 6 consecutive months after therapy has ceased, adequate follow-up necessitates continued urine cultures every 3 to 6 months for the next year and probably yearly thereafter.

Renal Tuberculosis

History and Symptoms. Renal tuberculosis has been referred to as the great imitator because there are no specific symptoms or aspects of the urologic history that can be called truly diagnostic or even strongly suggestive of the disease. The earliest symptoms of this condition may simply be gross or microscopic hematuria. If the renal tuberculosis has extended down the ureter to involve the bladder (tuberculosis of the bladder is virtually always secondary to renal tuberculosis), the symptoms may be those of lower urinary tract inflammation or infection and the presence of renal tuberculosis will only become apparent following a thorough urologic investigation. Inasmuch as renal tuberculosis is generally considered to be secondary to pulmonary tuberculosis, the symptoms may indeed be those of pulmonary tuberculosis or even of a widely disseminated tuberculosis, but this is a very uncommon finding nowadays.

Etiology. Renal tuberculosis is generally considered to be secondary to pulmonary tuberculosis and it is very probable that renal tuberculosis does not exist on a primary basis. The source of spread from the pulmonary focus to the kidneys is hematogenous. Renal tuberculosis probably occurs universally, but it seems to have a much higher frequency among the lower socioeconomic classes and its occurrence clinically is generally limited to a very few patients per year in large general hospitals. There are probably no more than several hundred new cases of renal tuberculosis annually in this country.

Physical, Laboratory, and X-Ray Findings. Physical findings, signs, and symptoms of renal tuberculosis are few and varied and may be as nonspecific as generalized malaise and lassitude or microscopic or gross hematuria. Individuals so afflicted will usually have no specific findings on examination, but the critical laboratory finding is the persistence of amicrobic pyuria. The repeated presence of white blood cells in properly collected urine specimens combined with the failure to obtain any organism from the urine should immediately suggest a possible diagnosis of renal tuberculosis. The method of general urine culture for aerobic and anaerobic organisms does not permit the growth of the tuberculosis organism and it will be completely missed unless specific cultures for the acid-fast organism are requested. If an individual with renal tuberculosis also has TB of the bladder, the symptoms may be those of bladder infection and inflammation, such as frequency and urgency of urination or dysuria. Amicrobic pyuria will be found and warrants specific acid-fast cultures (preferably the first voiding in the morning for at least three or four separate collections).

X-ray findings in renal tuberculosis are usually characteristic except in the early stages of the disease when x-ray interpretation may still be normal. However, even more advanced renal TB does not produce any pathognemonic urographic changes but rather produces changes that are strongly suggestive of TB. In x-ray films (plain) of the kidney, ureter, and bladder, renal calcification or calculi are found in about 20 percent of patients with renal TB; ureteral calcification is not nearly as common. The excretory urogram is helpful only if the disease, which primarily affects the renal parenchyma, has broken into the collecting system; then a calyceal irregularity, often described as "fuzzy, feathery, or moth-eaten," may be seen. This caliceal irregularity is strongly suggestive of renal tuberculosis and is produced by an erosion of the renal pyramids with a cortical necrosis. Calycectasis, an earlier and frequent finding in renal tuberculosis, is caused by the infundibular stricturing that results when the pathologic process involves that portion of the collecting system (Fig. 2–2). Dilatation of the renal pelvis may occur as the result of a stricture distal to it, and this ureteral stricturing or beading may also occur in more advanced renal tuberculosis. It should be noted that the process of scarring or stricturing in the renal collecting system is not produced by the active disease process alone, but is a natural occurrence during the healing process of tuberculosis when the patient is under therapy.

Diagnostic Methodology. Diagnostic methodology for renal tuberculosis is based on isolation and identification of *mycobacterium tuberculosis*. It should be emphasized that this procedure can be extremely difficult and is rarely accomplished on examination of a solitary urine specimen. The usual procedure is to have the patient bring to the laboratory a specimen of the first voiding of the morning on three or four separate occasions over a 2-week period. A smear is taken of each urine specimen in order to look for the tuberculosis organism. The urine is also cultured on an appropriate medium; guinea pig innoculation may be necessary as an adjunct to the culturing procedure. Renal tuberculosis may certainly be suspected when there is an antecedent history of pulmonary TB and when standard culturing techniques reveal a persistent amicrobic pyuria (many white cells without any bacterial growth). Finally, an intermediate strength skin test (5 TU purified protein derivative, PPD) should be placed on the patient's forearm. If this test is negative, as determined by the absence of induration in 48 to 72 hours, the likelihood of renal tuberculosis is extremely remote. If there is still strong clinical suspicion that the patient has tuberculosis, skin testing with a second strength of PPD (250 TU) is warranted. A positive result on either of the skin tests is by no means conclusive proof of renal tuberculosis or even pulmonary tuberculosis although many chest physicians work-

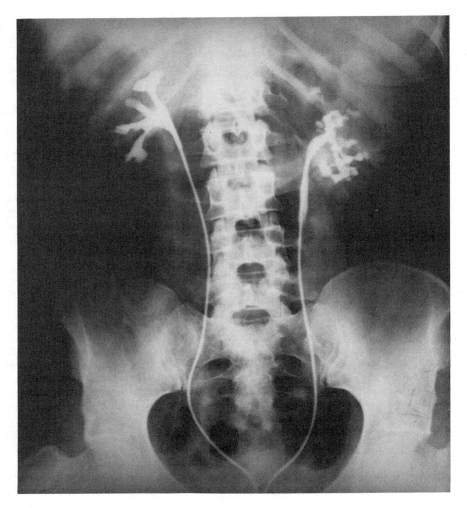

Figure 2-2. Renal tuberculosis. Bilateral retrograde ureteropyelograms, with the left kidney showing the typical findings of renal tuberculosis, best described as "moth-eaten," with numerous pinched-off calyces that are secondary to infundibular stricturing. The right kidney is normal.

ing in the field of tuberculosis now recommend long-term antimicrobial therapy for any individual whose skin test is positive. In the absence of any organism identification, however, the physician is probably not justified in assuming that renal tuberculosis exists on the basis of a positive PPD test alone; however, a positive skin test in the presence of roentgenographic findings strongly suggestive of renal tuberculosis warrants numerous and repeated tests using the patient's urine for culture and animal innoculation and may very well even justify anti-TB medication.

Management. The management of renal tuberculosis is not unlike that of pulmonary tuberculosis. When a definitive diagnosis has been made, acceptable therapy for this condition consists of a two-drug regimen of isoniazid (INH) in a dosage of 300 mg once daily for 1 year beyond the date of the last positive urine culture and rifampin 450 to 600 mg (dependent on the weight of the patient) daily for the same time period beyond the date of the last positive urine culture.

Acute Glomerulonephritis

There are many forms of acute glomerulonephritis, but by far the most common is the acute poststreptococcal variety. Although this disease may and certainly does occur in adults, it is far more common in children and is therefore discussed in detail in the chapter on pediatric urology (Chapter 5). There are many other forms of glomerulonephritis found in adults, all of which may produce signs and symptoms quite similar to those found in acute poststreptococcal glomerulonephritis. It is worthy of note that, taken together, the various forms of glomerulonephritis (with acute poststreptococcal glomerulonephritis being by far the most common) are the etiologic factors in over half of all patients coming to end-stage renal disease and requiring either dialysis, transplantation, or both.

LOWER TRACT INFECTION AND INFLAMMATION

Mention has already been made of the fact that patients with infection or inflammation of the entire genitourinary tract comprise the single most common category of urologic disease seen by the primary care physician and the urologist as well. Although infection of the upper urinary tract is much more serious, infection or inflammation of the lower urinary tract is by far more common and it produces concerns and anxiety far out of proportion to its morbidity.

The problems of lower urinary tract infection and inflammation are seen in both sexes and over the entire age spectrum. In women, cystitis is probably the most common urinary tract infection and the inflammatory conditions of urethritis or urethrotrigonitis are probably at least as common as cystitis. In elderly women, urethritis and urethrotrigonitis are perhaps the most distressing problems involving the lower urinary tract.

In men, the signs and symptoms of genitourinary tract infection or inflammation comprise what is far and away the most common category of urologic disease causing visits to the physician. As males become sexually active, the incidence of urethritis, epididymitis, and epididymoorchitis skyrockets; the symptoms of prostatitic "disease" are also common causes for physician visits. These diseases may remain troublesome throughout the relatively early years of adulthood. In males 40 years and older, there begins a marked increase in the frequency of bladder infections, often secondary to bladder outlet obstruction and the retention of residual urine postvoiding.

It must be noted that the terms "infection" and "inflammation" are not interchangeable nor are they synonymous and the distinction between them must clearly be understood if proper therapy is to be offered to the patient. Inflammation often exists without infection but infection is invariably accompanied by inflammation. The symptoms produced by each of these conditions are very similar and it is usually not possible to differentiate between them based on symptoms alone. Inflammation of the lower urinary tract in women may be caused by chemicals entering the bladder from below, as, for example, from a highly chlorinated swimming pool or from a bubble bath. Inflammation of the urethra, bladder neck, and even the trigone can readily occur secondary to the "pounding" and the "trauma" related to vigorous and prolonged sexual intercourse (recall that the urethra is only separated from the anterior vaginal wall by a thin layer of tissue). Inflammation of the bladder in the absence of any infection can also occur secondary to radiation (radiation cystitis), to chemotherapy (Cytoxan cystitis), or to a foreign body (such as a stone) in the bladder. What must be clearly understood is the fact that the differentiation between inflammation alone and inflammation accompanied by infection *cannot* usually be made from a history alone. It is absolutely imperative that cultures of the appropriate substance (i.e., urine, urethral discharge, prostatic secretions, etc.) be made before a final determination is reached regarding whether or not infection is contributing to the symptoms of inflammation. If appropriate, these cultures should include anaerobic and tuberculosis cultures before a definite determination is made regarding the etiology of the patient's symptoms. This differentiation is crucial because therapy is totally dependent upon it. The use of antimicrobial drugs in the absence of any bacterial organisms is inappropriate therapy at best and potentially very harmful, as the patient may suffer a drug reaction. Patients without bacterial infection but with all the symptoms of inflammation need a very different therapeutic approach from patients with true bacterial infections. Conversely, patients with a bacterial infection require appropriate antibiotic therapy and this cannot always be readily determined without appropriate culture and sensitivity studies.

Cystitis

History, Etiology, and Symptoms

Female Adult. The woman with a urinary tract problem requiring a visit to the primary care physician is most likely afflicted with lower urinary tract symptoms. The woman with classic cystitis may have a broad spectrum of symptoms, which runs from mild, suprapubic discomfort to marked discomfort on voiding (dysuria) accompanied by a feeling of having to void much more often than usual (frequency). Although there is frequent desire to void, only a small amount of urine is obtained at each voiding and it may or may not be grossly bloody. It is also fairly common for the patient with cystitis to complain of the fact that when she has the urge to void, she feels that she has to void "right now" or else may lose her urine involuntarily (urgency). When the infection is limited to the bladder, the patient usually feels well in general and rarely has a temperature in excess of 99° or 100°F. There is additional variety in the symptoms of women with lower urinary tract infections. Some complain of discomfort only *during* voiding whereas others may complain of discomfort or pain in the urethra or bladder at the end of voiding. Still others may complain of "stinging" or "tingling" at the actual time of voiding or may just complain of "feeling funny" during voiding. Most of these latter symptoms are usually variations produced by inflammation with or without infection in the urethra. When the inflammation or infection is limited to the trigone of the bladder the classic symptom is discomfort at the very *end* of voiding; a variation may be discomfort throughout voiding, with exaggerated pain at the very end.

The usual etiology of lower urinary tract infection or inflammation in women is ascending infection from the outside. Virtually all of the organisms causing bacterial infection in the female urinary tract are normal inhabitants of the intestinal tract that migrate from the perianal area along the perineum to the vaginal introitus.

Inasmuch as this bacterial migration and colonization in the introitus is a fairly universal phenomenon, there has been, until recently, considerable confusion as to why some women seem to develop bladder infections so much more frequently than others. In a recent series of experiments, women who frequently suffered from urinary tract infections were compared to a control group. The *number* of bacteria present in the vaginal introitus of women in the former group was significantly greater than in women in the control group, who rarely suffered recurrent infections. The presence of this greater number of bacteria within the introitus of those women suffering from recurrent infections appears to be due to a difference in the vaginal mucosa between the infected and the control group, in that there was a greater adherence of bacteria to the vaginal mucosa (epithelial cells) in the infected group than the control group. In all other appropriate ways, such as frequency of sexual activity, age, race, and so on, the infected group and the control group were matched. What has *not* as yet been determined is *why* the epithelial cells in the vaginas of some women are different than the epithelial cells in the vaginas of other women.

The marked increase in bacterial adherence within the vaginal introitus predisposes certain women to recurring lower urinary tract infections and it is most often sexual intercourse that serves as the agent by which the bacteria are actually introduced into the bladder. During sexual intercourse vaginal bacteria are transferred from the vaginal introitus in great numbers to the urethral meatus by the movements of the penis and, additionally, penile trauma to the anterior vaginal wall which borders on the urethra superiorly may possibly decrease the urethral resistance to bacterial invasion.

The young female patient with acute postcoital ("honeymoon") cystitis will often be embarrassed or uncomfortable about seeking medical attention for a condition that she is certain has resulted from sexual intercourse. It is important for the physician to reassure this patient that what has occurred is very common and not the result of any unusual or abnormal activities. The sympathetic physician can explain to these patients that the "woman above" position will result in the least possible amount of trauma to the anterior vaginal wall and the urethra and is least likely to result in bladder infections since the woman is able to keep the penis contained within the vagina and not permit it to slip into frequent contact with the urethral meatus, thereby dragging bacteria into proximity with the meatus. Ideally, the physician should also discuss the prophylactic merits of voiding before and after intercourse. This will deprive bacteria that are introduced into the bladder from having a hospitable medium in which to grow and will also serve to flush bacteria that have been introduced into the bladder back to the outside following intercourse. (Recall that most individuals produce 2 ounces of urine every hour, so voiding before and after intercourse is very feasible.) By conveying an air of comfort and ease, physicians can lessen the patient's embarrassment, assure the patient that her problems are not at all unusual, and help the patient to understand the reasons for her difficulties and learn techniques that she can use to minimize them.

One may wonder why such infections in women are not *more* prevalent. Although bacterial adherence is undoubtedly of great significance in the pathogenesis of recurrent urinary tract infections, there are certainly other factors that play a significant role. For example, host resistance to bacterial infection probably varies from individual to individual in much the same manner that susceptibility to colds varies among individuals. It has been documented experimentally that if pure strains of bacteria are introduced into normal human bladders, male or female, the resulting bacteriuria disappears spontaneously within a few hours, the bladder urine becomes sterile, and the patient is asymptomatic. From this it may be concluded that there is an intrinsic defense mechanism within the bladder that helps to prevent infections. It appears that this mechanism is within the bladder mucosa and it may well be centered in one of the mucopolysaccharidase known as glycosaminoglycans (GAGS). Thus it appears that host resistance in general and specific resistance of the bladder to bacterial invasion both play a role in recurrent urinary tract infections. Some women virtually never get bladder infections whereas others get them frequently. In addition to the bacterial adherence, and to differences in systemic and bladder resistance to infections, what other factors impact on the frequency of urinary tract infections? If, in fact, sexual intercourse is usually the triggering factor in an infection, why is it that some women get infections only occasionally even though they have a fairly consistent and frequent pattern of sexual intercourse? The answer may well lie within three interrelated variables: (1) the condition of the bladder mucosa at the time that the bacteria are introduced into the bladder (that is at the time of sexual intercourse); (2) the strains, numbers, and virulence of the bacteria that are introduced into the bladder (and this will, of course, be affected by the relative bacterial adherence in a given individual vaginal mucosa); and (3) the duration of intercourse, how vigorous or traumatic it is, whether the bladder has urine in it at the time and how soon after intercourse voiding takes place.

A bladder mucosa that has been altered away from its normal state, such as by chronic outlet obstruction or stone, is more susceptible to infection than a normal bladder mucosa. This is probably because of interference with or a disruption of the normal bladder defense mechanism that is located in the bladder mucosa. Even with a bladder that is anatomically and physiologically normal, however, there may be other variables determining the degree of normalcy of that bladder's mucosa. For example, the blood supply to the bladder is derived primarily from the paired inferior vesical arteries, which are branches of the hypogastric arteries, and these vessels arborize through the walls of the bladder so that as the bladder distends, the blood vessels become compressed. Now if an individual customarily and normally voids infrequently, for example, every 4 to 5 hours, the intravesical pressure between voidings can get very high, not withstanding the obvious variations that can be produced by the amount of fluids ingested, perspiration, insensible water loss, and so forth. Even assuming that the individual empties the bladder completely at each voiding it is entirely possible that the high intravesical pressure between voidings compresses the blood vessels supplying the bladder as they branch and travel within the bladder wall to the extent that the bladder mucosa is deprived of its normal blood supply. If large amounts of bacteria are introduced into the bladder through sexual intercourse in close temporal proximity to the deprivation of its normal blood supply, the situation may be conducive to development of an infection. Although the above may be a somewhat theoretical hypothesis that might be difficult to prove clinically, in the author's experience infrequent voiding is indeed one of the most common findings in women who are predisposed to recurrent urinary tract infections, and, far more often than not, changing these voiding habits brings about a prompt improvement in the frequency of documented infections. The question always comes up as to why infrequent voiding is so critical a factor when women have sexual intercourse frequently but only acquire a urinary tract infection a few times each year. I feel that the reason for this can usually be understood by a very methodical and careful history-taking session with the patient where, more often than not, it can be established that the intercourse that precipitated the present infection followed a day in which the woman's schedule was such that she had virtually no time to urinate and indeed voided much less frequently than her own norm. Careful questioning may also elicit the fact that intercourse on that particular evening was more prolonged or more repetitive than usual.

Although the large majority of urinary tract infections in women are related to sexual intercourse, it must be kept in mind that this is not always the cause. The possibility of asymptomatic infection in the upper urinary tract seeding bacteria into the bladder must always be considered. Additionally, although most uncommon, there is the possibility of a hematogenous spread of infection from a distant focus as well as the remote possibility of lymphatic spread of bacteria from the large bowel to the bladder. There are always occasional individuals who have never been properly taught how to clean themselves following bowel movements, that is, from the front towards the rear, and wrongly reverse the procedure, thereby bringing bacteria normally found in fecal matter into close proximity with the vagina and urethra.

Some women who do indeed void frequently and whose bladder mucosa is relatively resistant to infection may nonetheless develop infection in the bladder by the introduction of bacteria during sexual intercourse. This may be considered a dose-related phenomenon. That is, large numbers of bacteria can overwhelm the intrinsic resistance within the bladder mucosa, as can very prolonged intercourse with repeated introduction of smaller amounts of bacteria into the bladder.

There is another not insignificant group of patients in whom the urethral meatus is in a relatively hypospadiac position; that is, it is almost on the anterior wall of the vagina. A meatus such as this is literally pushed down into the vagina at the time of the downward plunge of the penis during sexual intercourse, allowing great numbers of introital bacteria to enter into the bladder. In an additional very small group of women the urethral orifice may be abnormally snug, thereby preventing complete bladder emptying by voiding. Their bladders carry residual urine that serves as a perfect culture medium in which infection can develop once bacteria are introduced. Such introduction is usually through sexual intercourse or on uncommon occasions by some other mechanism.

Male Adult. The adult male is seldom afflicted with cystitis. In view of his relatively long urethra it is very rare for ascending bacteria to reach the bladder in sufficient numerical strength to set up a focus of infection. When a man does develop a bladder infection, the clinician should consider the possibility that a bladder mucosal abnormality exists that decreases the natural resistance to infection. Such abnormalities may result from bladder outlet obstruction, neurogenic bladder, stone, and so forth. Accordingly, it is particularly important that the signs and symptoms of an acute bladder infection in a man are never ignored and that the patient is never told to "wait until the next infection" before any investigatory steps are taken. Sometimes, even in the presence of a perfectly normal bladder mucosa, chronic bacterial prostatitis may present an overwhelming number of bacteria into the bladder by means of the numerous prostatic ducts and this may be sufficient to produce acute bladder infection. In fact, recurring bladder infections in a man with no other discernible abnormalities of the urinary tract are probably caused by chronic bacterial prostatitis more often than by any other single entity, although, in the author's opinion, chronic bacterial prostatitis is a very uncommon disease, and not infrequently a bladder outlet obstruction is found to coexist with chronic bacterial prostatis and to be largely responsible for the recurring infections. Acute bacterial prostatitis is invariably accompanied by bacterial infection of the bladder, but this disease process is also uncommon and readily diagnosed by its more obvious signs and symptoms. Symptoms of men with cystitis (regardless of the etiology) are usually not unlike those of women so afflicted. Frequency, urgency, dysuria, suprapubic discomfort, the inability to void more than small amounts, and occasionally hematuria are the most common symptoms of acute cystitis in men and their temperature rarely goes over 99° or 100°F if the infection is limited to the lower urinary tract.

Physical, Laboratory, and X-Ray Findings. Acute cystitis in adults is distinguished by its paucity of physical findings. In the suprapubic area there may be tenderness to deep palpation or even to percussion; however, the absence of any tenderness in no way rules out a diagnosis of acute cystitis. Rectal examination of men with acute cystitis is indicated for the purpose of defining the size of the prostate gland. As already noted, an enlarged prostate gland that leads to bladder outlet obstruction and retention of residual urine is one of the prime causes of acute cystitis in men beyond the age of 50 years. As is pointed out in Chapter 7, however, the absence of a palpably enlarged prostate gland on rectal examination does not rule out prostatic enlargement as the cause of the bladder outlet obstruction nor does a palpably enlarged prostate prove conclusively that it is causing bladder outlet obstruction.

When acute cystitis exists, the peripheral hemogram may be normal or there may be a modest leukocystosis with a slight shift to the left. Urine examination, however, is essential for establishing the diagnosis; the centrifuged urine sediment will almost always contain at least 3 to 5 white blood cells per high power field and usually a great deal more. Yet it must be remembered that a virtual absence of white blood cells may be found in some patients with bona fide bacterial cystitis. There may also be some red blood cells per high power field and some nonrenal protein may be present due to the blood in the urine sediment. Bacteria may or may not be visible on examination of the urine sediment.

The critical test in establishing a diagnosis of acute bacterial cystitis is the urine culture showing greater than 100,000 colonies of an organism per milliliter of urine, provided the specimen has been properly collected (see Chapter 15). However, these numbers really refer to the properly collected "clean-catch" specimen for a woman. In a circumcised male, or a male whose foreskin has been retracted and whose glans has been thoroughly cleansed with soap and water, a midstream urine having 25,000 or 50,000 colonies of an organism per milliliter of urine very probably indicates bacterial infection and a count over 1,000 colonies or so in a catheterized urine is almost conclusive evidence of the presence of bacterial infection. In fact, if the catheterization has been performed under sterile conditions *any* bacterial colony count is probably indicative of infection. It must also be borne in mind that in the early stages of acute bacterial cystitis the natural defense mechanism of the bladder mucosa may be functioning to keep the colony count well under 100,000. Therefore, in general, bacterial colony counts between 10,000 and 100,000 in either sex should always be viewed as at least suggestive of bacterial infection, particularly if the symptoms of infection are present as well. It is also worth noting that the numbers of colonies just discussed really refer to gram-negative organisms; gram-positive organisms present in a *symptomatic* patient in colony counts between 1000 and 100,000 should definitely be considered evidence of an infection.

It is amazing how often women with symptoms of cystitis are treated with antimicrobials without a urine culture being obtained. In some of these individuals a urine culture would make it patently obvious that no bacteriuria exists. The proper diagnosis might be abacterial inflammation of the bladder neck or urethra, for which antimicrobial therapy is not indicated, or, perhaps, chlamydial infection, which requires a special culture technique and very specific therapy (see below). Additionally the presence of numerous white cells but no bacteria in the urine sediment of individuals with symptoms suggestive of acute cystitis (and this can only be determined by appropriate cultures) should alert the clinician to the possibility of tuberculosis of the urinary tract. This condition is certainly very uncommon in most areas and in most socioeconomic groups but must be kept in mind. It is certain to be missed unless urine specimens that failed to show any bacterial growth in standard culture media are recultured appropriately for the tuberculosis organism. It must also be remembered that less than 5 percent of lower urinary tract infections are caused by anaerobic organisms that would be missed completely if proper collection and culturing techniques for these delicate organisms were not carried out.

There are no other laboratory studies specifically indicated when a diagnosis of acute cystitis is considered beside the above mentioned cultures and, obviously, the appropriate sensitivity studies that should be run along with the cultures. The blood urea nitrogen and creatinine levels may be obtained if there is any reason to suspect underlying urinary tract disease and particularly if it is felt that the underlying infection may be related to bladder outlet obstruction, which can result in decreased glomerular filtration with elevation of the blood urea nitrogen and creatinine levels. Also, in older men in whom outlet obstruction due to prostatic carcinoma is a possibility, acid and alkaline phosphatase studies are warranted and I generally obtain these in men over 45 years of age.

X-ray findings in acute cystitis are uniformly unrewarding. Although the presence of acute bladder inflammation may be suggested on the excretory cystogram phase of the excretory urogram, this test by no means provides a conclusive diagnosis and should not be undertaken for this reason alone. In men with acute cystitis, however, an excretory urogram is warranted because the cystitis is almost always secondary to an underlying abnormality of the urinary tract; abnormalities such as prostate gland enlargement, prostatic calculi, or upper urinary tract disease can often be detected by means of an excretory urogram. Although excretory urograms in women for an initial episode or even for recurrent episodes of cystitis are generally unrewarding and not indicated, they may nevertheless be helpful for the occasional woman with recurrent cystitis that appears to be absolutely unrelated to sexual intercourse and for whom no logical etiology can be uncovered. In such patients, excretory urograms may disclose potential causes of cystitis such as a large residual urine, a bladder stone or other foreign object in the bladder, kidney stones or other abnormalities of the upper urinary tract that could contribute to infection.

Diagnosis and Management. As with so many other disease processes, the diagnosis of acute cystitis in adults is based on a combination of history, symptoms, and laboratory findings, with the last the sine qua non for the diagnosis. The proper collection of the midstream urine specimen is mandatory and a definitive diagnosis can be made if more than 100,000 colonies of a pathogen are present per milliliter of urine. When the colony count is between 10,000 and 100,000 organisms per milliliter, cystitis should be strongly suspected if the history and the symptoms are appropriate. This is particularly true in the male, for, with proper cleansing of the glans penis, the likelihood of bacterial contamination of the urine is slight. However, in women who have no symptoms whatever of urinary tract infection, a colony count of between 10,000 and 100,000 per milliliter of urine should probably be considered as a contaminant and the test repeated. Definitive diagnosis in some very occasional patients may rest with the results of a catheterized urine for culture and in this type of specimen *any* bacterial colonies growing in the culture medium are probably indicative of bacterial infection.

Male Adult. The man with acute cystitis should have a complete urologic workup after the first episode because, as discussed previously, careful investigation often uncovers an underlying abnormality of the urinary tract that is causing the infection. In men under 40 or 45 years old cystitis is most often due to chronic bacterial prostatitis (which itself is very uncommon) and in men over that age the cystitis is most often due to benign prostatic hyperplasia producing bladder outlet obstruction and residual urine in patients who may or may not also have chronic bacterial prostatitis. Excretory urography and cystoscopy are the absolute minimum requirements in the evaluation of males who have had acute cystitis, but careful attention should also be paid to obtaining prostatic secretions for culture in order to determine if bacterial prostatitis is the etiologic factor. Management of the man with acute cystitis is similar to that of the woman as far as selection and use of antimicrobial therapy. After the acute episode is over, urologic investigation should be undertaken and completed. Management of the patient at that point depends on the findings. The patient with bladder outlet obstruction secondary to benign prostatic hyperplasia probably requires surgical correction. Urethral strictures are another not uncommon cause of cystitis, particularly in the lower socioeconomic groups, since untreated gonorrhea is a leading cause of urethral strictures and seems to be more prevalent in these individuals. Periodic dilatation or surgical correction of these strictures must be considered seriously.

Should chronic bacterial prostatitis be the cause of the acute cystitis and should there additionally be an element of bladder outlet obstruction, then the obstruction should be surgically managed. If no outlet obstruction is present, then long-term antimicrobial therapy may be attempted, although it is often unsuccessful because it is extremely difficult to introduce adequate concentrations of antimicrobial agents into the prostatic acini. In very rare cases, transurethral resection of an unobstructing but chronically infected prostate gland may help the patient by promoting drainage of the surgically unroofed prostatic ducts.

Female Adult. In the woman with a seemingly straightforward case of acute cystitis, adequate management warrants antimicrobial therapy for 5 to 7 days notwithstanding the fact that the advocates of 1-day therapy or even single-dose therapy claim results as good as when the more conventional duration of therapy is chosen. The specific antimicrobial is obtained by sensitivity testing against bacteria found to be growing in the urine, but between 12 and 48 hours (depending on whether the culture and sensitivity testing is done in the physician's office or in a hospital laboratory) is required before these determinations can be made. Logic would dictate that the patient not be without treatment during this interval and an excellent antimicrobial to select pending the results of the sensitivity studies is one of the sulfa drugs such as sulfasoxazole (Gantrisin) or sulfamethoxazole (Gantanol). As is true before prescribing any drug, the clinician should inquire about possible allergy. Sulfasoxazole in a dosage of 2 g immediately and 1 g four times per day is the preferred regimen and is effective in about 90 percent of patients with uncomplicated acute cystitis. The antimicrobial can always be changed to a more appropriate agent should the sensitivity determinations so dictate. If the patient has a known allergy to sulfa drugs, or if there is another reason not to use these agents, then nitrofurantoin (Macrodantin) 100 mg four times per day, cinoxacin (Cinobac) 500 mg twice per day, or cefaclor (Ceclor) 250 mg twice per day are also satisfactory choices. A follow-up culture should be obtained 1 to 2 weeks after cessation of therapy in order to be certain that the patient's urine is sterile.

The desirable features sought in an antibacterial agent are activity against a broad spectrum of organisms, the ability to concentrate at the site of the infection, high urinary concentrations, ease of administration, and low incidence of side effects and toxicity. Obviously there are many antibacterials on the market today that meet these criteria for the treatment of urinary tract infections, but to the above list I feel that cost should be added, as it is a major factor for most patients. It is for this reason that my first choices, as noted above, are Gantrisin and Gantanol, which are probably the least expensive agents for the treatment of acute lower urinary tract infections. Gantanol has the advantage of twice per day administration compared with Gantrisin, which must be taken four times per day, but the costs are comparable for a course of treatment. The costs of Macrodantin, Cinobac, and Ceclor are roughly comparable and between two and three times as expensive as one of the sulfa drugs per course of therapy. They are all equally good, having perhaps a slightly wider spectrum of activity than a sulfa drug, and I generally use one of these drugs in the patient with a sulfa allergy or with an organism that I know to be resistant to sulfa. Trimethoprim/sulfamethoxazole (Bactrim or Septra), which is an excellent antimicrobial agent, was originally designed in the late 1960s to be used for organisms resistant to the more commonplace antimicrobials and I still choose to save this drug for that purpose.

The woman with acute cystitis who has had one or more similar episodes within the previous year should be treated as already noted (except in such instances where the patient may know that sulfa has been ineffective in treating her infection). If the patient is quite certain that her infections are unrelated to sexual intercourse, then a complete urologic investigation is probably warranted to rule out the possibility of an underlying pathologic condition such as chronic pyelonephritis, kidney stone, or even a urethral narrowing. Such a urologic workup would include, at the minimum, an excretory urogram and a cystoscopy that includes a urethral calibration and dilatation if necessary. Any underlying abnormalities can then be appropriately remedied. It is particularly important to initiate this complete urologic investigation in the case of women whose recurrent infections have included hematuria, although sound medical judgment would warrant a thorough approach to the problem even in the absence of this frightening finding. For the woman whose recurrent cystitis is definitely related to sexual intercourse, excretory urograms are probably not indicated unless the various therapeutic methods outlined below are proven to be unsatisfactory. Cystoscopy can probably be similarly deferred.

The etiology for the vast majority of uncomplicated lower urinary tract infections in women is sexual intercourse, as has already been discussed. Little can be done about the introduction of bacteria into the bladder during intercourse; thus, management primarily depends on the condition of the bladder and the number and virulence of the microorganisms present in the vaginal introitus at the time of intercourse.

Treatment of the sexually active female with recurrent urinary tract infections that are seemingly related to intercourse consists of urging her in the strongest possible terms to void every 1½ to 2 hours (except when sleeping), as well as immediately prior to and after intercourse. It is also very helpful for the patient to scrub her perineum daily with phisoHex- or Betadine-impregnated sponges in an effort to minimize the number of fecal bacteria colonizing the introitus. Ideally, this should be done in a shower following the bowel movement and prior to intercourse. Additional measures such as the control of vaginal infections whenever possible are also helpful. Other variables include host resistance, tissue immunity, and bacterial adherence (to vaginal epithelial cells), and these are factors over which the patient and the physician have little control. In the final analysis, however, women placed on the regimen just outlined will have a significantly decreased incidence of lower urinary tract infections. Some women, regardless of any prophylaxis, will continue to have infections resulting from intercourse. These women are often best served by putting them on an antimicrobial regime that is intended to minimize the bacterial colonization within the vaginal introitus, thereby minimizing her risk each time she has intercourse. Many drugs have been advocated for this prophylactic purpose and the author has had particularly good results using nitrofurantoin (Macrodantin) or cinoxacin (Cinobac). For women who have very frequent intercourse (daily or almost daily), 50 mg of Macrodantin or 250 mg of Cinobac at bedtime each night will work very well, and for women who have intercourse less frequently the same dosage of each medicine immediately following intercourse and repeated the following morning is similarly quite efficacious.

Urethritis and Urethrotrigonitis in Females

A significant number of women have symptoms strongly suggestive of acute cystitis, but repeated culture of their urine fails to reveal significant bacterial growth. Pyuria is usually present. These women should have urine cultures done anaerobically, aerobically, and for the tuberculosis organism as well; however, the majority of these patients still continue to show entirely sterile urine. Excretory urography shows perfectly normal structures. Cystoscopy is necessary, however, in order to arrive at a definitive diagnosis, which often is a granular urethrotrigonitis and may range from mild to quite severe. The appearance of the urethra when seen endoscopically is similar to that of a red cobblestone road. This is not a diagnosis of exclusion but one that can be made based upon the endoscopic examination. Recent studies have suggested that there may well be chlamydial colonization of the urethra in a significant percentage of women with urethrotrigonitis and these women often respond to tetracycline therapy, 250 mg four times per day for 2 weeks, or to one of the synthetic tetracyclines such as Minocin or Vibramycin. Women with the granular urethrotrigonitis that is sometimes referred to as "the female urethral syndrome" have sterile urine (other than the chlamydia that may be present in the urethra) and urine cultures are invariably negative. Even with chlamydia present, the urine cultures are still negative because chlamydia will only grow in a cell culture technique and not on any of the conventional culture plates. The important point to stress in the management of patients with this "female urethral syndrome" is that they do not have bacterial cystitis, the urine cultures are invariably negative, and the usual form of antimicrobial therapy that is used for cystitis inevitably fails. It should be obvious, therefore, that omitting the urine cultures and proceeding with straightforward treatment as if the patient had a bacterial cystitis are likely to yield poor results. The author feels strongly that patients with lower urinary tract symptoms should virtually never be treated for cystitis without a clean-catch midstream urine for culture first being obtained, although it is obviously not necessary to wait for the results of the culture before instituting therapy.

The "female urethral syndrome," which is also known as urethritis or granular urethrotrigonitis, can be most distressing to the patient and its treatment is certainly not as easy or as straightforward as that for bacterial cystitis. If chlamydia is not the etiologic agent then the tetracycline therapy (which can be used empirically if the facilities for a chlamydial culture are not available) will certainly not work. In some women an associated cicatricial urethritis that may be secondary to low circulating estrogen levels in older women (somewhat comparable to atrophic vaginitis) may be treated successfully with dilatation of the urethra and topical or systemic estrogen therapy unless contraindicated for some reason. Urethral dilatation helps to open the periurethral ducts and thereby promotes drainage from the inspissated glands. An extremely valuable adjunctive treatment is the local application of urethral inserts, and the author has found that 1 percent Protargol inserts are particularly beneficial for this purpose. These are not generally manufactured commercially because the process is not particularly profitable but are available from most colleges of pharmacy, which can make them on request. The use of one of these urethral inserts daily for about 2 weeks very frequently result in a gratifying relief of symptoms, although a second and even a third course of treatment may be necessary. When the disease process is entirely refractory to this or any other therapy thus far mentioned, the patient, under general anesthetic, may sometimes be helped by the highly specialized technique of transurethral fulguration of the various granular areas present in the urethra and bladder neck or by unroofing the periurethral glands and ducts to promote their drainage. The patient may feel worse for a few days following the therapy but long-term and even permanent relief may result after that initial period. If the etiology of the patient's urethral inflammation is related to the trauma of intercourse a change in the position during the sexual act may be helpful. Specifically, if the woman assumes the above position, she will be able to determine the depth of penetration and the "pounding" that she receives during intercourse; control of these factors may help to greatly ameliorate her symptoms.

Acute Bacterial Prostatitis

Acute prostatitis is caused by a sudden infusion of large amounts of bacteria into the prostate gland. In the author's experience, this disease entity is extremely uncommon and the author personally has seen a maximum of one or two such cases each year, even when working in a very large university population. The most frequent portal for these bacteria is by direct extension into the prostatic ducts from a focus of infection in the posterior urethra. With increased patient awareness and sophistication regarding urethral infections, however, treatment is usually promptly sought and received, so that the infection rarely spreads to the prostate gland. The organism within the urethra that enters the prostatic ducts and causes acute prostatitis may be virtually any that is pathogenic to the urethra, including the gonococcus bacteria as well as many of the gram-negative and gram-positive organisms. It must be borne in mind, if for no other reason than to save a patient the embarrassment of being accused of having had recent urethritis, that acute prostatitis may result from a hematogenous spread of bacteria from a distant focus of infection such as the teeth, tonsils, ears, or skin. In these cases the offending organism is usually of the gram-positive group.

Symptoms. The symptoms of acute prostatitis vary with the etiology of the condition. Most of the time the acute process is due to a direct spread of bacteria from a focus in the urethra; thus the majority of patients with acute prostatitis have an antecedent or a concurrent history of urethral discharge, burning on voiding, tingling in the urethra, and perhaps a known recent bout of gonorrhea. If the etiology of the acute process is a hematogenous dissemination of bacteria from a distant focus, there is no antecedent history of urethral infection. The actual onset of acute prostatitis is usually typical of any severe generalized infection, that is, a high fever, accompanied by chills, prostration, and acute toxemia. On defecation, there is usually moderate to severe rectal distress, with pain that may be referred to the lower lumbar region, genitalia, or thigh. Pain originating in the acutely inflamed prostate gland may also be referred to the suprapubic region and the lower abdomen and may simulate the pain of acute appendicitis or ureteral colic. If the seminal vesicles are involved as well, the pain is commonly in the groin, due to vasitis or peritoneal irritation. Again, if the urethral infection precedes the acute prostatitis, there may still be residual symptoms of dysuria with or without any urethral discharge; but if the infection is hematogenous in origin there may or may not be any symptoms specifically referable to the lower urinary tract.

Edema of the prostate gland may cause considerable enlargement of the gland and produce symptoms of bladder outlet obstruction that on occasion may progress to complete urinary retention. This may occur regardless of the etiology of the condition. This is a not uncommon finding when the inflammatory process within the prostate gland progresses to extensive abscess formation involving an entire lobe or the entire gland. This may be suspected if the acute process lasts for several weeks.

Physical, Laboratory, and X-Ray Findings. There are definite physical findings of acute prostatitis. The diagnosis is based on the physical finding of a "mushy" or "boggy" prostate gland upon digital rectal examination, with the gland feeling like a waterlogged sponge. This digital rectal examination is usually accompanied by exquisite prostatic tenderness and the physician must be cautious not to prolong the examination or massage the prostate gland in any manner for fear of introducing the prostatic bacteria into the general circulation and increasing the symptoms of bacteremia. Some concomitant low abdominal tenderness to deep palpation may also be present, but this is not a consistent finding.

The laboratory work usually shows a leukocytosis with a shift to the left and the urine sediment, particularly if it is collected following prostatic examination, usually shows numerous white cells per high power field. In virtually all patients with acute bacterial prostatitis, the midstream urine culture shows a significant bacteriuria, usually over 100,000 colonies of the offending organism per milliliter of urine. X-ray findings are not contributory to the diagnosis of acute prostatitis.

Diagnosis and Management. Acute prostatitis may be strongly suspected on the basis of history, symptoms, and physical findings as outlined above. A significant bacteriuria confirms the diagnosis. Management of this condition is, in part, symptomatic—the patient is most comfortable with bed rest during the acute episode, which may last for a few days or a week or so. Aspirin for a temperature of over 102°F will make the patient comfortable and because he may be in considerable distress medication may be required for the relief of pain. At times, stronger analgesia may be indicated and this can be provided with the use of Tylenol with codeine or even Percodan. Of prime importance, whether the patient is treated at home or in the hospital, is the generous use of antibiotics. Trimethoprim/sulfamethoxazole (Bactrim or Septra) is probably the drug of choice in an outpatient setting and it may be given in a dosage of two regular strength tablets (80 mg, 400 mg) twice per day or one double-strength tablet twice per day. If the patient is ill enough to require hospitalization, and this is a clinical judgment based on examination of the patient, either Gentamycin or Tobramycin is probably the antibiotic of choice, 3 to 5 mg/kg per day given intramuscularly in three equal doses, with 2 g of Ampicillin given intravenously every 6 hours. Failure of the acute process to resolve within several weeks usually means that the condition has progressed to abscess formation. In this case, prostatotomy is usually indicated and this may be done preferably by the transurethral route or alternatively by the open perineal approach. It should be noted that progression to abscess formation is most uncommon.

Chronic Bacterial Prostatitis, Chronic Nonbacterial Prostatitis (Prostatostasis), and Prostatodynia

The symptoms of all three of these entities, particularly the first two, can be very similar but the first is caused by bacterial invasion within the gland whereas the latter two are not.

The etiology of chronic bacterial prostatitis is somewhat obscure. It may well represent a residual infection following an inadequate clearing of an episode of acute prostatitis. In the author's experience, patients seen with this entity more often than not can recall a definite past history compatible with acute bacterial prostatitis. However, this entity may also be caused by small amounts of bacteria periodically invading the prostate gland either from a focus in the urethra or from a hematogenous dissemination. This persistent but minimal bacterial invasion can result in an infection within the prostate gland that is not of sufficient magnitude to produce a full-blown acute prostatitis but may cause the symptom complex that we think of as chronic bacterial prostatitis. Additionally, due to the known antibacterial action of prostatic fluid, virulent bacteria might be prevented from producing acute prostatitis but still lead to subacute or chronic prostatitis. In older patients with bladder outlet obstruction and resulting bladder infection it is also possible that infected urine traversing the prostatic urethra may leave sufficient bacterial implants within the prostate gland, by way of the prostatic ducts, to produce the symptoms associated with chronic prostatitis.

Nonbacterial prostatitis (prostatostasis) is very much akin to chronic bacterial prostatitis in its symptomatology but is not related to any bacterial infection within the prostate gland. Although the etiology of this condition is obscure and may ultimately be demonstrated to depend on various, presently unknown factors, it is the author's belief that nonbacterial prostatitis (prostatostasis) is caused by congestion and secondary inflammation (but not bacterial infection) within the prostatic acini that are due to inadequate and incomplete emptying of the acini and ultimately lead to engorgement and congestion of the prostate gland. The prostate gland is a veritable maze of poorly drained recesses and it may be visualized as something akin to the type of sponge that is used to wash dishes or cars. When the sponge (or in this case the prostate gland) is "wrung out" it is emptied of fluid and no longer congested or engorged and this "wringing out" of the prostate gland is what occurs during each ejaculation. However, in some individuals the prostate gland is subjected to prolonged congestion and incomplete emptying and this leads to the symptoms of chronic nonbacterial prostatitis. These symptoms most often arise when a man's sexual life has changed from frequent or regular intercourse to little or none, as, for example, might occur due to prolonged illness of a wife, a divorce, and so on.

Prostatodynia, which literally means "pain" in the prostate gland, is of very obscure etiology and may be related to a tendonitis of the central tendon of the perineum, a pelvic floor myalgia, or some entity yet to be described. It is not caused by any disease process within the prostate gland.

Symptoms. The symptoms described by a patient with either chronic bacterial prostatitis or chronic nonbacterial prostatitis (prostatostasis) are strikingly similar and
can best be summarized as being annoying, uncomfortable, and perhaps even worrisome, but only very rarely of any severity. These symptoms usually consist of a
vague feeling of discomfort or sometimes a dull ache in the perineum or "up inside
the rectum" most commonly noted when the patient is sitting, an itching or a sense
of discomfort in the posterior urethra or just "deep inside," a mild discomfort on
voiding, with or without frequency, and very occasionally a minimal urethral discharge of clear, whitish fluid. It should be noted that all of these symptoms can
be caused by an inflammation withing the posterior urethra alone without involvement of the prostate gland, and it is the author's opinion that the diagnosis of chronic
bacterial prostatitis is probably made far more frequently than this condition actually occurs.

The symptoms of prostatodynia are usually those of discomfort or a dull ache
in the perineum or "up inside the rectum" and some or all of the above symptoms
may additionally be present.

In the case of chronic bacterial prostatitis it is evident that the presence of bacterial infection within the prostatic acini may conceivably produce additional symptoms of systemic discomfort such as fever, chills, or a generalized malaise. Although
this is a most uncommon and unusual occurrence it may exist if the prostatic bacteria are present in sufficient virulence and numbers to gain access to the bloodstream and it then, in fact, becomes an acute prostatitis (see above). Patients with
chronic bacterial prostatitis or nonbacterial prostatitis (prostatostasis) will additionally often say that the symptoms of which they currently complain have been present
more than once before, often many times, with intermittent periods of relief followed by recurrence. It is very obvious on carefully interviewing these patients that
they are far more psychologically than physically upset and specific questioning will
often elicit the fact that they are scared to death that whatever is causing their
symptomatology may cause sterility, impotency, benign prostatic hyperplasia, or
even cancer. It is additionally often obvious that the symptoms in some patients
arise from a sense of guilt over some antecedent indiscretion such as an extramari-
tal adventure.

Virtually all patients with a genuine history of chronic bacterial prostatitis will
also give a history compatible with chronic urinary tract infection, and it is extremely unlikely that a patient *without* this history of recurrent chronic bacterial cystitis
has any sort of bacterial infection in the prostate gland.

Physical, Laboratory, and X-Ray Findings. Physical findings of chronic bacterial prostatitis, chronic nonbacterial prostatitis (prostatostasis), and prostatodynia are most
unrewarding. The author has little patience for physicians (and this includes urologists as well!) who perform a digital rectal examination of the prostate gland in
a patient with the symptoms noted above and then diagnose prostatitis based upon
an enlarged or a "boggy" prostate gland. This is absolutely fallacious reasoning because the "softness" or "bogginess" of the prostate gland in most younger men (the
age group affected with this symptom–disease complex is almost always under 40
or 45) depends entirely upon the frequency of recent ejaculations. Recall that the
prostate gland is full of numerous acini that produce about 90 percent of the fluid
present in the ejaculate and that the prostate gland itself is spongelike. If an individual who customarily ejaculates several times per week has a sudden change so
that he ejaculates weekly or less frequently, it is obvious that the prostate will feel

somewhat larger and somewhat softer than the norm because it is engorged with prostatic fluid. In short, the palpatory finding of a somewhat enlarged or some- what "boggy" prostate gland on digital rectal exam should suggest *only* that the prostate gland is engorged because of infrequent ejaculations and should absolutely *not* cause the examining physician to proclaim that the patient has "prostatitis."

In patients in whom chronic bacterial prostatitis or chronic nonbacterial pros- tatitis (prostatostasis) is suspected, vigorous "stripping" of the prostate gland by means of massage sometimes produces several drops of fluid at the urethral meatus; these may be examined microscopically. With true chronic bacterial prostatitis the pros- tatic fluid normally shows 10 to 20 (or possibly more) white blood cells per high power field and these may be clumped. There is also an increase in the number of oval fat bodies (fat-laden macrophages) and there may be a marked decrease or even an absence of "lecithin granules," which are normally abundant in the pros- tatic secretions of asymptomatic men. Unfortunately, under the microscopic examination, these expressed prostatic secretions (following prostatic massage) are identical in patients having nonbacterial prostatitis (prostatostasis), and the only way to differentiate between the two is by culturing the expressed prostatic secre- tions. Bacteria are found in the secretions of patients having bacterial prostatitis and no bacteria are found in the secretions of patients having nonbacterial prostatitis. In the patient with prostatodynia (and also in any normal and asymptomatic pa- tient) there are fewer than ten white blood cells per high power field, not in clumps, and the oval fat bodies are rarely seen whereas the "lecithin granules" are commonly seen. In the author's experience, it is usually not possible to obtain any expressed prostatic secretions in many individuals following "stripping" of the prostate gland even though these secretions are pooling in the prostatic urethra. An alternative method of differentiating bacterial prostatitis from nonbacterial pros- tatitis (prostatostasis) or from prostatodynia is by means of a specific technique used for localization of lower urinary tract infection. The patient is asked to initiate his stream in a glass marked "1" and then, without interrupting the stream produce a couple of ounces in a glass marked "2" and then, again without interrupting his stream, finish voiding into the toilet while still consciously retaining some urine in the bladder. Then, following the vigorous "stripping" of the prostate gland, the pros- tatic secretions will have been expressed into the prostatic urethra and pooled there even though they may not have reached the urethral meatus. The patient is then asked to initiate his stream again and place an ounce or two of urine into a glass marked "3" and then finish emptying his bladder into the toilet. Before a definitive diagnosis of chronic bacterial prostatitis can be made, there must be at least a ten- fold increase in the bacterial colony count obtained from glass "3" as compared with glass "1" while glass "2" (the midstream specimen) must be sterile. The bacterial counts alluded to here are not in the order of the customary 100,000 colonies per milliliter but rather are in the order of hundreds to thousands of colonies. If the bacterial colony count is the same in glass "1" as in glass "3" or if the colony count is greater in glass "1" than in glass "3" then the patient probably has a urethritis. To reiterate, it is absolutely erroneous to diagnose a chronic bacterial prostatitis unless either (1) the bacterial colony count in glass "3" exceeds the colony count in glass "1" by a factor of at least 10 or (2) the expressed prostatic secretions yield a positive bacterial culture and the colony count is tenfold higher than the bacterial colony count in glass "1." Should the bladder urine (glass "2") be infected, the en- tire bacterial localization test must be repeated after the urine has been sterilized with nitrofurantoin (Macrodantin) 100 mg four times per day or with oral penicillin G 250 mg every 6 hours (these antimicrobial agents are used because they do not diffuse into the prostate gland). As a matter of fact, if the glass "2" (midstream) culture is positive for infection (greater than 100,000 colonies per milliliter of urine), then the diagnosis of chronic bacterial prostatitis is very likely. Conversely, in the absence of any positive bladder urine cultures it is extremely doubtful that chronic bacterial prostatitis exists or ever did exist.

Obviously the above bacterial localization test can be used to differentiate chronic bacterial prostatitis from prostatodynia as well as from nonbacterial prostatitis (prostatostasis), but the expense of the localization tests can be avoided if one is able to obtain prostatic secretions for microscopy, as this alone can differentiate prostatodynia from the other two conditions.

Virtually all other laboratory studies are usually normal with chronic bacterial prostatitis or nonbacterial prostatitis (prostatostasis) and there are no specific x-ray findings diagnostic of either of these conditions or of prostatodynia.

Diagnosis and Management. From a purely medical standpoint, the diagnosis and management of acute and chronic prostatitis and prostatostasis are straightforward in many ways. However, because these conditions are accompanied by heavy psychosomatic overtones they frequently require that the primary care physician or the urologist function as a psychotherapist in order to treat the distressed patient adequately.

Chronic bacterial prostatitis, chronic nonbacterial prostatitis (prostatostasis), and prostatodynia can all produce similar symptoms. It is the author's feeling that chronic bacterial prostatitis is a very uncommon condition that is vastly overdiagnosed, to the great detriment of the patient. Moreover, as stated above, it is extremely poor medical practice to make a diagnosis of chronic bacterial prostatitis based upon the findings of a digital rectal examination unless the bacterial localization test as outlined above confirms the validity of this diagnosis. The reasons that the author feels so very strongly about the importance of correctly diagnosing this entity are as follows: (1) Telling a man that he has "prostatitis" is tantamount, in most patients, to giving him a medical problem from which he will suffer for many, many years to come. To most men, the prostate is a genital structure; to suggest a disorder of a genital structure is to cause anxiety, fear and concern for future potency, sterility, cancer, benign prostatic hyperplasia (BPH), and general well-being that lasts for many years. (2) Having made a diagnosis of "prostatitis" the physician then quickly places the patient on antimicrobial therapy on which he will remain for anywhere from several weeks to many, many months. Antimicrobials are not innocuous and more than one patient has suffered severely from the side effects of an ill-prescribed antimicrobial which was definitely not indicated in the first place. However, for the very uncommon patient in whom the bacterial localization test *does* demonstrate a true chronic bacterial prostatitis (these patients will virtually always have a history of recurrent bladder infections), the treatment of choice is trimethoprim/sulfamethoxazole (Bactrim or Septra) in a dosage of one double-strength (or two single-strength) tablet twice a day. This therapy will help a significant number of patients and should be continued for at least 1 month and combined with efforts to "empty" the prostate gland by intercourse, masturbation, or prostatic massage.

Nonbacterial prostatitis (prostatostasis) is invariably the disease process that is occurring most of the time that the patient is told that he has "prostatitis." Antimicrobials are not indicated for this condition, although the author would not quibble with a 1- to 2- week antibiotic trial. These patients should not be told that they have "prostatitis," but rather an engorgement of the prostate gland that is due to insufficient emptying of that gland because of a pattern of ejaculation that is not frequent enough for that individual at that period in time. Telling a patient that the best treatment for his problem is frequent intercourse or masturbation is, in the author's experience, far more rewarding and more beneficial to the patient than telling him that he has "prostatitis." Additionally, prostatic massage may sometimes be employed once or twice per week for 3 to 4 weeks (this is particularly helpful in patients for whom intercourse and/or masturbation are not options) and this also will promote emptying of the prostatic acini. Nonbacterial prostatitis (prostatostasis) may safely be diagnosed based upon the findings of the prostatic secretions and the negative cultures of the prostatic fluids or the urine that is voided immediately after prostatic massage.

Prostatodynia is a condition that probably has no relationship to the prostate and may best be treated symptomatically with hot Sitz baths, muscle relaxers and reassurance. It is probably caused by pelvic myalgias or other perineal disorders. Some recent and very interesting work from England suggests that certainly prostatodynia and possibly even nonbacterial prostatitis represent a symptom complex caused by osteitis pubis, and satisfactory treatment with Butazolidin has been rendered. Because of the not uncommon and very unhappy side effects of Butazolidin, the author prefers the use of Motrin or Clinoril and has occasionally achieved salutory effects with these drugs.

By far the biggest problem confronting the physician who is treating a man with bacterial or nonbacterial prostatitis or with prostatodynia is the patient's truly morbid fear that his condition will lead to impotence, sterility, BPH, or even cancer of the prostate gland. It is a severe test of the physician's counseling abilities to convince the patient that none of these sequellae can result from any of these conditions and that the patient's interests would be better served if he would cease to concern himself with his symptomatology. It is also the physician's responsibility to convince the patient that minor dysfunctions of the genital tract should be treated with the same lack of concern as minor discomfort anywhere in the body once an appropriate physical examination has ruled out the possibility of serious pathology.

Urethritis in Males

History, Etiology, and Symptoms. Urethritis is far more prevalent than chronic bacterial or nonbacterial prostatitis or prostatodynia and is probably the most common genitourinary tract problem bringing male patients to the primary care physician and even to the urologist. As with chronic bacterial or nonbacterial prostatitis the mental anguish exhibited by the patient far outweighs the severity of the pathologic process. The author has long marveled at the fact that the vast majority of men will not be the least bit concerned if they have a runny nose for a period of days or even weeks; however, let one small unexplained drop emanate from the urethral meatus and there is not a man alive who will not go scurrying off to his physician for an explanation, a prompt cure, and possibly even some confession! If an explanation and cure are not rapidly forthcoming, the vast majority of afflicted men become fixated on the interior of the penis and the pathologic process going on therein and they develop enormous anxiety over the present and future course of this pathologic process.

Symptoms of *posterior urethritis* are virtually the same as those of chronic bacterial or nonbacterial prostatitis. This is easy to understand if one recalls that anatomically the posterior urethra is precisely in the center of the prostate gland (Fig. 2–3) and has direct communication to and from that gland by means of the prostatic ducts. The probable reason that posterior urethritis does not lead to infection in the prostate more often is the previously noted antibacterial action of prostatic fluid. Posterior urethritis usually produces itching and discomfort sometimes described as being at the "base of the penis" or "way up inside." There may also be a vague discomfort or itching on urination and there is commonly a minimal urethral discharge noted at the meatus on arising in the morning or as a small yellow or brown stain on the shorts at the end of the day. The patient rarely if ever has any systemic symptoms accompanying posterior urethritis. The symptoms of *anterior urethritis* may be indistinguishable from those of posterior urethritis with regard to the vague discomfort or itching sometimes related to urination but the patient is often able to localize the source of his discomfort as being in either the penile urethra (anterior urethritis) or "way up inside" (posterior urethritis). The gonococcus organism is the likeliest etiology of anterior urethritis and it almost always attacks the anterior urethra initially, tending to produce a copious green, yellow, or white discharge. If untreated, it usually spreads to involve the posterior urethra. It should be noted that, uncommonly, gonorrhea may be present with only a scanty, watery discharge and, very rarely, with virtually no discharge at all. With the exception of gonococcus the various organisms that are capable of producing urethral infection and symptomatology may affect the anterior as well as the posterior urethra, but clinically the latter seems to be the area that is almost always involved. Invariably (with anterior or posterior urethritis), there is an antecedent history of vaginal, anal, or oral sexual contact. A diagnosis of anterior or posterior urethritis in the absence of any sexual contact or self-instrumentation is generally unwarranted.

Although anterior urethritis is almost exclusively caused by the gonococcus organism, posterior urethritis may be caused by almost any other organism that may enter the urethra independently or at the same time as the gonocuccus organism. Chlamydia is far and away the most common organism causing nongonococcal urethritis (NGU) or nonspecific urethritis (NSU) (the term used for all cases of urethritis that are *not* caused by the gonococcus organism) and mycoplasma is probably the second most common organism responsible for nonspecific urethritis. Numerous other sorts of bacteria and viruslike organisms that inhabit the vagina, the anus, and particularly the mouth (oral intercourse is a very common cause of urethritis because the mouth harbours more bacteria of greater potential virulence than does the vagina or even the rectum) can lead to posterior urethritis.

Not infrequently inflammation of the urethra may occur after a specific infecting organism has been successfully treated simply because a very anxious patient will insist on "stripping" his urethra several times a day searching for the urethral discharge that he hopes is no longer present. The inflammation and extreme irritation produced in the delicate mucous membrane of the urethra by this action is more than enough to produce all the symptoms of bona fide bacterial urethritis. This very common occurrence in anxious male patients most frequently occurs after genuine urethritis has been adequately treated with antimicrobial agents and it helps to perpetuate the symptoms long after they otherwise should have ceased.

Another etiologic factor in the production of the symptoms of posterior urethritis is a persistently alkaline urinary pH that results in a significant precipitation of calcium phosphate crystals with resultant urethral irritation upon voiding. In this un-

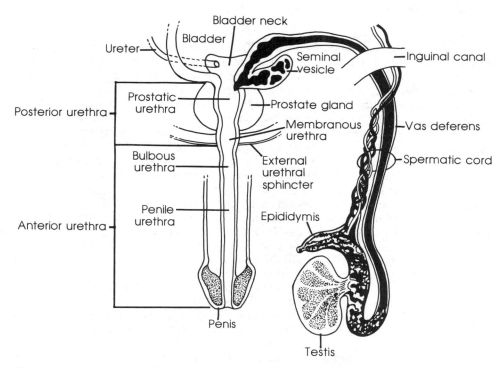

Figure 2-3. Schematic illustration showing the anatomic relationships between parts of the male reproductive system.

common condition a urine pH that is almost continually at 6.5 or higher will lead to an inability of the urine to keep its calcium phosphate crystalline material in solution; the presence of these calcium phosphate crystals that are not truly in solution will produce urethral irritation during and after every voiding. Persistent alkalinity of the urine does not necessarily represent any pathologic condition but may merely reflect dietary vagaries such as an unusually high intake of citric acid fruit juice (recall that citric acid is metabolized to bicarbonate and produces alkaline urine) or the absence of meats in the diet.

Physical, Laboratory, and X-Ray Findings. Urethritis is another unrewarding clinical entity insofar as actual physical findings. Inspection of the distal urethral mucosa may reveal marked erythematous changes. Laboratory studies are helpful in establishing the condition if there is an actual urethral discharge that can be cultured. If no discharge is present, a culture swab can be inserted into the distal 2 to 4 cm of urethra and rotated, after which it is streaked on an appropriate culture plate or placed in an appropriate culture medium. Also the first portion of the urinary stream usually has significant pyuria and possibly bacteriuria as well if the urethritis involves the anterior urethra, and the third portion of the voided stream has similar findings if the affected portion is in the posterior urethra (see above and Chapter 15 for details of the three-glass urine collection and its significance in localizing urinary tract infection).

Diagnosis and Management. The diagnosis of posterior urethritis is readily made based on the symptoms and physical findings of a very small drop, watery in appearance, noted at the urethral meatus either during the actual physical examination or as reported by the patient. Unless the physician can be certain that gonococcal urethritis is definitely not present (and such certainty is quite difficult to establish), a culture for gonorrhea should definitely be made either by culturing the urethral discharge or by using a sterile swab inserted into the distal 3 cm of urethra in patients without a discharge and the culture should be placed directly onto a chocolate agar culture plate and incubated in an atmosphere of 5 to 10 percent CO_2.

Far more common than gonococcal urethritis, however, is nonspecific (nongonococcal) urethritis, and cultures for these organisms may be done using a costly and tedious cell culture technique. In clinical practice, however, cultures for these organisms are generally not indicated (unless, of course, the clinician is doing a bacterial localization test to differentiate urethral from prostatic infection) because tetracycline is the treatment of choice for *both* chlamydia and mycoplasma and these entities probably cause 80 percent or more of the cases of nonspecific urethritis. Tetracycline is used in a dose of 1 g daily in four divided doses for 2 to 3 weeks for the treatment of nonspecific urethritis due to chlamydia or mycoplasma. Alternatively, a semisynthetic tetracycline derivative such as minocycline (Minocin) 200 mg initially and then 100 mg every 12 hours for 2 weeks may be used. For the treatment of gonorrhea the treatment of choice is still probably aqueous procaine penicillin G (4.8 million units) and this should be preceded by 1 g of Probenecid given orally 30 minutes before the penicillin. Alternatively, a single dose of 2 g spectinomycin may be given intramuscularly. Still another effective treatment for the reliable patient is oral tetracycline 0.5 g four times per day for 5 days (10 g total). For the patient in whom therapy is unsatisfactory or in whom the physician has reason to believe the offending organism to be other than chlamydia, mycoplasma, or the gonococcus, a general culture of any urethral discharge present or of the distal urethra itself can be made.

An uncommon cause of nonspecific urethritis that involves a very small fraction of individuals with these symptoms is persistently alkaline urine, a phenomenon that may be due to dietary irregularities. This condition may be readily diagnosed if the urine is examined after centrifuging and 2 to 3 cm of calcium phosphate sediment is at the bottom of the test tube. The pH of the urine is consistently around 6.5 or higher. Acidification of the urine by means of 2 to 4 g daily of ascorbic acid (vitamin C) will force the crystals back into solution and often greatly ameliorates the symptoms. A change in dietary habits may be necessary to effect a more permanent cure. It should be noted that ascorbic acid therapy should be used with great caution if the individual has any past history of uric acid or cystine lithiasis since these stones tend to precipitate in an acid urine; thus therapeutic acidification of the urine may cause stone formation. It should also be noted parenthetically that very long-term use of extraordinarily high doses of vitamin C (megavitamins) will inevitably result in the elevation of the urinary oxalate level and an increased risk of calcium oxalate lithiasis.

"Chronic urethritis" may be said to exist when the patient's symptoms of urethral irritation or minimal urethral discharge (usually noted as a persistent yellow to brownish 2 cm stain seen inside the shorts at night) persists beyond about 1 month. More often than not, the persisting minimal symptomatology results from the very anxious patient "stripping" his urethra every time he voids to see if the discharge is still present. As noted previously, such "stripping" of the urethra invariably produces urethral inflammation and irritation, thus perpetuating the symptoms thought to be from the nonspecific urethritis. Efforts must be made to convince the patient to desist from this "stripping" activity.

Of equal importance to the antimicrobials in treating nonspecific urethritis is reassuring the patient that his disease is self-limited and will not lead to any dire complications such as impotence, sterility, benign prostatic hyperplasia, or cancer of the prostrate.

Acute Epididymitis, Epididymoorchitis, and Orchitis

History, Etiology, and Symptoms. Acute epididymitis, epididymoorchitis, and orchitis are conditions that can produce varying degrees of intrascrotal discomfort, from mild to excruciating pain. With epididymitis and epididymoorchitis the patient usually notices a sudden onset of mild discomfort that may be located in the inguinal canal and perhaps the lower quadrant of the abdomen but much more commonly within the scrotum. Within a few hours to a day or two, the pain is definitely located within the scrotum and specifically in one or both testes. This pain exists whether the epididymis alone is involved (epididymitis) or the infection and inflammation have spread to involve the testis as well (epididymoorchitis). With epididymitis and epididymoorchitis there is frequently an antecedent history of urethritis and recent studies have shown the chlamydia organism to be the most common etiologic agent. In view of the fact that chlamydia is the most common organism causing nonspecific urethritis (NSU), this is not surprising. Other patients may give a history of an antecedent or concurrent focus of infection elsewhere in the body, for example, the teeth, throat, ears, or skin, and this could result in hematogenous spread of bacteria to the epididymis. In men over 40, epididymitis is most often secondary to infection within the bladder, which in turn is related to bladder outlet obstruction. The offending organism in this age group is most likely one of the gram-negative bacilli.

Pure orchitis, which is relatively uncommon, is secondary not to urethritis but rather to a focus of a *viral* infection elsewhere in the body with spread to the testis (hematogenously), whereas epididymitis and its common sequella epididymoorchitis are usually secondary to *bacterial* infection, either in the urethra or at a distant focus. Orchitis usually produces a dull ache in the testis that starts as a very mild discomfort and may become moderately severe. The patient usually has had a viral-type illness within the previous week or two and this may be nothing more remarkable than a generalized malaise. Mumps, both clinical with parotid involvement and subclinical with no localizing signs, is the most frequent viral etiology of pure orchitis and the one that produces the greatest degree of testicular edema. The resulting testicular pain is severe and far worse than any usually encountered with any other viruses that cause this condition. As a general rule the pain produced by a bacterial epididymitis or epididymoorchitis is much worse than the pain secondary to a viral orchitis.

Physical, Laboratory, and X-Ray Findings. Physical findings in epididymitis, epididymoorchitis, and pure orchitis are paramount in making any of these diagnoses. All produce abnormalities on examination of the scrotum and its contents. Acute epididymitis generally produces an exquisitely tender, frequently enlarged, and sometimes indurated epididymis; the entire epididymis or merely a portion of it may be involved. When the disease process is limited to the epididymis the adjacent testis will be palpably normal and above the epididymis when the patient is supine. Palpation of the cord superior to the testis with the patient still in the supine position may reveal a slight thickening and tenderness of the cord structures, which is caused by a vasitis, a not uncommon extension of the disease process. On occasion, the discomfort from that vasitis may extend into the inguinal canal. When the epididymis in a patient with epididymitis is carefully palpated, there is no doubt of its tenderness and enlargement and no doubt that it is responsible for the patient's pain. There is nothing subtle about the classic physical findings in epididymitis. Some patients, however, with very minimal epididymitis may complain of pain in the scrotum, but one cannot accurately make a diagnosis of epididymitis because palpation of the epididymis in these cases produces a sensation of reasonably normal structures. As with any inflammatory process, a variety of degrees exist and on occasion only a very minimal or segmental tenderness and enlargement may be palpable. In most patients with acute epididymitis, most or all of the epididymis is indeed palpably enlarged, sometimes up to five or ten times the normal size.

Inasmuch as many patients with epididymitis tend to develop an extension of the disease process to the ipsilateral testis within a very few days after the onset of the condition, resulting in epididymoorchitis, it is therefore only in the early stages of epididymitis or in less severe conditions limited to the epididymis that the testis remains palpably normal. As the adjacent testis becomes involved it too becomes exquisitely tender and may enlarge to two, three, or four times its normal size. With progression of the disease process, it is often impossible to differentiate the indurated and enlarged epididymis from the indurated and enlarged testis and the intrascrotal contents on the affected side are perceived as one large hard and often exquisitely tender mass that may be anywhere from the size of a golf ball to that of a large lemon.

A pure or acute orchitis almost always follows an antecedent viral infection. Physical examination of the affected testis in these individuals reveals a tender and uniform testicular enlargement with a perfectly normal epididymis palpable beneath the testis (with the patient in the supine position). In mild cases the patient's testis is minimally enlarged and tender and appears to be of normal consistency throughout. In severe cases, as may follow a clinical case of mumps parotiditis, the testis may be exquisitely tender, very firm, and again the size of a golf ball, a lemon, or even larger. The increasing tenderness of the enlarging testis is caused by the edema of the seminiferous tubules and the interstitial cells pressing outward upon the rigid tunica albuginea. In advanced cases of acute orchitis it is not always possible to make a correct diagnosis and the condition may be mistaken for an advanced case of acute epididymoorchitis.

These two conditions (epididymoorchitis and pure orchitis) may be indistinguishable from each other and the important things to look for in either of these inflammatory conditions involving the epididymis, the testis, or both is induration and enlargement of the affected parts accompanied by moderate to severe tenderness. It is extremely rare for these acute inflammatory processes to exist in their early phases with the absence of pain and tenderness on palpation. However, in the advanced and healing stages of each of these conditions, usually 1 week or more after onset, a great deal of induration or edema may remain but the pain and tenderness can be surprisingly minimal.

Other physical findings with these acute intrascrotal conditions are not significant and laboratory findings may or may not be helpful. If these conditions had been related to an antecedent urethritis and the urethral discharge is still present, culture and sensitivity studies should be done. When these conditions are hematogenous in origin, the urine is perfectly sterile and there is no urethral discharge. In suspected cases of viral orchitis, examination of the urine, the blood, and particularly the feces may often reveal one of the enteroviruses. The peripheral hemogram may or may not show a leukocytosis with a relative shift to the left and x-ray findings are not at all helpful in the diagnosis of these conditions.

Diagnosis and Management. Diagnosis of epididymitis, epididymoorchitis, and pure (viral) orchitis is based on the history and physical examination, and management is symptomatic in large measure. With any of these conditions, the patient is more comfortable when the scrotum is elevated, as this tends to move the weight from the epididymis, testis, and cord. Elevation can be accomplished by means of an athletic supporter or a Bellevue bridge if the patient is in bed. Although the author has preferred in the past to use antimicrobial therapy only where there was a temperature elevation or where the clinical symptoms were severe, recent studies showing chlamydia to be the most common etiologic agent in the production of epididymitis with or without concomitant orchitis seem to argue for placing these patients on antichlamydial therapy, specifically a course of tetracycline, 1 g daily in four divided doses for 2 to 3 weeks. Ice packs applied to the inflamed and tender epididymis or testis may offer some symptomatic relief but probably does not alter the pathologic process significantly.

If the patient is first seen before there is significant epididymal enlargement and induration, injection of 3 to 4 ml of 1 percent Xylocaine around the spermatic cord at the level of the external ring may completely eliminate the pain normally associated with this condition. Even when the patient is seen after the condition has become well developed, the use of a local anesthetic in this manner may bring about several hours of relief, with the possibility that the pain may not recur with as much severity as was present initially. Analgesics such as Tylenol with codeine or Percodan may be offered because the discomfort associated with these conditions in the first few days can be quite severe.

In cases of severe viral orchitis, such as may be seen as a sequella to mumps parotiditis, it may be necessary to use steroids to suppress testicular edema and very rarely surgical incisions in the tunica albuginea are warranted to relieve the extraordinary pressure on the tunica caused by edema of the seminiferous tubules. If untreated and severe enough, a pressure necrosis of the seminiferous tubules with atrophy of the testis may result.

The natural history of epididymitis and its frequent sequella, epididymoorchitis, leads to complete resolution of the induration, pain, and edema within 1 week to 2 to 3 months. The orchitis that accompanies epididymitis generally subsides and presents a palpably normal testis in 2 to 4 weeks after onset, as does the pure orchitis that is viral induced. However, inasmuch as most of these infections are usually seen in young men, it is important to recognize that any one of these conditions may be masking a coexisting cancer of the testis. Proper management, therefore, absolutely requires that the patient be examined approximately weekly. If the testis has not returned to a completely normal palpatory "feel" within 2 to 4 weeks after the onset of the disease process (regardless of any residual induration of the epididymis, which may be present for up to 3 months), surgical exploration should be considered.

It is also of the utmost importance that the surgical emergency of testicular torsion be considered in the differential diagnosis of epididymoorchitis, and pure (viral) orchitis (see Chapter 11).

REFERENCES

Evans A: Infections of the kidney and bladder in the adult. In Kendall AR, Karafin L (eds), Urology. Philadelphia, Harper and Row, 1983, vol 2, chap 14

Lattimer JK, Ehrlich RM: Genitourinary tuberculosis. In Kendall AR, Karafin L (eds), Urology. Philadelphia, Harper and Row, 1981, vol 1, chap 17

Rous SN: Urology in Primary Care. St. Louis, Mosby, 1976

Rous SN: Understanding Urology. Basel, Karger, 1973

Rous SN: Symptomatic treatment of selected cases of urethritis: A new method. NY State J Med 71:2865, 1971

Rous SN: The female urethral syndrome and urethritis and prostatitis in the male. Med Coll Virginia (MCV) 14(2):65, 1978

Slachta G, Conger KB: Inflammatory diseases of the male genital tract. In Kendall AR, Karafin L (eds), Urology. Philadelphia, Harper and Row, 1977, vol 1, chap 15

Stamey TA: Pathogenesis and Treatment of Urinary Tract Infections. Baltimore, Williams and Wilkins, 1980

3

Infection and Inflammation: Gram-Negative Sepsis and Gram-Negative Shock

EDUCATIONAL OBJECTIVES

1. List the symptoms and findings and common urologic causes of gram-negative sepsis (shock).
2. Describe the management of patients in gram-negative shock.
3. List the criteria for making the diagnosis of gram-negative sepsis (shock).

Bacteremia or sepsis exists when microorganisms (aerobic or anaerobic) are present in the bloodstream. Gram-negative bacteremia or sepsis is the most common type in the urologic patient because the overwhelming majority of organisms causing urologic disease are gram negative. There are probably between 70,000 and 300,000 cases each year of gram-negative bacteremia, and in about 40 percent of these cases shock complicates the picture, with a resultant mortality of 40 to 90 percent. It may therefore be roughly estimated that gram-negative bacteremic shock results in approximately 20,000 to 60,000 deaths each year in the United States, although by no means are all of these in urologic patients.

Invasive infection with gram-negative bacteria (or with many other kinds of bacteria, fungi, or viruses) can result in the release of a large number of potential mediators of the septic shock syndrome in addition to the bacterial endotoxin that seems to play a major enhancing role in virtually all of the deleterious effects of septic shock syndrome. The specific inciting factors of this syndrome are not well known, nor are the modes of action of its various potential mediators. It is known, however, that the infecting organism can activate certain protein systems, resulting in the formation of active mediators from inactive precursors (such as the complement, kinin, or clotting systems); the invading organism can promote the release of active mediators from cellular sites (such as histamine or prostaglandins) and in some instances the invading organism can directly contribute to the damage of vessel endothelial cells and compromise tissue blood flow.

Shock secondary to sepsis is caused by a sequestering or a maldistribution of a normal or a high cardiac output to different body compartments. Therefore the hypotension in septic shock occurs when a decreased systemic vascular resistance is not fully compensated for by increases in cardiac output. The inadequate blood flow to the affected parts of the body is manifested by development of lactic acidemia, which occurs in response to tissue hypoxia, and inadequate peripheral use of oxygen leads to end organ dysfunction, such as kidney, brain, and liver failure. It must be emphasized that the cause of this peripheral vascular insufficiency is not understood completely but it is probably related to systemic release of vasoactive mediators that produce selective vasodilation of certain vascular beds, leukocyte clumping caused by activated complement components, and vascular endothelial cells. These can result in interstitial fluid accumulation, producing a high flow of blood to nondamaged vascular beds and a decreased or absent flow in vascular beds where endothelial injury is severe.

Careful observation of patients with gram-negative septic shock has revealed consistent patterns of hemodynamic change that have been documented to occur. Early in the course of the disease there is a marked diminution in peripheral resistance, increased or occasionally normal cardiac output, decreased central venous pressure, hyperventilation, and lactate accumulation. Respiratory alkalosis usually occurs but metabolic acidosis may occur occasionally. As the shock progresses there is a continued diminution in cardiac output, peripheral vasoconstriction with increased systemic resistance, and metabolic acidosis with additional lactate accumulation. In other words, the early hemodynamic changes of gram-negative shock are those of an expanded circulatory bed not adequately compensated for by increases in cardiac output and circulating blood volume. In these early stages progressive volume expansion is the treatment of choice. If this does not result in improvement, then vasoactive agents should be administered to increase cardiac output without reducing peripheral vasoconstriction. If these therapeutic efforts are not successful, renal or respiratory failure, or both, is the usual cause of death because the small vessels of the kidneys and lungs are particularly susceptible to the changes occuring in gram-negative shock.

ETIOLOGY

In nearly every series of patients studied, *Escherichia coli* has been the most frequent etiologic agent, usually accounting for about one third of patients. *Klebsiella*, *Enterobacter*, and *Serratia* are next in frequency, each accounting for about one fifth of patients, and *Pseudomonas* and *Proteus Providencia* species account for about 10 percent of patients. Bacteroides and other anaerobic bacilli are common causes of bacteremia originating from the female genital tract but are very rarely isolated from bacteremia secondary to urinary tract infections.

Gram-negative bacteremia and bacteremic shock generally occur in older patients and when the urinary tract is causative there is usually a history of urologic instrumentation, or of obstruction, or of a foreign body somewhere in the urinary tract. Probably the most common cause of gram-negative sepsis and shock is iatrogenic, resulting from placement of a catheter in the urethra, a simple sounding of a strictured male urethra, or an endoscopic procedure, especially in patients with infected urine. A very common and frequently overlooked cause is an urethral catheter that becomes obstructed and no longer drains adequately. In addition, obstruction anywhere along the urinary tract from the renal nephron to the urethral meatus can cause sepsis and shock. Benign prostatic hyperplasia, bladder neck obstruction, and urethral stricture can also be initiating factors in this dreaded complication. Urinary tract calculi can predispose to gram-negative sepsis and the asymptomatic staghorn calculus, in particular, is a potentially lethal presence because of its association with infection and because of the extreme rapidity with which a patient can progress from a state of good health to one of sepsis and shock when a staghorn calculus is present. Pyelonephritis, renal tuberculosis, and malignancies impinging upon or obstructing urinary tract drainage can also predispose to this condition. Other causes of obstruction to the urinary tract can be vesicoureteral reflux, retroperitoneal fibrosis, pregnancy, and cysts of various origin that can compress the ureter.

SYMPTOMS AND SIGNS

The first thing to bear in mind is that the patient with gram-negative bacteremia may appear quite well clinically, but very subtle findings such as a change in mentation (minimal confusion, slight stupor, minimal agitation, and so on) or even only a fever should alert the clinician to the possibility of gram-negative bacteremia. If, additionally, there is frank mental confusion and shaking chills, the possibility of this entity should be strongly considered and if, further, the patient is known to have an infected urinary tract, or has hyperpnea or tachypnea, he or she should probably be treated as if gram-negative bacteremia existed. A diminished urinary output may frequently be present and nausea and diarrhea may also be found. It is of the utmost importance to recognize that the blood pressure may or may not fall initially because of the compensatory outpouring of epinephrine and norepinephrine, and therefore the clinician should not delay in making the diagnosis or instituting treatment simply because the patient is still normotensive. If gram-negative bacteremia is suspected it would be a most serious and perhaps even a fatal error to wait until hypotension ensued before initiating appropriate therapy. A patient with the sort of urologic history or any of the signs or symptoms discussed above should be immediately considered as having gram-negative bacteremia and should be treated for presumptive gram-negative sepsis. One may err in treating these individuals when there is no actual sepsis, but little damage is done. Delayed treatment of gram-negative sepsis, however, usually leads to gram-negative shock, with a resulting mortality rate of 50 percent or higher. By the time the profound fall in blood pressure is noted and very high fever occurs (in some patients the high fever may never occur), the patient may possibly already be beyond salvation.

TREATMENT

As soon as gram-negative bacteremia is suspected, blood should be obtained on three or four occasions at roughly 30-minute intervals for culture and sensitivity studies and antimicrobial therapy should be started immediately pending the results of the blood culture and sensitivity studies. Urine cultures, via catheter for women patients, should also be sent to the laboratory promptly. When the urinary tract is believed to be the site of origin of the bacteremia, the author prefers to start therapy with an aminoglycoside such as gentamicin or tobramycin, 5 mg/kg/day, divided into three or four equal doses. Additionally, the simultaneous use of cefazolin (Kefzol), 1 g every 8 hours, is indicated and both of these intravenously administered antibiotics should be continued for 7 to 10 days or until a negative blood and urine culture is obtained, thereby ruling out the provisional diagnosis of gram-negative sepsis. If the diagnosis is confirmed, however, the patient is usually switched to an oral agent such as cephalexin (Keflex), 500 mg every 6 hours, for another 10 days after the intravenous antibiotics have been stopped.

The other cornerstone of therapy, in addition to intensive antibiotic therapy, is volume expansion, as the early hemodynamic changes in this condition are those of an expanded circulatory bed that is not adequately compensated for by cardiac output and circulating blood volume. Aggressive fluid replacement is the basis of the hemodynamic treatment of septic shock and combinations of a physiologic salt solution such as normal saline or Ringer solution (without lactate) and dextrose and water are recommended. Plasma expanders such as albumin or plasma protein factors should be given to supplement these fluids and fluids should be administered at the rate of 300 to 500 ml each 30 minutes, with careful monitoring of the response to volume using either a large-bore central venous pressure catheter or, preferably, a flow-directed pulmonary artery catheter (Swan–Ganz). The latter catheters have the advantage of allowing sequential determinations of pulmonary capillary wedge pressure, cardiac output, and systemic vascular resistance changes in response to fluid infusion and other therapeutic measures. Large volumes of fluid are usually necessary during the first hours to reestablish a hemodynamic state, and this volume expansion is continued until the blood pressure improves, as indicated by persistent venous pressure values above 120 mm of water or pulmonary capillary wedge pressures equal to or greater than 18 mm of mercury, or there is evidence of either impending fluid overload or cardiac decompensation. Clinical evidence of adequacy of tissue perfusion should include changes in skin characteristics, mental state, and urinary output.

If this aggressive program of volume expansion does not result in improvement of the patient's blood pressure and overall condition, then vasoactive agents should be administered to increase cardiac output. Dopamine is probably the agent of first choice and in low doses of 2 to 5 micrograms per kilogram body weight per minute it increases cardiac output without producing peripheral vasoconstriction. Unfortunately, however, higher doses of Dopamine are often used to increase the blood pressure, and at these doses, greater than 10 $\mu g/kg/min$, significant α-adrenergic effects develop, with subsequent vasoconstriction similar to that caused by norepinephrine. This latter drug is a potent vasoconstrictor and, although it may increase blood pressure, it also often results in significant tissue hypoperfusion secondary to the vasoconstriction; its use therefore is not indicated. Alternatively, Dobutamine may also be helpful. This drug is a synthetic catecholamine that serves to increase cardiac output but does not selectively dilate the renal and mesenteric vessels, as does Dopamine. The usual dosage range for Dobutamine is 2 to 15 $\mu g/kg/min$.

The value of corticosteroids in the treatment of gram-negative bacteremia and shock is still controversial, with no clear conclusions as to whether or not these agents are beneficial. If used, they should be given as a single large dose. The intravenous infusion of dexamethasone 6 mg/kg/min or methylprednisolone 30 mg/kg/min may be of some benefit in stabilizing cell and lisosomal membranes, thereby limiting cell premeability and damage. It must be emphasized, however, that the role of corticosteroids in the treatment of gram-negative sepsis and shock remains controversial. Finally, the use of large amounts of intravenous fluids as noted above is absolutely essential, and as many as 18 liters of solution in a 24-hour period may be necessary in some individual patients, albeit under close monitoring. Corrections must be made for electrolyte depletions that are noted and especially for the acidosis that usually accompanies severe prolonged shock. Sodium bicarbonate is used for base replacement.

SUMMARY

If one overriding thought can be left with the reader as regards the care of the patient with gram-negative bacteremia and sepsis, it is that this condition is extraordinarily subtle in its early stages and the clinician must be very astute to suspect it and to diagnose it early enough in its natural history to assure successful results.

REFERENCES

Carson CC: Gram-negative sepsis and urinary tract infections. Drug Ther 41–48, 1982

Gleckman R, Esposito A: Gram-negative bacteremic shock: Pathophysiology, clinical features and treatment. S Med J 74:335, 1981

Holloway WA, Reinhardt: Septic shock in the elderly. Geriatrics 39:48, 1984

McCabe WR, Treadwell TL: Gram-negative bacteremia. In Stamey TA (ed), 1983 Monographs in Urology. Princeton, NJ, Custom Publishing Services, 1983

Parker MM, Parillo JE: Septic shock. JAMA 250:3324, 1983

Rous SN: Urology in Primary Care. St. Louis, Mosby, 1976

4
Infection and Inflammation: Antibiotics

EDUCATIONAL OBJECTIVES

1. List the common and preferred antimicrobials against *Escherichia coli*.
2. List the common and preferred antimicrobials against coagulase-negative staphylococci.
3. List the common and preferred antimicrobials against *Proteus*.
4. List the common and preferred antimicrobials against *Pseudomonas*.
5. List the common and preferred antimicrobials against *Enterococcus*.

Antibiotics are beneficial only when bacteria are present; a corollary of this statement is that antibiotics are contraindicated in the absence of bacteria. Although these statements might seem to be perfectly obvious, the fact remains that many physicians use antibiotics much too liberally in the absence of any documentation regarding the presence of bacteria. Specifically, women with symptoms of lower urinary tract infection or inflammation are often placed on antibiotics before the physician has first obtained a culture of the urine, and it is equally common for men to be diagnosed as having "prostatitis" and placed on antibiotics for weeks or months at a time without a positive bacterial localization test confirming the diagnosis. However, it *is* sound medical therapy to place a symptomatic patient on antimicrobials pending the culture results, with appropriate action taken after the results are available. At the risk of sounding dogmatic, the author cannot strongly enough condemn the continued and long-term use of antimicrobials in the absence of any urine cultures or in the presence of negative aerobic, anaerobic, and acid-fast urine cultures. Some general comments and observations about the bacteria commonly involved in urinary tract infections and the antimicrobial agents used in the clinical treatment of patients harboring these bacteria are warranted.

MOST COMMON MICROORGANISMS IN UROLOGIC PRACTICE

Escherichia coli is probably the offending organism in 80 to 90 percent of acute infections of the urinary tract in men, women, and children. In the very recent past, coagulase-negative staphylococci (*S. epidermis* and *S. saprophyticus*) have edged out *Klebsiella* in the second place position and perhaps account for somewhere in the neighborhood of 5 percent of acute urinary tract infections. *Klebsiella* runs a very close third, followed by indole-negative *Proteus* (*P. mirabilis* sp), the miscellaneous *Enterobacteriaceae* group, which includes indole-positive *Proteus*, and then *Enterococcus* and *Pseudomonas* close out the list of commonest microorganisms affecting the urinary tract.

DRUGS OF CHOICE

Escherichia coli
Just about any antimicrobial will be effective when *E. coli* is the offending organism. The author perfers Gantrisin as the drug of first choice because it is effective better than 90 percent of the time and it is about the least expensive agent that can be used. If a sulfa allergy or some other reason precludes its use, then nitrofurantoin (Macrodantin) or cinoxacin (Cinobac) or cefaclor (Ceclor) are drugs of choice.

Coagulase-Negative Staphylococci
The findings of significant bacteriuria with one of the coagulase-negative staphylococci such as *S. epidermis* or *S. saprophyticus* had usually been treated as an insignificant contaminant not representative of true infection in years past. It is only quite recently that workers in the field of infectious disease have become convinced and have convinced most practicing physicians that bacteriuria due to either of these organisms represents genuine infection that merits treatment.

Trimethoprim/sulfamethoxazole (Bactrim or Septra) is efficacious and one of the sulfonamides (e.g., Gantrisin) may work equally well. Nitrofurantoin (Macrodantin) is yet another good antimicrobial for these coagulase-negative staphylococci.

Klebsiella
This group of organisms, which, until recently, was considered the second most common cause of urinary tract infections (to *E. coli*) now runs a close third to the coagulase negative staphylococci and the *E. coli*. Any first-generation cephalosporin, such as Keflex, would be a drug of choice, as would be trimethoprim/sulfamethoxazole (Bactrim or Septra). Should the patient require injectable antibiotics, intravenous Bactrim or Septra, or any of the aminoglycosides would be indicated.

Indole-Negative *Proteus* (*Mirabilis* Sp)
This not uncommon organism is often associated with staghorn calculi in the kidney because of its ability to split urea and to produce a very alkaline urine. Along with *Klebsiella* and the other organisms noted below, *Proteus* is much more likely to be found in the patient who has a complicated or recurrent problem with urinary tract infections rather than in the patient with a single (or even repeat) episode of an acute, uncomplicated type. A first-generation cephalosporin, such as Keflex, or trimethoprim/sulfamethoxazole (Bactrim or Septra), or ampicillin is probably the drug of choice in treating this organism, and a second- or third-generation cephalosporin or an aminoglycoside is also highly efficacious when injectable medications are required.

Miscellaneous *Enterobacteriaceae*, Including Indole-Positive *Proteus*
This group of organisms is infinitely more resistant to antimicrobial therapy than any of the organisms discussed thus far and a third-generation cephalosporin such as cefotaxime (Claforan) or moxalactam (Moxam) is probably the drug of choice.

Of the oral medications, trimethoprim sulfamethoxazole (Bactrim or Septra) is probably the drug of choice. Also indicated for this group of organisms are the injectable aminoglycosides.

Enterococcus (Streptococcus faecalis)

This gram-positive coccus is sensitive to the various penicillins, as are virtually all of the gram-positive cocci. Either ampicillin or amoxicillin is the treatment of choice.

Pseudomonas

Traditionally considered to be one of the more resistant type of organisms involving the genitourinary tract, *Pseudomonas* is indeed resistant to many antimicrobials. The antibiotics of choice against this organism are the aminoglycosides and the semisynthetic penicillins, carbenicillin, ticarcillin, piperacillin, and azlocillin. It is worth noting that different strains of *Pseudomonas* may be resistant to one or more of the listed antimicrobials, particularly the aminoglycosides, and definitive therapy is often based on in vitro susceptibility data.

Anaerobic Organisms

The anaerobic gram-negative bacilli, in terms of pathogenicity, consist of *Bacteroides* species and the *B. fragilis* group. Penicillin G is the drug of choice for the *Bacteroides* species and, in case of penicillin allergy, a cephalosporin, chloramphenicol, clindamycin, or metronidazole may be used. For the *B. fragilis* group, clindamycin (Cleocin) is the drug of choice, with chloramphenicol also effective, as is metronidazle (Flagy). It cannot be emphasized enough that anaerobic organisms are responsible for a small percentage of urinary tract infections, certainly under 5 percent and probably in the range of 1 to 2 percent, but that the diagnosis of these infections will be missed completely unless the urine is collected meticulously (by suprapubic aspiration or catheterization) in a special container with carbon dioxide and nitrogen replacing the oxygen within the container. The container should be opened only long enough to fill it with the fluid (urine) and then rapidly capped. It must then be incubated in an atmosphere that is virtually void of any oxygen. Unless these steps are followed meticulously, the presence of anaerobic organisms can be missed entirely.

CULTURE MEDIA FOR GRAM-POSITIVE ORGANISMS AND GRAM-NEGATIVE ORGANISMS

Bacterial growth in urine can be missed entirely if appropriate culture techniques are not carried out. The blood agar plate is used to monitor universal growth, and both gram-positive and gram-negative organisms will grow on it. To specifically identify and isolate gram-negative organisms, MacConkey agar is the medium of choice, although EMB (eosin-methylene blue) may still be used in some laboratories. To selectively grow gram-positive organisms, a CNA plate is used. This means that the culture medium is treated with colistin and nalidixic acid to suppress the growth of any gram-negative organism, thereby allowing the gram-positive organisms to be identified.

The foregoing is mentioned particularly for the physician doing his or her own office cultures because the very occasional patient having a gram-positive or an anaerobic organism that is producing a urinary tract infection will be missed completely unless the appropriate culture techniques are followed.

LONG-TERM SUPPRESSIVE THERAPY

Long-term suppressive therapy should be differentiated from what was earlier described as prophylactic therapy. The latter applies, for example, to the woman who tends to get recurrent lower urinary tract infections secondary to intercourse. Long-term supressive therapy is used here to refer to the attempts of the physician to keep the urine sterile in patients who either have a foreign body within the urinary tract (i.e., a suprapubic tube, a urethral catheter or a nephrostomy tube) or who have an underlying abnormality of the urinary tract, such as a neurogenic bladder, with a resulting inability to empty the lower tract at each voiding. In the author's opinion, the presence of a permanent foreign body within the urinary tract essentially precludes the possibility of keeping the urine sterile and the author does not generally even try to do this. As long as there is no vesicoureteral reflux present and as long as there is no evidence of any renal involvement with the infectious process (as evidenced by temperature elevations above 101° or 102°F and flank pain and bacteriuria), the author does not try to keep the bladder urine sterile, assuming the bladder is kept empty by a permanent indwelling catheter. If and when the patient develops the signs and symptoms of a urinary tract infection, then treatment is certainly warranted and should be continued for several days or until the urine becomes sterile. However, to keep a patient with a foreign body in the urinary tract on permanent antibiotics would only create a bacterial resistance in the patient to one antibiotic after another and would still not, in the long run, keep the urine sterile. Obviously the goal is to remove all foreign bodies from the urinary tract. If this cannot be done, it is very doubtful that the urine can be maintained in a sterile state. On the other hand, if the patient is free of any foreign bodies but does not have a totally intact urinary tract (as one might find with a neurogenic bladder secondary to a spinal cord lesion), then long-term suppressive therapy with agents such as methenamine mandelate (Mandelamine) and ascorbic acid (to acidify the urine) might be of some benefit. Methenamine mandelate is metabolized to formalin in the presence of urine in which the pH is lower than 6.0, with maximum efficacy occurring at pH 5.5 or less. The formalin that is produced then directly kills any bacteria that may be present, and inasmuch as this is not a true antibiotic there can be no bacterial resistance developed. Successful methenamine mandelate therapy, however, depends on maintaining the urine at a very acid pH, and this is impossible to do without taking a potent acidifying agent such as ascorbic acid. If this latter is taken in a dosage of 2 to 4 g daily, the desired effect may well be obtained but it must be verified by means of regular use of litmus or nitrazine paper for pH checks of the urine. It should be noted that the risk of long-term ascorbic acid therapy is the precipitation of uric acid crystals or stones (due to the low pH) in the urinary tract and the elevation of urinary oxalate levels (because one of the byproducts of ascorbic acid metabolism is oxalate), which may lead to calcium oxalate lithiasis.

RENAL FAILURE

Patients with less than normal renal function or with frank renal failure pose a specific problem when antimicrobial therapy is necessary. Many of the antimicrobial agents in common usage are probably contraindicated in patients with decreased renal function for a variety of reasons. However, it is either because of a direct toxic effect on the kidneys or because of the toxic effects of byproducts of the antibiotic that accumulate because of the inability of the poorly functioning kidneys to excrete them. Regardless of this potential danger, patients with decreased renal function who develop a urinary tract infection must be treated. Probably the best antimicrobial to use for these patients is one of the penicillins or one of the cephalosporins, since it is generally not necessary to adjust their dosages in patients with decreased renal function and toxicity is minimal. Aminoglycosides are potentially extremely toxic in patients with decreased renal function and must be used with great care by appropriately adjusting the dosages for the decreased function of the kidneys and then measuring blood levels of the drug on a regular basis. The two drugs that should probably be avoided *completely* in patients with decreased renal function are trimethoprim/sulfamethoxazole (Bactrim or Septra) and tetracycline, the former because it is extremely difficult to monitor blood levels of this drug in the patient with renal impairment and the latter because it is notorious for accentuating renal failure and precipitating an accompanying severe acidosis. If one of the tetracyclines *must* be used, doxycycline is probably the safest.

ANTIMICROBIALS

Sulfa Drugs

This group of drugs is probably still the most commonly used in the treatment of acute urinary tract infections and certainly remains extremely effective and very inexpensive. In adults, Gantrisin is given in a dosage of 2 g immediately and 1 g four times per day for about 1 week. In children the dosage is weight related, with a recommended dosage of 100 to 150 mg/kg/day in four divided doses and an initial dose that is one half the 24-hour dose. Gantrisin, as well as the other systemic sulfa drugs, is a bacteriostatic agent; its action on bacteria is by competitive inhibition of the bacterial synthesis of folic acid from para-aminobenzoic acid. Resistant strains of bacteria are capable of utilizing folic acid precursors or preformed folic acid. The sulfa drugs have a wide spectrum of bacteriostatic activity and are often effective against *E.coli*, *Klebsiella*, staphylococci, *Proteus mirabilis* (indole negative) and, occasionally, *Proteus vulgaris* (indole positive). Excretion of all of the sulfa drugs is chiefly by the kidneys, with glomerular filtration as the primary mechanism. Therefore, in patients with impaired renal function, the sulfa drugs must be used under reduced dosage schedules; it is probably best not to use them at all if other antimicrobials such as penicillins or the cephalosporins are appropriate. Sulfa drugs are not recommended in infants less than 2 months old or in pregnant women.

Trimethoprim Sulfamethoxazole (Bactrim or Septra)

As noted above, sulfonamides competitively inhibit the bacterial synthesis of folic acid from para-aminobenzoic acid. Trimethoprim competitively prohibits the activity of bacterial dihydrofolate reductase. In combination, the two agents act in a synergistic bactericidal manner by blocking the bacterial production first of folic acid and then of folinic acid, which is necessary for the microbial production of DNA. This synergistic bactericidal effect, which may not be present when either agent is used alone, is affective against many gram-positive and gram-negative bacteria. The combination drug (Bactrim or Septra) is available in both oral and intravenous forms, but the oral form is much more commonly used. The combination drug is highly effective against the enterobacter group, *E. coli*, *Klebsiella*, *Pro-*

teus, and *S. epidermis*, among others. It is notably lacking in efficacy against *Pseudomonas* and it has virtually no effect against anaerobic organisms. It is indicated in the treatment of chronic and recurrent urinary tract infections caused by susceptible bacteria but it is probably "too good" an agent to be used for the patient with the first-time, acute lower urinary tract infection, a situation that might be analogous to using an elephant gun to shoot a mouse! It is normally used in a dosage schedule of two Bactrim (or Septra) tablets every 12 hours for 7 to 10 days or one Bactrim DS (double-strength) tablet every 12 hours for 7 to 10 days. In children, the dosage is one fifth of a teaspoonful of the pediatric suspension (which contains 40 mg trimethoprim and 200 mg sulfamethoxazole per teaspoonful) per kilogram per 24 hours given in two divided doses every 12 hours for a week.

For the patient with upper urinary tract pyelonephritis in whom intravenous therapy is warranted, Bactrim or Septra is an acceptable agent. Oral Bactrim or Septra is highly effective in acute bacterial prostatitis when susceptible organisms are demonstrated and it is probably the drug of choice in chronic bacterial prostatitis, if this diagnosis is certain. It is also an effective alternative therapy for uncomplicated gonococcal urethritis, but it is ineffective against syphilis.

Bactrim or Septra, as noted above, may interfere with folic acid metabolism and should therefore only be used during pregnancy if the potential benefit justifies the potential risk to the fetus.

Trimethoprim (Trimpex or Proloprim)

Trimethoprim (Trimpex or Proloprim) selectively interferes with bacterial biosynthesis of nucleic acids and proteins and it has a spectrum of activity that includes the common gram-negative urinary tract pathogens as well as the coagulase-negative staphylococcus species but it has no activity against *Pseudomonas*. Its advantage in this form over the combination form (Bactrim or Septra) is that the possibility of allergic manifestations caused by sulfonamides in susceptible individuals is eliminated, as is the "big gun" synergistic effect of the combination form, which unquestionably represents an overkill when used for patients with uncomplicated urinary tract infections. The usual oral dosage of trimethoprim is 100 mg every 12 hours for 7 to 10 days. It is not recommended in pregnancy or in patients with decreased renal function.

Nitrofurantoin

The nitrofurantoins are available as Furadantin or Macrodantin, the latter being a macrocrystal preparation that is absorbed and excreted more slowly than the former and is less irritating to the digestive tract. In vitro, it is bacteriostatic in low concentrations and it is considered to be bactericidal in higher concentrations, with its presumed mode of action based upon its interference with several bacterial enzyme systems. In general, bacteria develop only a limited resistance to nitrofurantoins, which are usually active against *E. coli*, *enterococci* (strep faecalis), and *Staphylococcus aureus*. Macrodantin is generally not active against most strains of *Proteus* and *Serratia* and has no activity against *Pseudomonas*. Some strains of enterobacter species and *Klebsiella* species are also resistant to Macrodantin. Inasmuch as bacteria seem to develop only a limited resistance to the nitrofurantoin family of drugs, these drugs are probably preferable to one of the sulfa drugs in cases of chronic or recurrent urinary tract infections when organisms such as *E. coli* have become resistant to the sulfa family of drugs. The low serum concentrations of nitrofurantoins after oral administration probably preclude its use for treatment of parenchymal upper urinary tract infections, particularly those associated with renal cortical or perinephric abscesses. Nitrofurantoin is not indicated in patients with decreased renal function because of impaired excretion of the drug, and it is contraindicated in pregnant patients as well as in infants less than 1 month old.

Overall, it is a splendid drug that is highly efficacious when used properly and is not excessively expensive. The dosage of Macrodantin is 50 to 100 mg four times per day in adults, and in children it is 5 to 7 mg/kg/day given in four equally divided doses.

Cinoxacin

Cinoxacin (Cinobac) is a synthetic compound belonging to the same class of antimicrobials as nalidixic and oxalinic acids. It is effective against all of the common gram-negative pathogens, with the notable exception of *Pseudomonas*. It is bactericidal and the mode of action has been shown to be inhibition of bacterial DNA replication. Inasmuch as this drug is eliminated primarily by the kidney, its use in patients with reduced renal function is less than ideal and its use in prepubertal children and during pregnancy is not recommended. Side effects in patients taking this drug are very minimal, and the usual dosage is 500 mg twice per day or 250 mg four times per day for 7 to 10 days. It is specifically indicated for the treatment of initial and recurrent urinary tract infections in adults caused by susceptible organisms.

The Penicillins

As a group, the penicillins are the most frequently and widely used of all antimicrobial agents because they are effective, low in toxicity, and relatively inexpensive. Their effectiveness is due to bactericidal action, excellent distribution throughout the body spaces, and a wide spectrum of activity. Alerginic reactions are the most frequent and serious problem associated with their use. The action of the penicillins depends on the presence of a bacterial cell wall and the ensuing inhibition of the cell wall production by the antibiotic. *Penicillin G* is one of the most frequently used naturally occurring penicillins and it may be used orally or parenterally. Its disadvantages are that it is degraded by gastric acid, destroyed by the enzyme penicillinase, and associated with a fairly high incidence of allergic reactions. It is the drug of choice in patients infected with the gonococcus organism (provided the organism does not produce penicillinase). It is also efficacious against *Bacteroides* (but not the *B. fragilis* group). When used orally it is given in a dose of 25,000 to 50,000 units per kilogram per day up to a maximum of 300,000 units per kilogram per day in divided doses and therapy should be continued for 10 days to 2 weeks.

Ampicillin, amoxicillin, carbenicillin, ticarcillin, mezlocillin, azlocillin, and *piperacillin* are semisynthetic penicillins that have been developed and have an extended spectrum of activity against aerobic gram-negative bacilli. They do not resist the action of penicillinase and are thus ineffective against some of the gram-positive or gram-negative organisms that produce penicillinase.

Ampicillin is an orally and parenterally administered agent active against several gram-negative species including many strains of *E. coli, Proteus mirabilis,* and *Haemophilus influenzae.* Most strains of *Klebsiella* and all strains of *Pseudomonas* are resistant, and resistant strains of bacteria such as *E. coli* have emerged in certain clinical situations. Ampicillin is more active than penicillin G against enterococci, and this may be synergistically enhanced by the concurrent administration of an aminoglycoside. Ampicillin is stable in gastric juices and thus is very suitable for oral use.

The usual adult dose of oral ampicillin is 500 mg every 6 hours; in children, 100 mg/kg/day is given in three to four divided doses. The parental dosage in adults is 500 mg every 6 hours and in children is 50 mg/kg/day in three to four divided doses. Although, based on in vitro testing, ampicillin is efficacious against selected urinary tract infections, the author prefers not to use it because of the more than occasional patient with an *E. coli* infection in whom there is no in vivo sensitivity to it and also because in some patients ampicillin seems to produce diarrhea and vaginitis.

Amoxicillin is closely related to ampicillin in its antibacterial activity and is only used orally. It has a much more complete absorption from the gut than ampicillin, leading to higher blood levels and less drug remaining in the intestinal tract, with a resulting lower incidence of vaginitis and diarrhea. Its dosage in adults is 250 mg every 8 hours and in children 20 mg/kg/day in three divided doses every 8 hours with much the same antibacterial activity as ampicillin.

Carbenicillin has an antibacterial range similiar to that of ampicillin but with a very important added activity against certain strains of *Pseudomonas*, the indole-positive *Proteus* species, and many *Enterobacter* species. *Klebsiella* species are generally resistant to carbenicillin, as are many *Serratia* organisms. This agent must be given parenterally because it is not well absorbed from the gut and it is usually given in doses of 200 mg/kg/day by intravenous drip, with a maximum adult dose of 40 g daily. The dose in children is variable according to weight.

Carbenicillin indanyl sodium is an oral form of carbenicillin that, because of its relatively high cost and the potential development of resistance, should be reserved for situations in which less expensive drugs are ineffective or inappropirate. In general, it should be reserved for the treatment of severe infections due to P. *aeruginosa, Proteus* species, and other gram-negative bacteria that are susceptible to it but resistant to other antibiotics. Carbenicillin is also used in combination with gentamycin to treat severe *Pseudomonas* infections because many strains are sensitive to the synergistic effect of this combination. However, because gentamycin is inactivated when in prolonged contact with *any* penicillin, the drugs must not be mixed in the same solution, but should be given at different times or sites. Finally, the oral form of carbenicillin (Geocillin) is one of the treatments of choice for chronic bacterial prostatitis caused by a susceptible organism. The usual dosage of this drug is two tablets four times daily.

Ticarcillin is similar to carbenicillin although it has more activity against P. *aeruginosa*. It is used as an alternative to carbenicillin in the treatment of serious gram-negative infections and it may only be given parenterally. The recommended dosage is 50 to 300 mg/kg/day, up to a total of 18 to 24 g/day in patients with *Pseudomonas* infections. Because ticarcillin delivers less of a sodium load than carbenicillin, it may be advantageous in patients with compromised cardiac or renal function.

Mezlocillin (Mezlin), *Azlocillin* (Azlin), *and Piperacillin* (Pipracil) are new, extended-spectrum semisynthetic penicillins that some refer to as the "fourth generation" penicillins. They have a wider antimicrobial spectrum, more anti-*Pseudomonas* activity, and less toxicity than the aminoglycosides and all are derived from the ampicillin molecule with side chain adaptations. These three agents together are collectively referred to as "ureidopenicillins" and they are all generally bacteriocidal, except against certain strains of *Pseudomonas*, *E. coli*, and *Klebsiella*. They act primarily by inhibiting cell wall synthesis of bacteria. They are not absorbed orally and hence are only administered parenterally. They are active against both gram-positive and gram-negative bacteria and have demonstrated activity against streptococci, enterococci, most Enterobacteriaceae, *Pseudomonas*, and many anaerobes, including *B. fragilis*. Piperacillin probably also has the greatest activity of the three drugs against *P. aeruginosa*. Recent reports, however, have indicated a considerable rate of resistance to these three drugs among the Enterobacteriaceae family and this would suggest that the use of this group of drugs as single therapy in suspected gram-negative sepsis is unwise. The major overall advantage of this group of drugs is their increased activity against *P. aeruginosa* and *Klebsiella*, although the enhanced anti-*Klebsiella* activity is limited to only about half of the various strains of this organism. The anti-*Pseudomonas* activity, however, covers 80 to 95 percent of strains. The dosage for this group of drugs is similar to that for ticarcillin and consists of 6 to 16 g intramuscularly (IM) or intravenously (IV) every 6 to 12 hours. Maximal adult dose is about 24 g/day.

Dioloxacillin (Dynapen) and Methicillin (Staphcillin)
These are penicillins that are highly resistant to penicillinase produced by staphylococcal organisms and are therefore indicated in highly selective circumstances.

Cephalosporins
Cephalosporin antibiotics are bacteriocidal against most gram-positive cocci and gram-negative bacilli of clinical importance. They are relatively nontoxic but, like the penicillins, may cause hypersensitivity reactions. All of the cephalosporins are semisynthetic derivations of an antibacterial compound elaborated by the fungus *cephalosporium*, which is closely related to penicillin in its structure and mechanism of action. Cephalosporin antibiotics are bacteriocidal and act by inhibiting cell wall synthesis by binding to bacterial enzymes located beneath the cell wall. The extraordinary ability of many gram-negative bacilli to develop bacterial resistance to antibiotics has spawned a whole progression of cephalosporins, each succeeding generation of which will usually have a greater efficacy against one or more gram-negative organisms than the preceding generation. A general rule is that the earlier-generation cephalosporin should be used whenever possible in order to prevent development of organisms resistant to the newer agents. The first-generation cephalosporins have good activity against most gram-positive cocci, but this activity, interestingly, is decreased with succeeding generations of these antibiotics. Cephalosporins are generally the agents of choice for treatment of infections caused by susceptible members of the Enterobacteriaceae family; of the first generation oral cephalosporins cephalexin (Keflex) is probably as well known as any and cefazolin (Kefzol) is the parenteral first-generation cephalosporin that has two major advantages: a substantially longer half life and much higher serum concentrations. Cephalexin (Keflex) is usually given in a dosage of 1 to 4 g daily in divided doses and cefazolin (Kefzol) is given in a dose of 500 mg to 1 gram every 6 to 8 hours IM or IV. The second- and third-generation cephalosporins only come in parenteral form and cefamandole (Mandol), a second-generation agent, is generally administered in a dose of 500 mg to 1 g every 8 hours IM or IV. Third-generation cephalosporins such as moxalactam (Moxam) are given in a dose of 2 to 4 g daily in divided doses and it is only these third-generation agents that have any significant inhibiting effect on *Pseudomonas*. The third-generation cephalosporins are extremely expensive, costing three to four times more than a first-generation parenteral

cephalosporin. They are also between two and three times as costly as a second-generation parenteral cephalosporin.

Aminoglycosides

The aminoglycosides in current clinical use for parenteral therapy include streptomycin, kanamycin, gentamicin, tobramycin, amikacin, and the newer ones, which are *netilmicin* and *sisomicin*. These agents are rapidly bacteriocidal through irreversible binding to the bacterial ribosome, thereby inhibiting protein synthesis and bringing about cell death. Gentamicin, tobramycin, and amikacin are indicated for serious, aerobic, gram-negative infections, including those in which *P. aeruginosa* is suspected of being an etiologic agent. All of these antimicrobials are used parenterally only and it should be noted that kanamycin has very limited efficacy at this time. Resistance to it is increasing among the Enterobacteriaceae family and its activity against *P. aeruginosa* is negligible. Gentamicin and tobramycin have very similar indications and spectrum of activity, with tobramycin perhaps slightly more active against some strains of *P. aeruginosa*. Amikacin is active against most gram-negative bacilli that are resistant to other aminoglycosides. This is because it is inactivated by only two of the eight common enzyme systems of bacteria, whereas gentamycin and tobramycin are affected by seven. Amakacin is clearly the aminoglycoside of choice when gentamycin resistance is prevalent. The two newer aminoglycosides, netilmicin and sisomicin, are quite similar to gentamycin in most regards and are not any more effective than gentamycin against resistant organisms. Unlike the penicillins and cephalosporins, the aminoglycosides may cause considerable toxicity and this may involve vestibular impairment, auditory toxicity or nephrotoxicity. There is probably little choice among the aminoglycosides in terms of overall toxicity produced. The usual dosage for gentamycin, tobramycin, and netilmicin is 3 to 5 mg/kg/day given IM or IV in divided doses every 8 hours. Amikacin, kanamycin, and streptomycin are given in a dosage of 15 mg/kg/day in divided doses every 6 to 12 hours. Streptomycin can only be given intramuscularly whereas the other aminoglycosides may be used either IM or IV. It is absolutely imperative that the kidney impaired patient be given reduced dosages on a careful schedule, with regular monitoring of the serum levels of the aminoglycoside.

Tetracyclines, Erythromycin, and Clindamycin

The *tetracyclines* are active in vitro against many urinary tract pathogens and are safe, inexpensive, and effective when prescribed properly. They should not, however, be used to treat urinary tract infections in pregnant women or in children under 12 years of age because of toxic side effects, particularly to the teeth. It is also extremely important that they not be used in patients having any sort of renal impairment because of the very real danger of increasing the azotemia and also producing a severe acidosis. Also, the tetracyclines are not really indicated for the treatment of acute pyelonephritis unless other more appropriate antimicrobial agents, such as the aminoglycosides, the semisynthetic penicillins, the cephalosporins, or trimethoprim sulfamethoxazole, are contraindicated. Specifically, the tetracyclines are the agents of choice for the treatment of urethritis caused by *Chlamydia* and ureaplasma ureolyticum and it is also indicated in the treatment of epididymitis which may be caused by chlamydial infection. Additionally, the tetracyclines may be used for the treatment of syphilis and gonorrhea in patients who are allergic to penicillin, but it is the author's firm belief that there are few, if any, additional uses for tetracycline in the care of patients afflicted with genitourinary tract disease. The usual dosage of tetracycline when used for one of the above disease entitites is 1 to 2 g daily in four divided doses for 2 weeks. If the synthetic oxytetracycline *doxycycline* (Vibramycin) is used, the dosage is 100 mg every 12 hours on the first day and then 100 mg daily thereafter for 2 weeks; if the semisynthetic tetracycline minocycline (Minocin) is used, the dosage is 200 mg initially followed by 100 mg every 12 hours.

Erythromycin has very limited usage in urology but it may be used for the treatment of gonorrhea and syphilis in patients who are unable to tolerate penicillin G or a tretracycline, as well as in those very few patients with chronic bacterial prostatitis caused by an organism sensitive to erythromycin. The dosage of this oral agent is 1 to 4 g every 6 hours for 2 weeks.

Clindamycin is the agent of choice for infections caused by the *B. fragilis* group or for the other anaerobic microorganisms in persons who are allergic to penicillin. Its oral dosage is 150 to 450 mg every 6 to 8 hours and it can also be given intramuscularly or intravenously (depending on the severity of the disease process) in dosages of 600 to 1200 mg/day in two to four equal doses.

Methenamine Mandelate and Methenamine Hippurate

Methenamine mandelate (Mandelamine) and *methenamine hippurate* (Hiprex) are sometimes used in the long-term management of patients with an impaired urinary tract, a foreign body in the urinary tract, or some other underlying reason for recurring urinary tract infection. Both work only in an acid pH and the urine must consistently be kept more acidic than pH 6, ideally around pH 5.5. This pH cannot be maintained unless the patient is given an acidifying agent such as ascorbic acid in amounts of 2 to 4 grams daily. At this acid pH, the methenamine component is hydrolyzed to formaldehyde, which has a direct bacteriocidal effect on both gram-negative and gram-positive organisms. Bacterial resistance cannot develop to formaldehyde, and when it fails to work it is usually because inadequate urinary acidification has been accomplished. It should be noted that this is not a particularly efficacious antimicrobial regimen for acute infection inasmuch as it is virtually impossible to acidify the urine in the presence of infection due to urea-splitting organisms. However, the maintenance of sterile urine in that state by the long-term use of one of these agents has occasionally produced gratifying results and patients can be kept on this regimen for 1 to 2 years or even longer with no untoward effects. The usual adult dosage of Mandelamine is 1 g four times per day and of Hiprex 1 g twice per day.

REFERENCES

Brugh R, Rous SN, Rosenblum R: Severe metabolic acidosis as a complication of intravenous tetracycline therapy. J Urol 117:395, 1977

Kostas C-I, Mobley DE, Rous SN, Schneider RE, Burt RAP: A multicenter double blind evaluation of two dosage schedules of cephalexin for the treatment of urinary tract infection in outpatients. Journal of Family Practice 17:135–140, 1983

Rous SN: Urology in Primary Care. St. Louis, Mosby, 1976

Rous SN: Cinoxacin in the treatment of acute urinary tract infections. J Urol 120:196, 1978

Rous SN: Bacterial infections of the urinary tract (male). In Conn HF (ed), Current Therapy, 32nd ed. Philadelphia, Saunders, 1980, pp 515–517

Rous SN: A comparison of cefaclor versus trimethoprim sulfamethoxazole combination in the treatment of acute urinary tract infections. J Urol 125:228, 1981

Rous SN: Bacterial urinary tract infection in males. In Edlich RF, Spyker DA (eds), Current Emergency Therapy—1985. Rockville, MD, Aspen Medical Publications, 1985

Stamey TA: Pathogenesis and Treatment of Urinary Tract Infections. Baltimore, Williams and Wilkins, 1980

Symposium on Antimicrobial Agents: Mayo Clin Proc 58:3, 1983

5
Pediatric Urology

EDUCATIONAL OBJECTIVES

1. Describe the "big bang" theory and explain the impact of this theory on the treatment of vesicoureteral reflux.
2. List the causes of enuresis.
3 Discuss the role of urodynamic studies in evaluating the enuretic child.
4. Discuss the management of functional enuresis.
5. Discuss the management of acute pyelonephritis in a girl and in a boy.
6. Discuss the management and therapy of chronic or recurrent pyelonephritis in a girl and in a boy.
7. Discuss the etiology of acute glomerulonephritis.
8. List the clinical symptoms occurring with acute glomerulonephritis.
9. List the physical and laboratory (urine and blood) findings of acute glomerulonephritis.
10. List the methods used in making a diagnosis of acute glomerulonephritis.
11. Discuss the short- and long-term management of acute glomerulonephritis.
12. Discuss the common causes of cystitis in little girls.
13. Describe the management of cystitis in little girls.
14. List the clinical symptoms associated with Wilms tumor.
15. List the most common causes of hematuria in children for the following age groups: neonates (first month of life); infants (1 month to 1 year of age); children (1 to 16 years of age).
16. Discuss the pros and cons of neonatal circumcision.
17. List the most common causes of abdominal masses in infants and children.
18. Describe what is meant by "a dysfunctional voider."

URINARY TRACT INFECTION AND INFLAMMATION

Introduction
In infants (less than 1 year of age), urinary tract infection is somewhat more prevalent in boys than in girls and it is related to such problems as congenital obstruction in the urinary tract, sepsis, and umbilical artery catheterizations and not usually to direct invasion of the urinary tract by bacteria. Nevertheless, upon urologic investigation, 75 percent of infants having urinary tract infection have been found to have vesicoureteral reflux. After 1 year of age far more girls than boys suffer from urinary tract infection; at any given point in time for any given community of girls (in the United States and Great Britain) between 1 and 2 percent have been found to have bacteriuria with or without symptoms of urinary tract infection. Between 13 and 30 percent of this 1 to 2 percent of girls already have renal scarring (secondary to vesicoureteral reflux) when they are first treated for the bacteriuria. In children of all ages, approximately 30 percent who have urinary tract infections are found to have vesicoureteral reflux when investigated.

Etiology of Urinary Tract Infections

Virtually all urinary tract infections in children (after the first year of life) result from fecal contamination, and the organisms causing the infection are normal inhabitants of the gastrointestinal tract. It is obvious that in children, feces and the resultant bacteria in the feces have frequent access to the perineum and the vaginal introitus (and therefore the urethra as well) because of the less than meticulous perineal hygiene maintained by most children, and it is equally obvious that the younger the child, the less meticulous the perineal hygiene! Nevertheless, only a distinct minority of female children actually contracts urinary tract infections and an even smaller minority contracts these infections on a recurring basis. There must be an explanation for the fact that while virtually all children at one time or another are exposed to fecal contamination and therefore to potential bacterial pathogens, only some children become infected.

Recent work strongly suggests that bacterial adherence to the vaginal introitus is one of the major reasons—and quite probably the single most important one. Simply stated, extensive studies have shown that the vaginal mucosa in children (and this applies to adult women as well) with recurrent urinary infections seems to allow more vigorous and extensive adherence of bacteria than that of normal children, thereby promoting and facilitating more frequent and numerically greater colonization by these bacteria. The vaginal introitus may represent the most important surface area in the pathogenesis of urinary tract infection in female subjects (adults as well as children) because colonization of this surface area has been experimentally shown to precede the development of bacteriuria, with the bacteria found on the vaginal epithelium proven to be the same organism subsequently responsible for the bacteriuria. Variations in the vaginal biology of female children (and adults) suffering from recurring urinary tract infections seem to allow for more vigorous adherence of bacteria, without any relation to the adhesive properties of the bacteria itself. These variations in the vaginal biology of affected children (and women as well) appear to be the predominant factors controlling bacterial adherence to the vaginal mucosa. Additional studies have suggested that the bacterial pili (fimbriae) play an important role in determining differences in bacterial adherence but it is most probable that variations in the receptiveness in the host vaginal epithelium remain the major factor in determining the extent of bacterial adherence in any given individual.

Vaginal secretory immunoglobulins have also been considered to be a factor in the prevention of bacterial colonization but their role is probably very secondary in the pathogenesis of urinary tract infections as compared with that of bacterial adherence.

Postvoiding residual urine is also responsible for urinary tract infections because residual urine in the bladder is either secondary to or soon leads to abnormalities in the bladder mucosa that render the bladder unable to defend itself against urinary tract infections; thus, residual urine does tend to ultimately lead to bladder infection. In children, residual urine is really only seen when there is congenital underlying disease producing severe obstruction or neurologic disease in the urinary tract. The underlying abnormality producing the residual urine must be corrected before the urinary tract infection can be prevented.

For many years it was thought that urethral stenosis predisposed girls (and women) to recurrent urinary tract infections, but it is likely that urethral stenosis, *unless it is so severe that it leads to residual urine*, is of little or no importance.

Symptoms of Lower Urinary Tract Infection

The female child is unique as regards lower urinary tract infections, both because of her anatomic predisposition to infection (due to her very short urethra and its proximity to the vaginal introitus) and the very real possibility of coexisting vesicoureteral reflux (see above). Bladder infections are therefore relatively common in girls and may present with episodes of involuntary loss of urine, frequency, foul-smelling urine, nighttime bedwetting (enuresis) in a previously trained child, occasional low abdominal pain, looking and acting "not quite right," and occasional involuntary loss of feces (encopresis). In the female child who is not yet toilet trained, the history or the complaints may simply be that the mother feels that the child is cranky or just "not being herself," although there are frequently no objective or subjective findings that indicate the presence of a bladder infection. It is fairly common, however, for little girls to "squat," particularly when they have marked urgency because the squatting position enables the child to dig her heel into her perineum thereby helping to retard the flow of urine. Little boys with urinary tract infections may have frequent "accidents," particularly during the sleeping hours, despite having previously been toilet trained. The child with a urinary tract infection also seems to need to void much more often than usual, and there may be a very short interval between his or her desire to void and an involuntary loss of urine (urgency and urgency incontinence). Some boys additionally have trouble with bowel control (encopresis) and others may simply be very cranky. If the male child has not yet obtained voluntary urine control, the symptoms may be more difficult to detect and may consist simply of foul-smelling urine (the ammonia odor resulting from the urea-splitting action of certain bacteria), low abdominal discomfort, or, again, just not feeling "quite right."

Symptoms of Upper Urinary Tract Infections

Acute pyelonephritis in children can be singularly confusing and may lead to diagnostic difficulties. Children the age of 10 years and under usually do not have pain specifically referable to the costovertebral angle but more characteristically, because of cross innervation by sympathetic nerve fibers, have symptoms suggestive of gastrointestinal tract disease. Abdominal pain, nausea, vomiting, and diarrhea are the typical symptoms of acute kidney infection in children and the younger the child the more the gastrointestinal tract symptoms predominate. These children usually also have a temperature elevation that may be as high as 105°F.

Undoubtedly, the majority of children who have lower urinary tract infections never develop acute pyelonephritis, although a significant number of children do indeed develop this additional problem secondary to vesicoureteral reflux (Fig. 5–1). This vesicoureteral reflux results from a structural abnormality at the vesicoureteral junction that allows urine free access from the bladder into the ureter and then into the kidney whereas, in normal children (and adults) it is not possible for urine to reflux from the bladder back up into the kidney. When there is no infection in the bladder, the reflux of sterile urine is generally considered to be a harmless phenomenon, and even the reflux of infected urine into the kidney is not always harmful as long as *intrarenal reflux* does not exist. This last named phenomenon allows the infected urine direct access into the renal parenchyma (from the renal collecting system where it would remain were there no intrarenal reflux) and leads to the renal scarring that is so often associated with vesicoureteral reflux and chronic pyelonephritis. Whether or not vesicoureteral reflux in a given individual will also

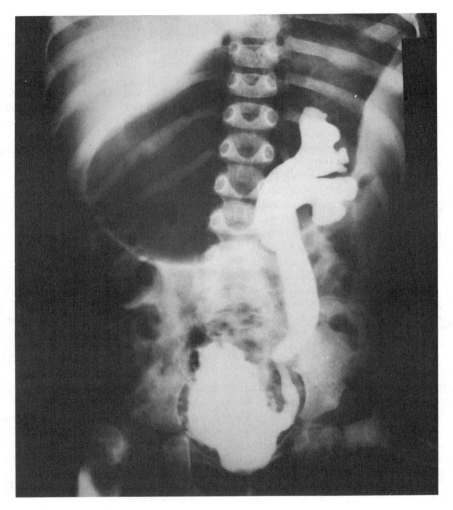

Figure 5–1. This is a retrograde cystourethrogram showing massive vesicoureteral reflux on the left, filling the entire ureter and renal collecting system and producing significant hydroureteronephrosis.

result in intrarenal reflux is determined by whether or not the kidney into which vesicoureteral reflux occurs has a normal or an abnormal configuration of one or more renal papillae. It is only the congenitally deficient renal papilla that allows vesicoureteral reflux to send urine directly into the renal parenchyma and that leads to the development of the so-called Big Bang Theory. This theory simply states that renal scarring will occur very rapidly in the face of vesicoureteral reflux of infected urine into a kidney with one or more deficient papillae so that intrarenal reflux follows the vesicoureteral reflux. This intrarenal reflux of infected urine with resultant parenchymal damage and ultimate scarring occurs rapidly—and probably on the very first occasion of vesicoureteral reflux of infected urine—so that there is little actually that can be done to prevent it. The theory also holds that vesicoureteral reflux is not particularly dangerous in the presence of perfectly normal renal papillae since intrarenal reflux cannot occur. This theory and its corollary are not necessarily accepted universally, and there are many who feel that reflux of infected urine, with or without normal papillae, is dangerous and may lead to scarring and therefore should not be allowed to occur. Most workers in the field, however, agree that vesicoureteral reflux of sterile urine (which is frequently never discovered because a urologic investigation is never precipitated) is relatively harmless assuming normal intravesical pressure. It is interesting to note that the renal "scarring" associated with pyelonephritis generally does not occur if the reflux of infected urine occurs after the child is 6 or 7 years or older because, to a large degree, renal growth has stopped by this age and continued growth of the kidney is necessary for visible (on x-ray) scarring to occur. This is because the scarring that is so characteristic of chronic pyelonephritis results from continued growth of the kidney around an area of scarring and fibrosis rather than retraction of a scarred or fibrotic area in the presence of a fully grown kidney.

Management of Urinary Tract Infection

In children afflicted with acute urinary tract infection, the diagnosis and management is not very much different than it is for the adults, with the exception of some very important diagnostic steps to determine whether or not the possibility of upper urinary tract damage exists because of vesicoureteral reflux. Little boys, like men, are rarely affected by acute bladder infection in the absence of any underlying pathology; therefore, a complete diagnostic workup is indicated after the first such infection. In addition to the excretory urogram with physiologic voiding films and retrograde cystourethrograms to look for vesicoureteral reflux, cystoscopy is probably indicated if any abnormalities of the lower urinary tract are seen on any x-ray studies. Proper management of the boy with bladder infection calls for treatment of the underlying entities that are found to be etiologic in the bladder infection and of course treatment of the infection itself.

As already pointed out, girls are affected with lower urinary tract infections far more frequently than boys, and because of this and the fact that these infections are often recurrent, it is absolutely essential to be certain that the lower urinary tract infections are not damaging the kidneys as a result of the presence of unilateral or bilateral vesicoureteral reflux. After their first lower urinary tract infection has been diagnosed, girls should have excretory urograms and retrograde cystourethrograms, both to evaluate the upper tracts and to establish whether or not vesicoureteral reflux exists. Ideally, the voiding cystourethrogram should be done under fluoroscopy because vesicoureteral reflux is sometimes only transiently present, and it may only be seen on fluoroscopy and not actually noted at the time that the spot x-ray films are taken. Vesicoureteral reflux alone does not warrant surgical correction of this condition, but it should serve as a red flag to the clinician that the particular child in question is at definite risk for upper urinary tract damage should lower urinary tract infections continue. Based on the "Big Bang" theory it is certainly possible that all of the damage to the kidney that might result in the presence of vesicoureteral reflux would have already been caused by the very first infection. This is not a universally accepted viewpoint, however, and it is therefore prudent to try to prevent further infections of the lower urinary tract in order to minimize damage to the upper urinary tract in refluxing children. If the diagnostic studies as outlined disclose entirely normal upper urinary tracts in the presence of vesicoureteral reflux, the child must be followed meticulously for an indefinite period of time, or until reflux ceases spontaneously, and should be maintained on prophylactic antimicrobial therapy so that the upper urinary tract is not put at risk by the presence of lower urinary tract infections. This prophylactic antimicrobial therapy can be with sulfasoxazole (Gantrisin), nitrofurantoin (Macrodantin), or one of the cephalosporins and generally consists of daily, or every other day, administration of between one fourth and one half the usual therapeutic dose of a given antimicrobial. This should be done in addition to making every effort to improve the perineal hygiene, teaching the child to clean herself from the front to the back following bowel movements, and, ideally, to keep the skin of the perineum properly cleansed by daily showers, which should preferably be taken after the bowel movement. While on antimicrobial therapy, the child should have a urine culture done every couple of months to be certain that a "silent" breakthrough and infection has not occurred. Careful monitoring of these children is necessary for an indefinite period of time, or until vesicoureteral reflux ceases spontaneously, which it does better than 80 percent of the time, usually by puberty, in those patients with normal upper urinary tracts as seen roentgenographically. If it is not possible to maintain the child's urine in a sterile status on antimicrobial therapy, then serious consideration should be given to surgical reimplantation of the ureter to prevent further vesicoureteral reflux. Although this surgery will clearly not have any effect on the recurrent lower urinary tract infections, it will prevent the reflux of infected urine into the kidneys.

If the diagnostic workup in these children with recurrent lower urinary tract infections reveals that there are already pyelonephritic changes or if there is significant dilatation of the ureter or even of the kidney, the odds are greater that these children will eventually come to reimplantation of the ureterovesical junction because spontaneous cessation of reflux is much less likely to occur in patients with dilated ureters. Also, x-ray evidence of upper tract damage is often a strong stimulus to intervene surgically to prevent additional damage, although it is highly unlikely that any damage that has occurred will resolve, regardless of the therapeutic modality chosen.

ACUTE GLOMERULONEPHRITIS

Acute glomerulonephritis is unquestionably the most common cause of hematuria (both gross and microscopic) in children between the ages of 6 and 18, and post-streptococcal glomerulonephritis is far and away the most common type of glomerulonephritis. There may sometimes be a history of an acute upper respiratory tract infection which classically involves a streptococcal infection of the throat or skin. At physical exam, the child may have a generalized edema or only a periorbital edema, with the latter either transient or persistent. Overall, the child may fit anywhere on a disease spectrum from perfectly healthy to acutely ill because of elevated blood pressure, renal failure, or anemia.

The etiology of acute glomerulonephritis in the majority of cases is thought to be one of the streptococcal organisms, often type 12 or 14, which cause infections of the throat or skin (it is not unusual, however, for infections with organisms other than streptococcus to ultimately lead to glomerulonephritis). Acute glomerulonephritis usually follows the streptococcal infection by several days. It is of particular importance to note that development of acute glomerulonephritis as a sequella to the initial streptococcal infection is apparently unrelated to the proper or improper treatment of the infection when it first occurs. In other words, whether glomerulonephritis develops is dependent on the offending organism and the virulence of that organism and is unrelated to the promptness or the excellence of the treatment of the initial infection. This is because once the invading organism has entered the body in sufficient numbers, and particularly in a sufficently virulent form, glomerulonephritis has already been established and it is too late for it to be aborted by any treatment.

Glomerulonephritis is thought by some to be an immune type of reaction that is in some way linked to the presence of the initial streptococcal (or other organism) infection; a subsequent streptococcal infection is not necessary for acute glomerulonephritis to result. In fact, the exact nature of the reaction causing glomerulonephritis is poorly understood and has been a subject of intense debate for many years. It is interesting to note that neither bacteria nor any toxins produced by bacteria have ever been isolated or identified from glomeruli affected by this condition.

In mild cases, there may be nothing more than microscopic or perhaps gross hematuria, and it must constantly be kept in mind that either of these findings in children should lead the clinician to suspect acute glomerulonephritis as the first and foremost etiology. In more severely ill patients, there may be edema (periorbital or generalized), elevated blood pressure, pallor that is secondary to anemia, and possibly findings compatible with renal failure. Laboratory findings inevitably include the previously mentioned hematuria, red blood cell casts in the urine (virtually always present), and proteinuria. There may also be a decreased creatinine clearance and an elevated serum creatinine level. Critical factors in establishing diagnosis of acute glomerulonephritis are depressed serum complement levels (C_3 and C_4); these usually return to normal within 6 weeks or so. Persistent depression of these levels beyond 6 weeks should suggest a membranoproliferative type of glomerulitis, which is much more serious, and a renal biopsy for prognostic purposes is usually then indicated. In addition to the depressed serum complement levels (which are not specific for poststreptococcal glomerulonephritis but rather indicate *any* kind of glomerulonephritis), the ASO titer will be elevated if the disease is poststreptococcal, as will the antihyaluronidase and anti-DNase B titers. Additionally, hyperkalemia may be present. Roentgenographic findings of acute glomerulonephritis are not diagnostic and normal excretory urograms are the rule. In chronic glomerulonephritis that has progressed to the point of end-stage renal disease, the kidneys as seen on excretory urography may be rather small, but there will be normal collecting systems.

It must be emphasized that although acute glomerulonephritis is most commonly seen in children, it can exist in adults and it must always be considered in the differential diagnosis of hematuria with and without proteinuria. On rare occasions, hypertension may be the only physical finding and it may or may not be accompanied by headaches or vomiting. Rarely, there may actually be a complete absence of any kind of hematuria and the urine sediment may be completely normal. Better than 95 percent of cases of acute glomerulonephritis are poststreptococcal and the clinician is thus justified in assuming this to be etiologic, but it must always be remembered that other organisms may produce this condition.

Renal biopsy is rarely indicated for confirmation of the diagnosis. It is, however, indicated in patients who have persistent hematuria for 6 months or more or in patients in whom the C_3 and C_4 levels do not return to normal in 6 weeks. It may also be indicated in patients for whom progressive deterioration continues. The reason for the biopsy is to determine whether or not a membranoproliferative type of glomerulitis exists because these are far more serious and carry a far graver prognosis than the more common and typical type of glomerulitis. Where unusual types of glomerulitis are suspected, immunofluorescent techniques may be necessary for a definitive diagnosis and renal biopsy may also be indicated for this reason.

The management of acute glomerulonephritis may be divided into a short- and a long-term aspect. The critical factor in the short-term management of this condition is the patient's blood pressure when he or she is first seen. If it is normal and there is no edema present, bed rest is probably not necessary. It must be stressed, however, that such individuals must be carefully watched because blood pressure elevation can be very rapid. Accordingly, these patients should probably have their blood pressure checked two or three times per week until recovery is underway. If blood pressure is normal when the patient is first seen but edema of any sort is present, it is likely that blood pressure may rapidly rise; therefore, it is advisable that such patients have bed rest until it is reasonably certain that there will not be any blood pressure elevation.

If blood pressure is elevated when a patient is first seen, bed rest is strongly recommended, even in the absence of edema, and should continue until blood pressure is normal and edema, if present, has subsided. During this time, the patient should have a restricted sodium and fluid diet and should be weighed daily. Blood pressure elevation may be treated with reserpine and hydralazine hydrochloride (Apresoline), which may be given intravenously, or a more potent antihypertensive drug may be used when there is severe blood pressure elevation. Patients ill enough to require bed rest and careful monitoring must be closely watched for any signs of renal failure, which must be treated immediately. The short-term management of acute glomerulonephritis may involve anywhere from a few days to many weeks, depending on the course of the disease in a given patient.

Long-term management of the patient with acute glomerulonephritis mainly involves careful follow-up of the individual. Gross or microscopic hematuria, usually the latter, may persist without proteinuria and microscopic hematuria may persist for up to 1 year even though healing has occurred. If both hematuria and proteinuria persist, the prognosis is much more severe. The patient's blood pressure must be watched carefully for several years after the original illness. The vast majority of patients suffering from acute poststreptococcal glomerulonephritis recover completely.

Steroid therapy is not necessary in either short- or long-term management of glomerulonephritis. The only one of the glomerulonephritides where steroid therapy is specifically indicated involves the relatively rare case of lupus nephritis. In the long-term management of acute glomerulonephritis, renal biopsy may occasionally be necessary to confirm the type of nephritis existing, as noted above. The patient suffering from acute glomerulonephritis may actually feel quite well and the physician may find it difficult to convince the patient and the parents that bed rest is the treatment of choice in certain cases. Most important in the management of these patients, however, is the necessity for the physician to be certain that appropriate long-term follow-up is obtained even when the patient and his or her family see no reason for this.

HEMATURIA

Hematuria in children is not common and it is helpful to the clinician to note that there are very specific conditions that are most likely to be causative of hematuria (gross or microscopic) whenever it does exist. In neonates, hematuria is extremely rare, but when it does occur, one third of the cases are idiopathic and all of these seem to do well. The other two thirds are either due to renal artery thrombosis, renal vein thrombosis, polycystic kidney disease, or obstructive uropathy with secondary infection. If meatitis is discounted, hematuria is extremely rare in children from 1 month to 1 year of age. Meatitis is seen not infrequently in circumsized children and it is secondary to prolonged contact of the unprotected glans penis with a urine-soaked diaper (ammoniacal dermatitis). Meatitis usually becomes evident from small amounts of blood on the diaper and it could not be called a true hematuria. In patients aged 1 to 16 years, the two most common causes of hematuria are glomerulonephritis and lower urinary tract infection. It is not very difficult to differentiate between them because lower urinary tract infections are invariably accompanied by symptoms of lower urinary tract inflammation. Whether or not acute glomerulonephritis is the most common overall cause of gross or microscopic hematuria in children is a moot point. It is certainly the most common cause of hematuria of upper urinary tract origin, as well as the most common cause of hematuria in both the otherwise asymptomatic child and the child who may have symptoms that are otherwise quite unrelated to the urinary tract itself. It is common enough that the author, given a child with hematuria and no other symptoms, will first consider and rule out acute glomerulonephritis before even considering an excretory urogram or cystoscopy.

Another cause for hematuria, which is found in teenage boys, is an acutely inflamed posterior urethra secondary to very frequent and repeated masturbation over a prolonged period of time. The posterior urethra becomes acutely inflamed secondary to the spasmodic contractions associated with orgasm and ejaculation and on cystoscopic examination the area looks very much like a piece of raw hamburger.

ABDOMINAL MASSES

Abnormalities of the kidney are probably the most common cause of abdominal masses in infants and probably in children as well; certainly abnormalities of the kidney are the most common cause of flank masses. Of these abnormalities ureteropelvic junction obstructions are the most common kidney lesions causing abdominal or flank masses, with multicystic dysplastic kidneys and Wilms tumors probably the next likeliest renal causes of such masses. Ureteropelvic junction obstruction, if unilateral, often produces very few symptoms and it is not at all unusual for these lesions to be diagnosed in infants only because of the mass produced by the lesion (and not because of any specific symptoms) and in older children and adults only because of an excretory urogram that was performed in the course of a workup for pyuria, hematuria, or infection, which may or may not have been related to the ureteropelvic juncture obstruction itself.

In some children, a borderline ureteropelvic junction permits adequate passage of fluid from the kidney to the bladder except when the junction is faced with an unusually large quantity of fluid, such as occurs during a brisk diuresis. The additional fluid load cannot pass the borderline ureteropelvic junction, resulting in a hydronephrosis with flank pain. There is invariably a complete resolution of the hydronephrosis and the pain when the diuresis has ceased (the so-called beer drinkers syndrome).

Multicystic dysplastic kidneys are characteristically nonfunctioning and asymptomatic (assuming a normal kidney on the contralateral side) and are generally only diagnosed because of the observed abdominal mass. Wilms tumor is the most common solid cancer found in children and usually occurs in children between 1 and 5 years old; it is extremely rare after the age of 8. It comprises about 5 percent of all renal cancers and about 500 new cases of Wilms tumor are reported each year in the United States. The tumor is most probably congenital in origin and there is moderately strong supporting evidence to back up the thesis that it develops from the metanephric blastema cells between the 8th and 34th weeks of gestation. The symptoms produced by Wilms tumor are virtually nil and this may well be because the afflicted children are too young to verbalize their complaints coherently. Hematuria, if present at all, is a very late finding since the disease is parenchymal and usually does not break into the collecting system to produce hematuria. The lesion is most commonly discovered by the pediatrician during a routine physical examination when an abdominal mass is palpated or by the child's mother who may notice an abdominal mass when she is bathing, changing, or dressing the child. Excretory urography is called for immediately on discovery of any abdominal mass and the diagnosis of Wilms tumor may often be made based on the urogram alone. A marked distortion of the collecting system and the greatly enlarged renal outline are the criteria for the diagnosis, which should be followed by ultrasound for diagnostic certainty. Occasionally, CT scans are also helpful in establishing the diagnosis. During the very brief interval between presumptive diagnosis of Wilms tumor and surgery, various staging procedures are carried out, such as chest x-ray, liver function tests, and peripheral hemogram. Radical nephrectomy is the treatment of choice and any palpable lymph nodes in the region of the renal pedicle and the adjacent great vessels should be removed. If the tumor has been totally confined within the renal capsule and completely excised, no radiation is given, but chemotherapy consisting of Vincristine and Actinomycin D is recommended. For advanced stages of carcinoma in which it is not felt that all of the cancer has been removed, treatment with radiation therapy is used in addition to the chemotherapy. Actinomycin D is probably the most efficacious drug but it is even more effective when given in combination with Vincristine. Both of these medications act directly on the the tumor cells; Actinomycin D binds to DNA to block RNA production, disorganizes and disrupts the cells, and thereby prevents protein synthesis; Vincristine destroys the mitotic spindle, thus producing mitotic arrest. These medications are given intravenously on a weight-related dosage schedule and are continued on an intermittent schedule for 15 months to 2 years following nephrectomy.

The survival, or "cure rate," for children with Wilms tumor depends primarily on the stage of the tumor at the time of initial therapy and on the age of the child. Inasmuch as this is considered to be a congenital lesion, it is readily understandable that the older the child, the longer the tumor has presumably been present and the worse the prognosis. The cure rate for stages 1, 2, and 3 for children under 2 years of age is better than 90 percent. Where more distant metastases are present at the time of diagnosis (stage 4) the cure rate is nearer to 50 percent.

VOIDING PROBLEMS (DYSFUNCTIONAL VOIDING)

If defined strictly, dysfunctional voiding would refer to any type of abnormal voiding, but it is most commonly limited to those causes of abnormal voiding in which the nervous system, as it relates to the act of voiding, is perfectly normal. When looked at in its simplest terms, the detrusor (bladder) is a smooth muscle organ that is innervated by the autonomic nervous system and it has two basic functions: to store urine and to evacuate urine. The dysfunctional voider fails either to store or evacuate urine adequately, and this may be due to a variety of nonneurologic factors. There are two urinary sphincters—the internal sphincter, which is composed of smooth muscle and is actually a part of the detrusor itself, and the external sphincter, which is composed of skeletal muscle. Abnormal function of either or both of these may also lead to dysfunctional voiding.

Urodynamics are tests (see Chapter 1) that are used to quantitate the act of voiding and to measure urine storage, urine evacuation, and the function of the two urinary sphincters in a manner that enables the physician to determine the specific problem that is leading to the dysfunctional voiding. If the specific problem can be accurately identified, it can often be successfully treated pharmacologically (see below) or, alternatively, it can be treated with intermittent catheterization, surgery, or psychologic consultation.

Although dysfunctional voiders are not common, they may often be recognized by "bizarre" findings that cannot be satisfactorily explained by any other means. For example, when the detrusor contracts normally the sphincters should relax, thereby permitting bladder emptying in an efficient manner. Failure of either or both sphincters to relax leads to a poor urinary stream, incomplete bladder emptying, and, frequently, recurrent infection. By means of urodynamic studies, a "detrusor–sphincter dyssynergia" may be discovered, and this can often be treated successfully. Diurnal enuresis, for another example, usually signifies increased bladder irritability, with difficulty in retaining urine. These are often the children classically known as "squatters" because they characteristically assume a squatting position so that the heel can dig into the perineum and act as a compressor of the urethra to help the child to avoid wetting herself. In little boys, grasping the penis and squeezing it has a similar purpose and a similar effect.

Perhaps the most common of this unusual and mixed bag of voiding problems is nocturnal enuresis, the etiology of which is often obscure but which nevertheless fulfills the criteria of "the dysfunctional voider" in that it is a problem of urine storage (or the lack of same) in the face of an apparently normal bladder innervation. Nocturnal enuresis may be considered to be both primary and secondary, with the former pertaining to those children who have never been able to sleep through the night without bed wetting, and the latter referring to those children who have been previously trained and then became bed wetters. Both primary and secondary enuretics may fulfill the criteria of "dysfunctional voider," although the secondary bed wetter group is also often related to a problem of infection or obstruction somewhere in the urinary tract or to psychologic trauma such as the birth of a new sibling. It is the primary group of enuretics, however, that fall under the catch-all heading of dysfunctional voiders and it is this group of patients that is most often helped by pharmacologic manipulation to promote bladder storage, diminish bladder irritability, and the like.

At the very least, the enuretic child should always have a urine culture; if this is negative it is very unlikely that significant urinary tract disease is causing the enuresis. If there is a question about any abnormality in the urinary tract, an excretory urogram with physiologic voiding films should be done. The absence of any abnormalities on these films rules out an organic urinary tract lesion as the cause of the enuresis. It should also be noted that if there are no symptoms at all of daytime voiding problems the odds are very high that there is no organic urinary tract lesion present. Bed wetting tends to be a familial problem (much more commonly seen in boys) and careful questioning of the distraught mother often reveals that the child's father (or mother) or other siblings or close relatives have had this problem, which is most often nothing more serious than a delay in maturation of the nervous system. This delay manifests itself by uninhibited bladder contractions (an "irritable" bladder), which almost always ceases spontaneously, usually before the child reaches the age 6 or 8 but sometimes much later. The principle of therapy is to "tide the child" over until his bed wetting ceases spontaneously, and the author has found the best means to do this is with the oral medication, Ditropan, which decreases the bladder "irritability," thus minimizing the uninhibited contractions. If Ditropan does not achieve the desired result, the author uses imipramine (Tofranil), which has the same action on the bladder as Ditropan and additionally tends to prevent too deep a level of sleep. If neither medication seems to work, another excellent alternative is a nocturnal alarm system in which the first few drops of urine waken the child so that he finishes voiding in the bathroom.

Pharmacologic drugs that alter the contractility of the bladder include the following: the cholinergic family of drugs, which stimulate bladder muscle contraction, an example of which is bethanechol chloride (Urecholine); the anticholinergics, which decrease the contractility of the bladder muscle, examples of which would be atropine and probanthine; and the musculotropic drugs, which seem to block the muscle function at the muscle fiber level, an example of which is oxybutynin (Ditropan). Additionally, diazepam (Valium) is commonly used to relax skeletal muscle and dibenzylene is often used to relax smooth muscle, particularly of the bladder neck and urethra. A drug that has the opposite effect of dibenzylene is ephedrine, which brings about a contraction of the α-adrenergic fibers that innervate the bladder neck and urethra. Use of one or more of these drugs, in properly selected patients who have dysfunctional voiding, can bring about striking improvement in a given set of symptoms.

Undeniably, the entire concept of "dysfunctional voiding" may be difficult to comprehend, and, happily, relatively few children are afflicted. However, there are children who appear to have an intact nerve supply to the bladder, the urethra, and the sphincters, but who nevertheless have voiding problems that are distressing or may even have serious urinary tract complications, such as huge residual urine amounts, or dilatation and damage to the upper urinary tracts. Also, as already mentioned, primary enuretics may be considered to be a type of dysfunctional voider. The important thing to realize from the foregoing is that these problems, though they may be uncommon, are real and do exist, and they exist in the *absence* of underlying neurologic disease. They may be much better understood by means of the various urodynamic studies that are available to the clinician, and successful results are often achieved using one of the therapeutic modalities mentioned.

EXTERNAL GENITALIA

One of the very commonly occurring problems in pediatric urology is whether or not a newborn should be circumsized. The arguments for circumcision (excluding religious ones) have always been that it prevents penile cancer and it facilitates penile cleanliness. There is no question that both of these statements are true, but, in the author's opinion, neither is a sufficiently good reason for routine newborn circumcision. Penile cancer is extraordinarily uncommon and accounts for barely 0.1 percent of all cancers in males and it is almost exclusively seen in the lower socioeconomic groups, where it is associated with poor penile hygiene and specifically with chronic infection and recurrent balanitis and balanoposthitis. It is very rarely, if ever, seen in individuals who practice retraction of the foreskin on a daily basis with thorough cleansing of the penis and the maintenance of penile hygiene. Unquestionably, for those individuals unwilling or unable to practice proper penile hygiene circumcision is indicated but it is doubtful if universal mass and routine newborn circumcision is indicated to prevent complications later in life in those few individuals unable to maintain proper hygiene, and it is equally doubtful that widespread newborn circumcision can be justified to prevent penile carcinoma in those few individuals who would otherwise contract it. Having mentioned the foregoing to indicate why routine circumcision is not *necessary*, the author would also point out specific reasons *against* routine neonatal circumcision. First, both accidental denuding of the penile shaft as well as serious thermal burns of the penile shaft are complications that occur more than rarely, and both of these misfortunes necessitate corrective plastic surgery, which is not always perfectly successful. Second, and probably the most common complication of circumcision, is the meatal stenosis that ultimately results in a fair number of individuals, and this is secondary to the meatitis that results because the unprotected (without the removed foreskin) glans penis (and meatus) is exposed to a continuously wet diaper, with a resulting inflammation of the meatus. The meatitis usually heals with a resulting meatal stenosis and this may or may not require a meatotomy. Third, there is considerable additional cost to the parents or to third-party insurance carriers resulting from the required additional hospitalization of the infant (and sometimes the mother as well) since circumcision is done on the fourth day postpartum, and mother and child might otherwise leave the hospital on the second or third postpartum day.

In summation, the author feels that neonatal circumcision should certainly not be denied to any mother requesting it and no attempt should be made to dissuade her from this if it is her intent; however, neonatal circumcision should *not* be carried out unless the mother specifically *does* request it. In this manner, a lot of needless surgery with its resultant expense and potential complications can be avoided.

UNDESCENDED TESTICLES (CRYPTORCHIDISM)

The incidence of an undescended testis is variable and in full-term infants it is probably between 2 and 3 percent. It is somewhat higher in premature infants. By 1 year of age the incidence is well under 1 percent because most testes, if they are going to descend normally, have done so by the end of the first year of the child's life. When a testis is undescended it does not ultimately undergo normal spermatogenesis even though it continues to make testosterone normally. For this reason, it is generally felt that the undescended testicle should be brought down as soon as possible (after the first year of life) and certainly before the start of school where the less than normally endowed child might be the subject of considerable teasing at the hands of his classmates. Ideally, surgery to bring down an undescended testis should be done to children when they are between 2 and 4 years of age and it is possibly worth a try at hormonal stimulation (with exogenous human chorionic gonadotropin) to cause spontaneous descent of the testis. In the author's experience, this is virtually never successful with unilateral incomplete descent of a testis because the presence of one intrascrotal testis pretty well precludes the possibility that inadequate hormonal stimulation was responsible for incomplete descent of the other testis. In the case of bilaterally undescended testes, hormonal therapy is very definitely indicated and is successful about one third of the time. It is important for the clinician to differentiate the true undescended testis from the *retractile* testis, which is notoriously difficult to find at the time of a physical examination but is, in fact, normally descended, very mobile, and frequently retracted into the upper reaches of the scrotum or even the area proximal to the external inguinal ring. Retractile testes do not require surgical correction. Perhaps the major reason for bringing down the true undescended testis, in addition to improving and increasing spermatogenesis, is the fact that the undescended testis has a greatly increased chance of undergoing malignant degeneration. Even though delivering it into its normal position in the scrotum does not alter this increased tendency for malignant degeneration it does make the testis more readily available to palpation by the patient and his physician, which helps in the detection of any developing malignancy at a very early stage.

When bilateral undescended testes are present, particularly in the presence of any degree of hypospadias, the possibility of an intersex problem must always be considered and consultation obtained.

VALVES OF THE PROSTATIC URETHRA

The neonate presenting with a low, midline abdominal mass probably has a distended bladder, as this is the most common cause of such abdominal masses in children (and in adults as well). The etiology of the bladder distension may well be obstructing valves within the prostatic urethra, a condition that in its most severe forms leads to a stillborn child secondary to obstruction of the bladder and upper urinary tract with resulting renal failure. In most patients with prostatic urethral valve disease, endoscopic destruction of the urethral valves ultimately leads to a normal urinary tract. This condition may be diagnosed on retrograde voiding cystourethrography and the obstructing valves can be seen and actually destroyed cystoscopically. If the diagnosis is made in neonates, cystoscopy may be deferred until the child is somewhat older because of the very considerable risk of producing permanent urethral stricture disease by passing a cystoscope into a urethra that is too small to accomodate it readily. If cytoscopy is deferred and the urethra severely obstructed due to these valves, temporary diversion of the urine by making a communication between the bladder and the skin (cutaneous vesicostomy) is usually done.

HYPOSPADIAS, CHORDEE WITH HYPOSPADIAS, AND EPISPADIAS

These congenital anomalies are beyond the purview of this text. It is pointed out that these are all congenital conditions in which neonatal circumcision is contraindicated because the foreskin must be preserved for its future role in the reparative surgery of these conditions.

Epididymitis, Epididymoorchitis, Orchitis, Torsion of the Spermatic Cord, Torsion of the Testicular Appendages, Varicocele, Hematocele, Hydrocele, and Testis Cancer

All of these conditions are discussed fully in Chapter 11.

REFERENCES

Gruskin AB: Pediatric nephrology for the urologist. In Kendall AR, Karafin L (eds), Urology. Philadelphia, Harper and Row, 1977, vol 1, chap 23

Haddy, TB, Bailie MD, Bernstein J, Kaufman DB, Rous SN: Bilateral, diffuse nephroblastomatosis: Report of a case managed with chemotherapy. J Pediatr 90:784, 1977

Hodgson NB, Durkee CT: Urinary tract infections in childhood. In Kendall AR, Karafin L (eds), Urology. Philadelphia, Harper and Row, 1982, vol 1, chap 21

Johnston JH, Williams DI (eds): Pediatric Urology, 2nd ed. London, Butterworths, 1983

Kelalis PP, King LR, Belman AB: Clinical Pediatric Urology, 2nd ed. Philadelphia, Saunders, 1984

Rous SN, Bailie MD, Kaufman DB: Hereditary nephritis—A poorly known entity. Urology 5:377, 1975

Rous SN, Bailie MD, Kaufman DB, Haddy TB, Mattson JC: Nodular renal blastema, nephroblastomatosis and Wilms' tumor—Different points on the same disease spectrum? Urology 8:599, 1976

Stamey TA: Pathogenesis and Treatment of Urinary Tract Infections. Baltimore, Williams and Wilkins, 1980

Turner WR Jr: Urinary tract infections in children. J S Car Med Assoc 78:658, 1982

6
Malignant Neoplasms of the Genitourinary Tract

EDUCATIONAL OBJECTIVES

1. List the clinical symptoms associated with hypernephroma.
2. List the symptoms of bladder cancer.
3. List a differential diagnosis for hard areas of the prostate gland as noted on rectal palpation.
4. List the symptoms of early carcinoma of the prostate gland.
5. List the causes of scrotal mass.
6. Discuss the management and prognosis of hypernephroma.
7. Discuss the relationship of estrogen and testosterone in carcinoma of the prostate gland.
8. List the late symptoms of carcinoma of the prostate gland.
9. Discuss the hormonal treatment of carcinoma of the prostate gland.
10. Palpate a significantly enlarged lower pole of a kidney.
11. Palpate a prostate gland that has hard nodular areas suggestive of carcinoma and identify it as such.
12. Palpate a prostate gland that is diffusely hard, as in carcinoma, and identify it as such.
13. Describe the diagnosis and management of carcinoma of the bladder.
14. List the symptoms of carcinoma of the testis.
15. Describe the diagnosis and management of carcinoma of the testis.
16. Discuss with a patient and his family the implications of surgery for carcinoma of the prostate gland, necessitating orchiectomy and treatment with Stilbestrol.

CANCER OF THE PROSTATE GLAND

The second leading cause of cancer death in men over 75 and the third leading cause of cancer death in men in the 55- to 74-age group, prostate cancer accounts for approximately 76,000 new cases in the United States annually with an estimated 25,000 deaths each year. It is also, on an overall basis for all age groups, the third leading cause of cancer deaths in men (behind lung and colon and rectal cancer). Overall, 10 percent of all cancer deaths in men are of prostatic origin. The overwhelming preponderance of prostate cancer is adenocarcinoma and its cause or causes are not known. In the vast majority of cases the carcinoma originates as one or more collections of malignant cells in the outer portion of the gland beneath the true capsule. These malignant cells then spread in any one or more of four ways: they may expand into a discreet and palpable nodule, penetrate through the fibers or true capsule, invade into the stroma or true tissue of the prostate gland, or me-

137

tastasize to parts of the body removed from the prostate gland itself. The age-adjusted death rate secondary to prostate cancer has remained fairly constant for the past 45 years and it is somewhere around 20 per 100,000 male population. However, it should be noted that the relative 5-year survival for this particular malignancy has increased significantly since 1960 when it was 50 percent for whites and 35 percent for blacks. It now approaches 70 percent for whites and 60 percent for blacks. This increase of the 5-year survival is not incompatible with the unchanged age-adjusted death rate for prostate cancer over the past 40 years and it probably represents earlier diagnosis and earlier treatment for this lethal condition.

Early Symptoms

There are no symptoms of early carcinoma of the prostate gland! If metastases occur very early in the course of the disease (in which case the term "early" would no longer be applicable), there might be pain at the site of the metastatic deposit. Symptoms of bladder outlet obstruction might result when and if the prostatic carcinoma invades from the periphery through the stroma of the prostate gland and into the lumen of the prostatic urethra so that the bladder outflow tract is obstructed. This is not at all common, however, and it is far more likely that bladder outlet obstruction in a patient known to have prostatic carcinoma is caused by coexisting benign prostatic hyperplasia insofar as the peak incidence of both conditions is in men of the same age group, which is over 60 years. Very uncommonly, prostatic carcinoma can arise deep within the "inner" portion of the prostate gland, in which case symptoms of bladder outlet obstruction can occur relatively early in the course of the disease. The unfortunate fact remains, however, that there simply are no symptoms of early carcinoma of the prostate in the vast majority of patients afflicted with this disease.

Late Symptoms

The late symptoms of carcinoma of the prostate gland are those of metastatic disease. This tumor spreads through lymphatic as well as venous channels, with a particular affinity for retroperitoneal lymph nodes of the obturator, and the external and internal iliac chains and also for the bony structures of the lower spine, pelvis, and proximal femurs. Lymph node involvement does not generally produce any symptoms but bone pain secondary to metastatic tumor is a very common late finding in this condition and its presence and persistence in an otherwise asymptomatic man should suggest metastatic cancer of the prostate gland as the cause. Very uncommonly, gross hematuria may be a symptom of late prostatic carcinoma if malignant invasion of the prostatic urethra has occurred. It is important to note that prostatic carcinoma as a cause of gross hematuria should be ranked low in any differential list of causes of hematuria, and particularly should be listed well behind the two leading causes of gross hematuria in men over 50, which are benign prostatic hyperplasia and bladder cancer. When bladder outlet obstruction does occur in the patient known to have advanced carcinoma of the prostate it is far more commonly caused by benign prostatic hyperplasia with or without coexisting carcinoma than by carcinoma alone. Finally, it should be noted that advanced carcinoma of the prostate gland not infrequently results in ureteral obstruction, either bilateral or unilateral, by direct extention of the tumor. If bilateral, it can produce uremia and electrolyte imbalance with resultant symptoms of weakness, lassitude, anorexia, vomiting, and even coma or death.

Diagnosis by Digital Rectal Examination

The digital rectal examination of the prostate gland remains the very best way to diagnose prostatic carcinoma in an early enough stage to permit possible curative surgery. This examination should be carried out annually in every man over age 40. The physician should carefully palpate the entire surface of the prostate gland, searching for areas that feel harder than other areas—findings that should immediately raise suspicions of prostatic carcinoma. Palpation of the bony prominence found at the base of the physician's thumb if the fist is tightly clenched should give a rough idea of the palpatory findings of prostatic carcinoma. Characteristically, these hardened areas take the form of nodules, but it is not at all unusual to find a large segment of one lobe, an entire lateral lobe, and sometimes even the entire gland rock hard; such an extensive spread of areas of hardness generally suggests advanced prostatic carcinoma. The differential diagnoses of such hard areas of the prostate gland—nodular or diffuse—are prostatic calculi, granulomatous prostatitis, tuberculosis, syphilitic gumma, or even benign adenomata of the prostate gland. It must be stressed, however, that hard areas within the prostate gland, nodular or otherwise, must be considered as carcinoma until proven otherwise.

Diagnosis by Prostatic Biopsy

When an area of the prostate that has been palpated is suspected of being carcinomatous or even felt to be slightly suspicious of carcinoma, biopsy should be carried out promptly. It can be performed with a traditional biopsy needle either by the transrectal or transperineal route or using the new technique, in which a "skinny needle" is used to obtain a prostatic aspirate for histologic study. The latter is obviously the simplest and the most comfortable one for the patient, but the risk of missing a very well-differentiated cancer is real, inasmuch as prostate cancer is diagnosed on the architectural pattern of the tumor as well as on the cellular architecture and the needle aspiration technique *only* provides aspirated cells for histologic examination, so that examination of the overall architecture is not possible. Prostatic biopsy using the skinny needle technique is done on an outpatient basis whereas biopsy using the transrectal or transperineal route is done on either an inpatient or an outpatient basis depending on the wishes of the patient himself and on the practice habits of the physician. Regardless of how the biopsy is carried out, the important point to be remembered is that some sort of prostatic biopsy is an absolute must in any patient felt to have a gland "suspicious" of adenocarcinoma based on digital rectal examination. Biopsy is also a must before any sort of definitive therapy can be undertaken, even in the patient whose prostate gland is "classic" for carcinoma.

Diagnosis by Laboratory, X-Ray, and Radionucleide Tests

Blood alkaline and acid phosphatase levels should be determined in individuals in whom the diagnosis of prostatic carcinoma is being considered. In recent years, newer radioimmunoassays, which are less likely to have false negatives and which are more specific for a prostatic origin of the acid phosphatase when the values are elevated, showed promise of greatly improving the sensitivity and specificity of acid phosphatase determinations. However, as these newer tests have been used extensively in clinical practice, it now appears that their sensitivity is not nearly as great as had initially been hoped, so that they are not absolutely satisfactory as "screening" tests for patients with prostatic cancer in its early stages. Furthermore, these tests have been found to have very worrisome, but false, elevations simply secondary to a signifcant mass of benign prostatic hyperplasia. The bottom line, therefore, appears to be that these newer radioimmunoassays offer very little over the old enzymatic assay method as far as diagnosing cancer of the prostate that is still confined within the prostate gland. It is probably best that blood samples for acid phosphatase not be drawn for at least 24 hours after digital rectal examination is done (and probably 48 hours after a prostatic biopsy is done), lest a possible false elevation of the serum acid phosphatase level be obtained. Acid phosphatase is an enzyme produced in the prostate gland (and in other tissues as well), and when prostatic carcinoma has spread beyond the confines of the true capsule of the gland, the prostatic fraction of acid phosphatase is usually released into the bloodstream in larger amounts than normal. Therefore the finding of an elevated blood acid phosphatase level is presumptive evidence that the carcinoma has already spread beyond the confines of the prostate gland. False positive elevations are relatively few; false negatives, however, do occur in a significant percentage of the cases in which metastatic spread has already occurred, but these false negative determinations are much less frequent with the newer radioimmunoassays than with the older enzymatic assay.

In summary, the newer radioimmunoassay methods of measuring acid phosphatase are much more sensitive than the older methods as far as measuring *only* that portion of the blood acid phosphatase made in the prostate gland and there are therefore, theoretically at least, fewer false positives and negatives. However, even the newer methods are not really able to detect (with any degree of accuracy) the relatively small cancer well confined within the prostate gland, nor can these newer methods distinguish between a prostatic carcinoma and a modest-sized benign enlargement of the prostate. When significantly elevated, in the patient known to have prostatic cancer, the acid phosphatase levels are helpful in documenting the likelihood of metastatic disease and in following the progress of therapy in metastatic disease.

The elevation of the blood alkaline phosphatase level is nonspecific and merely means that there has been bone destruction with the laying down of new bone (it may also be elevated in liver disease, but this can usually be ruled out or verified by other tests of liver function). The cause of the alkaline phosphatase elevation may be metastatic carcinoma of the prostate gland but it may also result from a number of other conditions; interpretation of elevated alkaline phosphatase levels must be made in this light. Bone x-ray studies and bone scanning are helpful in determining the presence of metastatic prostate gland disease (see Figs. 1–13, 1–31). Bone x-ray films, however, may not reveal osteolytic or osteoblastic lesions for many months after metastatic spread has occurred. Bone scanning is of particular use when the bony x-rays are normal since changes in the bone suggestive of metastatic disease will appear in bone scans 3 to 6 months before any changes will be visible on bone x-rays. The radioisotope used for bone scanning is technetium-99m-MDP (diphosphonate) and this isotope is taken up by bone in its reparative phase. In other words, any bone destruction because of metastatic cancer, bone disease, trauma, arthritis, or the like is followed by a reparative process in the bone, and it is this process that is being measured by the increased uptake of the radioisotope. Unfortunately, the reparative process is the same regardless of the etiology of the bone damage, with the bone scans appearing the same whether the destructive process is secondary to metastatic disease, trauma, or inflammatory disease; therefore a positive bone scan does not constitute firm evidence of metastatic disease, although it is certainly strongly presumptive of this in the face of a known primary prostatic cancer.

What is really desperately needed is a good screening test for prostatic carcinoma—one that can be done inexpensively, without false positives or false negatives, and intended primarily for the totally asymptomatic individual without any palpable prostatic nodules. Thus far, such a test has been most elusive.

Grading and Staging of Carcinoma of the Prostate Gland

Grading and staging of carcinoma of the prostate is probably much more important than it is with most other cancers because the prognosis and the treatment are intimately related to the grade and stage of the tumor. Stage A carcinoma of the prostate, sometimes referred to as "occult" prostate cancer, is that cancer that is not detectable by digital rectal examination of the prostate or by any presently known diagnostic step, whether roentgenographic, radionucleide, or using the patient's urine or serum. In other words, it is prostate cancer that is only diagnosed by serendipity. This usually means a surprise finding of carcinoma in the surgical specimen after the patient has had a transurethral resection or an enucleation prostatectomy for symptoms of benign bladder outlet obstruction. The totally unexpected finding of carcinoma in the surgical specimen following such surgery can occur up to 10 to 15 percent of the time. Looked at another way, approximately 15 percent of all patients seen clinically because of a diagnosis of carcinoma of the prostate will have had the diagnosis made as a result of surgery for symptoms of what was thought to be benign bladder outlet obstruction. All urologists are fully conversant with the fact that some of the patients found in this manner to have Stage A carcinoma of the prostate seem to do well for many, many years after the diagnosis has been made without having any treatment at all. On the other hand, urologists are equally aware that some patients in this Stage A group deteriorate rapidly and die within 1 to 2 years following discovery of the Stage A prostate cancer. In an attempt to determine which Stage A prostate cancer patients will do well without any further treatment and which will not, extensive retrospective studies of patients with Stage A prostate cancer were undertaken. The results suggest that, for prognostic and therapeutic purposes, these patients are better considered in separate categories of A_1 lesions and A_2 lesions. The patient with Stage A_1 prostate carcinoma is one in whom fewer than three chips of prostate carcinoma are found following the transurethral prostatic resection and these chips are uniformly of low grade (grade 1 or 2). The patient is felt to have a Stage A_2 prostatic carcinoma if the cancer is in more than three chips that have been removed or it is a high-grade tumor (grade 3 or grade 4). It is *only* the Stage A cancers that are detected serendipitously following prostate surgery for what is thought to be benign disease. Stages B, C, and D are, by definition, all suspected or diagnosed based on digital rectal findings, bone pain, or elevated acid phosphatase levels.

Stage B carcinoma of the prostate is also divided into B_1 and B_2 lesions, and all Stage B lesions are palpable on digital rectal examination. B_1 lesions are smaller than 1 cm and confined to one lobe of the prostate, whereas B_2 lesions are larger than 1 cm or are found in both lobes of the prostate gland.

A Stage C carcinoma is one that seems, on digital rectal examination, to involve one or both seminal vesicles or the base of the bladder or to have come through the true capsule of the prostate gland.

A Stage D cancer is one in which the disease has definitely escaped the confines of the prostate itself; a D_1 lesion is one with local metastases whereas a D_2 lesion is one with distant metastases.

For all of the tissue-diagnosed stages of prostatic carcinoma, the histologic grade is reported by the pathologist and is of great prognostic and therapeutic importance, probably more so even than the stage of the cancer. The grading system refers to the overall architectural pattern of the tumor as well as the histologic appearance of the individual cells. On a scale of 1 to 4, grade 1 is the most differentiated and the least malignant and grade 4 is the most poorly differentiated and the most malignant.

Treatment of Carcinoma of the Prostate Gland

Stage A. By definition, Stage A tumors are those that are discovered serendipitously, usually following a transurethral resection of the prostate (TURP) for symptoms of bladder outlet obstruction. These tumors are neither suspected nor diagnosed preoperatively. If the pathologic report of the surgically removed prostate tissue is that of an A_1 tumor (see above), then it is important to be certain that all of the tumor has been removed and that there is not, in fact, additional tumor remaining within the prostate gland. The author therefore prefers to do a second TURP on these patients as soon as is practicable; if no additional tumor is found in the surgical specimen the patient is considered to have an A_1 tumor. No further therapy for this condition is needed, but it is recommended that the patient be followed yearly with random needle biopsies of the prostate to ensure the tumor does not recur. If the repeat TURP shows additional cancer in the prostate, then, by definition, the patient goes into the category of an A_2 prostate cancer. If the *initial* TURP is reported as an A_2 prostate cancer (as defined above), then the patient requires vigorous and definitive therapy because A_2 cancers are far more lethal than A_1 cancers. The author feels that patients with A_2 cancer should have a radical prostatectomy provided that there is no evidence of tumor spread anywhere as determined by bone scans and acid phosphatases and provided the lymph nodes are negative for any cancer. The examination of the lymph nodes is called "staging" of the cancer and is done by selectively removing lymph nodes bilaterally from the obturator and the external and internal iliac chains. If any lymph nodes are grossly positive, then the cancer is automatically staged as a "D" and radical prostatectomy is not carried out. If all of the nodes are negative, then radical (removal of the *entire* prostate gland) prostatectomy is carried out.

Stage B. For Stages B_1 and B_2 cancers of the prostate, radical prostatectomy is the treatment of choice, again following the examination for any metastatic disease as just noted and the "staging" lymphadenectomy. If all the nodes examined are negative, radical prostatectomy is carried out.

Stage C. Stage C cancers of the prostate may or may not be benefited by radical prostatectomy and this may possibly be the one place for radiation therapy in the treatment of carcinoma of the prostate.

Stage D. Stage D carcinoma of the prostate is probably not going to be helped by either radical surgery or radiation therapy. These carcinomas are treated palliatively (there is no known cure for Stage D cancer) and the cornerstone of palliative therapy for metastatic cancer of the prostate remains hormonal manipulation. Inasmuch as the vast majority of prostatic cancers are androgen dependent, acceptable palliative therapy includes androgen deprivation (castration), the administration of exogenous estrogens, or both. It has been well documented that the survival of patients with Stage D prostatic cancer is not prolonged by hormonal manipulation; patients, however, subjectively "feel" better and have less discomfort when under hormonal therapy. By no means, however, is there any sort of general agreement among urologists as to whether the optimum time to institute hormonal therapy is when the diagnosis of Stage D (metastatic) cancer is made or when the patient becomes symptomatic from his cancer (bone pain). The author personally prefers to withhold therapy until the patient is symptomatic because hormonal manipulation offers the patient an excellent therapy for symptomatic relief from pain but one that cannot be beneficial if it has been "used up" by being employed as soon as the diagnosis is made. Chemotherapy is used at times in Stage D carcinoma of the prostate, and various agents have been studied over the years. Cyclophosphamide (Cytoxan), methotrexate, and, perhaps, cis-platinum are chemotherapeutic agents that have been used extensively and with beneficial palliation in some patients. However, to date there is no chemotherapeutic modality that can be counted upon to prolong the life of the patient with prostatic cancer.

Radical prostatectomy, while undeniably the treatment of choice for patients with carcinoma that is localized to the prostate gland (Stages A, B, and possibly C), is not without risks, and probably up to 5 percent of patients having this procedure done will be incontinent postoperatively. Until recently, the vast majority of patients undergoing radical prostatectomy were also impotent postoperatively but newer surgical techniques for doing radical prostatectomy appear to have considerably lowered the incidence of impotence. The role of radiation therapy in the treatment of carcinoma of the prostate, in the author's opinion, is modest indeed, and the author feels strongly that long-term survival is infinitely better after radical prostatectomy than after radiation therapy. Furthermore, there is no evidence to suggest that radiation therapy is of any benefit once the carcinoma has spread outside the prostate gland, and the complications of radiation therapy are considerable. Radiation proctitis and particularly cystitis combined with a 40- to 60-percent impotence rate from the radiation therapy might all still be acceptable if the survival rate of irradiated patients were comparable to that of patients undergoing radical prostatectomy. However, it is not, and the author personally limits the use of radiation therapy to some patients with Stage C carcinoma of the prostate and to patients with Stages A_2 and B lesions whose general medical condition precludes radical prostatectomy.

The palliative therapy of Stage D carcinoma of the prostate is best described as androgen deprivation and this can be established in many ways. Removal of the testes will accomplish this; the hypothalamus can be turned off by giving exogenous sex steroids in the form of diethylstilbestrol or the sex steroid receptor at the nuclear level can be blocked with agents such as flutamide or cyproterone acetate. The author personally prefers removal of the testes because it eliminates the possibilities of unpleasant side effects such as gynecomastia, and it clearly eliminates the very considerable risk to the cardiovascular system posed by estrogens. Also, when oral medications of any sort are given, the question of compliance arises. This is obviated if removal of the testes is the treatment. Obviously, if the patient refuses castration then exogenous estrogens are used.

Treatment of cancer of the prostate gland by castration is quite obviously horrifying to most patients. These individuals are usually already terrified by having had a prostatic cancer recently diagnosed; to then be denied what may be the most important part of their lives (the ability to have intercourse) only compounds their distress. This can be greatly softened by an understanding approach. The physician should elicit from the patient what his understanding is of the contemplated surgical procedure (castration) and his concepts of how he will function postoperatively and then be able to explain in detail exactly how the patient's condition will be altered by surgery. It is important to explain that the patient's beard will not cease to grow nor will his voice change, but that he will probably (not always) lose the ability to have erections and intercourse. The physician must offer support and reassurance in these circumstances so that the patient's integrity as a man is not destroyed completely. In those patients who may equate the inability to perform sexually with being homosexual, the clinician must dispel this concept. It is also important that the clinician help the patient to realize that the proposed androgen deprivation that is the cornerstone of palliative therapy for carcinoma of the prostate may enable him to live more comfortably than he would otherwise. To patients for whom sexual intercourse is still important, the physician should explain something about the different types of penile prostheses (see Chapter 14) that may be used should normal erections become impossible following castration or the use of exogenous estrogens.

Survival Rate

The overall 5 year survival rate for appropriately treated prostatic cancer in Caucasians is 63 percent and this includes all stages of the disease at the time of diagnosis. If the disease is definitely localized to the prostate, the survival is 77 percent and if it has spread beyond the confines of the prostate it is 39 percent. In blacks, the overall survival rate is 51 percent for all stages, 66 percent for patients presenting with localized disease, and 33 percent for those presenting with disseminated disease. It is important, however, to realize that 5-year survival of patients with prostatic carcinoma cannot be equated with a cure of this condition and that the survival rate continues to decrease after the 5-year point.

CANCER OF THE BLADDER

By far the most common cancer of the urinary tract (not the genital tract), bladder cancer, occurs with a frequency of about 39,000 new cases annually in the United States, with the male-to-female ratio something under 3:1. Nearly 11,000 people die each year of this disease, with the ratio of males to females again just under 3:1. Histologically, the vast majority (well over 90 percent) of bladder cancers are transitional cell carcinomas and the remainder are fairly well divided between squamous cell carcinomas and adenocarcinomas, with the former slightly more common than the latter. Bladder cancer is perhaps unique in that it is one cancer in which specific chemicals can be incriminated as causative agents. Although only a small minority of the total number of cases of bladder cancer have in fact been found to be related to a specific chemical cause, the fact remains that we do know that chemicals such as betanaphthylamine, xenylamine, and benzidine are all carcinogenic for the bladder. Of these, the worse is betanaphthylamine, which is a byproduct in the aniline dye manufacturing process. It is also quite certain that a definite increase in the incidence of bladder cancer exists in cigarette smokers and we further know that certain metabolites of triptophane, an essential amino acid, have a carcinogenic effect on the bladder when they are present in the urine. Additionally, there has been much in the lay literature about the possible relationship of cyclamates and saccharin to bladder cancer. Well-controlled studies, however, have pretty well demonstrated that cyclamates and saccharin do not have any role in the etiology of bladder cancer. It is also known that chronic infection in the bladder that is long-standing is associated with an increased incidence of bladder cancer.

Symptoms and Signs

The most common symptom or sign of bladder cancer is hematuria, either gross or microscopic. It is fallacious, however, to think that gross hematuria signifies a higher grade or a higher stage of carcinoma than does microscopic hematuria. Classically, the hematuria of bladder cancer is gross, total, and painless, and its presence mandates a thorough and complete urologic investigation, as does the presence of documented microscopic hematuria. Bladder cancer typically produces intermittent rather than continuous gross hematuria, and it is usual and common in the natural history of this condition for the patient to have noted an episode of gross total painless hematuria, after which his or her urine remained grossly clear for several weeks or even months before the hematuria recurred. Another, much less common presentation of bladder cancer is that of the "irritable" bladder in which the patient complains of frequency, urgency, and dysuria or any combination of these symptoms. This should alert the clinician to the possibility of bladder carcinoma, particularly in the presence of a negative urine culture. Sometimes a large, necrotic tumor is present in the bladder and may serve as a nidus for infection, thereby producing those symptoms classically found with infection and also yielding a positive culture. It is important for the physician to recognize that hematuria, even in the presence of symptoms suggestive of acute cystitis and unrelated to the results of a urine culture, might be caused by carcinoma of the bladder.

Physicians will be greatly aided in maintaining a high level of suspicion regarding bladder cancer in patients with microscopic or gross hematuria if they recall that bladder cancer is either the most common or the second most common cause of gross and microscopic hematuria in men over 50 years of age. Benign prostatic hyperplasia, it must be noted, is the other leading cause of hematuria in this age group. It should be obvious, however, that whether bladder cancer or benign prostatic hyperplasia is the likely etiologic factor, a thorough diagnostic workup is mandatory in the presence of documented microscopic hematuria or following the first episode of gross hematuria. In women over 50 years, infection and bladder cancer are the two likeliest causes of hematuria and so a thorough investigation in the female is also warranted.

Laboratory Studies

In addition to the confirmation of blood in the urine by a microscopic examination of the urine sediment, the most important laboratory study is probably a cytologic examination of the urine. This has justifiably achieved an important and prominent place in the diagnosis of bladder cancer as well as in the postoperative follow-up of the patient known to have bladder cancer. The success of urine cytology examinations is directly dependent upon the skill of the cytotechnician and the cytopathologist in preparing and examining the specimen. Abnormal cancer cells are definitely present in virtually all carcinomas of the urothelium, making the cytologic examination important in the detection not only of bladder cancers but of ureteral cancers or cancers of the renal collecting system. The problem is that the cancer cells are not always detected or recognized as such in the examination of the specimen. It is well known that urine cytologies may become positive as long as 2 years before a visible tumor appears within the bladder; nevertheless, the presence of a positive urine cytology mandates vigorous and meticulous diagnostic studies until the carcinoma is found. In trying to predict whether a given bladder tumor will recur or become more invasive, some benefit may be obtained by studying the surface antigens of the tumor cells inasmuch as there is evidence to suggest that these surface antigens are lost in those tumor cells in which a more aggressive behavior may be forthcoming. A new diagnostic test using a monoclonal antibody-based enzyme-linked immunoassay for detecting urinary fibrinogen degradation products, shows great promise as a screening test for bladder cancer.

Diagnostic Methodology, Including X-Rays

At the very least, excretory urograms and cystoscopic examination must be carried out. Bladder carcinoma can almost invariably be diagnosed cystoscopically (the excretory urogram is to evaluate the upper tracts as a possible source of the hematuria), except in those relatively uncommon cases of squamous cell carcinoma or in situ carcinoma where the bladder mucosa neither appears normal nor has the classic appearance of a transitional cell carcinoma. In cases of visible tumor, excisional biopsy with the patient under a general anesthetic is carried out for the purpose of determining the stage and grade of the tumor. CT scans of the pelvis are sometimes helpful in determining the depth of invasion of a bladder tumor and whether or not the tumor has already spread beyond the confines of the bladder. However, these CT scans are not always highly accurate for the purpose of determining the extent of the tumor; this should be kept in mind especially if this diagnostic step is being considered as a determining factor in whether or not to proceed with a laparotomy and a possible definitive operation.

The detection of carcinoma in situ can be particularly difficult and a recently developed technique using intravenous hematoporphyrin followed a short time later with fluorescent lighting and cystoscopy has shown considerable promise in allowing endoscopic visualization of the carcinoma in situ.

Staging and Grading of the Tumor

The two most important factors affecting the prognosis and the treatment for the patient with bladder cancer are whether or not the tumor is invasive (Stage) and what the histologic appearance of the tumor is (Grade). Tumors that are confined to the mucosa are considered a Stage 0; tumors invading into the lamina propria (submucosa) are considered Stage A; tumors invading into the muscle are considered a Stage B and they are referred to as B_1 if they invade into the superficial muscle and B_2 if into the deep muscle; tumors reaching the serosa of the bladder and involving it with or without perivesical fat also being involved are referred to as Stage C; tumors that have spread totally outside the confines of the bladder are referred to as Stage D, and those that have spread to adjacent organs or pelvic lymph nodes are called D_1 tumors whereas those with distant metastases in any site are called D_2 tumors. The actual staging of the tumor is carried out by means of a deep transurethral resection of the tumor such that the tumor and its underlying muscle are removed en bloc for pathologic examination and in this manner the depth of invasion of the tumor can be readily determined.

The histologic grade of the tumor is measured on a 1 to 4 scale, with 1 being a well-differentiated tumor and 4 being a poorly differentiated tumor.

Treatment

For those tumors that are superficial (Stage 0 or A) and low-grade (1 or 2) the treatment of choice is transurethral resection of the tumor with fulguration of the tumor base. The patient is then sometimes put on a course of chemotherapy with intravesical Thio-tepa. These patients need to be followed cystoscopically every 3 to 6 months for several years because bladder tumors tend to recur. Most recently surgery using laser beams has shown promise, particularly in the superficial tumors. For patients with tumors that are invasive into the bladder musculature (Stage B), treatment depends upon the histologic grade of the tumor. Occasionally, tumors that are invasive into the bladder musculature can be treated with deep transurethral resection, intravesical Thio-tepa, Mitomycin, or BCG (tuberculosis vaccine has been found beneficial for some bladder tumors) and follow-up over a protracted period of time with cystoscopic examinations. Often, if a tumor is invasive into the muscle, particularly if it is high grade (3 or 4), it is best treated by segmental resection of that area of the bladder involved with the tumor or even by a total cystectomy and diversion of the urine. The more deeply invasive into the bladder muscle the tumor is, the greater the indication is for a cystectomy. There may additionally be some merit to a course of preoperative radiation therapy.

Stage C bladder tumors are probably best treated by cystectomy and urinary diversion, and even Stage D tumors may often best be handled in this manner because the natural history of bladder tumors as they get more extensive is to cause a great deal of hematuria and bladder spasm, both of which can be quite debilitating to the patient.

The role of radiation therapy in the treatment of bladder carcinoma is variable and it certainly represents a viable alternative to cystectomy but the main problem is that bladder radiation leaves the patient as a virtual urologic cripple because the ensuing radiation cystitis will produce severely distressing symptoms of frequency, urgency, nocturia, and dysuria. In patients felt to have incurable bladder cancer by virtue of extension beyond the confines of the bladder, urinary diversion may be carried out so as to obviate the complications of radiation cystitis, after which the bladder can be radiated extensively for palliation.

The role of chemotherapy in the palliation of bladder cancer is a real one, and remarkable remissions have occurred, particularly with the use of cis-platinum. The other chemotherapeutic agent that has been of some benefit, when given with cis-platinum has been Adriamycin. A totally nonspecific type of systemic immunotherapy using BCG (bacillus Calmette–Guerin) and administering live organisms that are immunogenic has met with considerable success in those centers where it has been used. It is indicated for the invasive and higher grade tumors for patients in whom cystectomy may not be indicated. Although these various forms of chemotherapy and immunotherapy are without doubt beneficial, they must absolutely be considered as palliative and not curative.

For those few patients having adenocarcinoma or squamous cell carinoma of the bladder, prompt cystectomy is the treatment of choice in these highly lethal tumors.

Survival Rates

For patients with low-grade and low-stage carcinoma, the 5-year survival rate approaches 90 percent. It is important to realize, however, that these low-grade and low-stage tumors often tend to recur, and about half the time the recurrences are of a higher grade or of a higher stage than the original tumor. When a bladder tumor is found at the time of diagnosis to be invasive into the bladder musculature, the 5-year survival rate drops and it drops precipitously if it is invasive into the deep muscle. If the superficial musculature alone is involved, the 5-year survival rate is somewhere in the neighborhood of 50 to 60 percent; if the deeper musculature is involved, the 5-year survival rate drops into the range of 20 to 25 percent. Once the tumor has extended all the way through the bladder wall, such that it is a stage C or a stage D, the 5-year survival rate is in the neighborhood of 10 percent.

CANCER OF THE KIDNEY

Between 16,000 and 18,000 new cases of kidney cancer are diagnosed each year in the United States and about 8,000 people die annually from this disease. Renal cancers occur about twice as commonly in males as in females and represent approximately 1.7 percent of all cancers found in males and about 1 percent of all cancers found in females. The death rate from all cancers of the kidney show male predominance in a ratio of about 2:1. These figures comprise all of the histologic types of renal malignancy, although there are four specific types of renal cancer that make up virtually all of this group. The most frequently encountered are renal cell carcinomas (adenocarcinoma of the kidney), which account for about 83 percent of all kidney cancers. Synonymous with renal cell carcinoma are the terms hypernephroma, Grawitz tumor, clear cell carcinoma, and dark cell carcinoma. Although there are some histologic differences between the last two named in this group, they are basically the same tumor and have the same symptomatology and treatment, but the prognosis is felt to be a bit better with the clear cell variation. Next in order of frequency after renal cell carcinoma are malignant tumors of the renal collecting system, with an incidence of about 7.7 percent of all kidney cancers. Wilms' tumor (also called nephroblastomas) account for 5.6 percent(and virtually all of these are in young children), and sarcomas of the kidneys account for about 3.3 percent of renal cancers.

Of all malignant genitourinary tumors occurring in males, kidney cancers as a group are third in frequency, preceded by cancers of the prostate gland and bladder, respectively. In females, bladder cancer is also more common than kidney cancer.

Renal Cell Carcinoma

Since renal cell carcinoma, also called hypernephroma, is by far the most common of the kidney cancers, it is the one that should be of greatest concern to the clinician and the medical student. The etiology of renal cell carcinoma is unknown.

Symptoms and Signs. Renal cell carcinomas have traditionally been classified with the great mimics encountered in clinical medicine and this is because they can present in a myriad of ways. Although the classic symptom triad of hematuria, flank pain, and flank mass is often mentioned in the literature as being the diagnostic criteria for this condition, it is a fact that no more than 10 of 15 percent of patients with renal cell carcinoma present with this triad. By direct pressure necrosis, hemorrhage, extension, and metastasis, renal cell carcinoma can produce the clinical picture of an amazing variety of maladies and the clinician must always be alert to the possibility of its presence even when none of the so-called classic triad is present. Gross hematuria may be the first symptom of renal cell carcinoma in perhaps a quarter to a third of patients with this disease, but it is found at some point during the course of the disease in about 70 percent of patients. Hematuria, which may be only microscopic, whether accompanied or unaccompanied by any other urinary tract symptoms should always provide ample grounds for suspicion of cancer. Microscopic or gross hematuria *always* warrants a full and complete urologic investigation without any delay. The second of the classic symptoms, flank pain, is often very vaguely localized and dull in quality and may be present in one third to one half of patients with renal cell carcinoma. Severe pain is rare and when it does occur it is usually caused by the movement of blood clots or a tumor down the ureter, thereby simulating the renal colic of stone disease. Severe pain may also be due to frank rupture of the tumor itself, an uncommon occurrence that has been reported. The third of the classic triad, a palpable mass, may be identified in perhaps one third of patients with renal cell carcinoma, and although such masses are most commonly detected in the flank region, they may also be felt in the anterolateral abdominal area.

The intriguing thing about renal cell carcinoma is its ability to mimic and simulate an infinite variety of disease entities, thereby contributing greatly to the confusion of the clinician, the bewilderment of the patient, and, most unhappily, an inevitable delay in arriving at the correct diagnosis. For example, fever has been reported as the sole symptom in 2 percent of patients with renal cell carcinoma and as the initial symptom in 11 percent of patients. As many as one third of individuals with renal cell carcinoma will have observed fever during the course of the disease and the recurrence of fever in the postnephrectomy course may be associated with metastases or residual tumor. Occasionally, gastrointestinal complaints such as anorexia, constipation, nausea, and vomiting are the first and only symptoms. Metastases to the skin are seen in 2 to 3 percent of individuals with renal cell carcinoma and may occasionally be the initial symptom.

In summary, symptoms of renal cell carcinoma are many and varied, with microscopic or gross hematuria probably being the single most common symptom that will occur at some time during the course of the disease process. Although the peak incidence of renal cell carcinoma is in patients in the 50- to 70-year age group, it is incumbent on the physician to consider the possibility of this disease in *any* patient who has any amount of blood in the urine, upper abdominal or flank mass, otherwise unexplained upper abdominal or flank pain or discomfort, fever of unknown origin, otherwise unaccounted for weight loss, otherwise undiagnosed subcutaneous nodules, or generalized malaise.

Diagnostic Methodology

Excretory Urogram. The initial step in the management of an individual suspected of having a renal cell carcinoma is the excretory urogram, preferably of the high-dose or infusion variety. A completely normal excretory urogram with full visualization of the collecting systems and normal renal contours bilaterally can pretty well rule out the existence of renal cell carcinoma. The excretory urogram in the vast majority of individuals with renal cell carcinoma will show a distortion of the collecting system because of the mass effect of the carcinoma within the paranchyma (Fig. 6–1) and enlargement or irregularity of the renal outline, a delay in visualization, or even complete nonvisualization (if the renal vein is filled with tumor). Distortions of the intrarenal architecture and enlargement or irregularity of the renal outline strongly suggest a mass lesion within the kidney, with the principal dif-

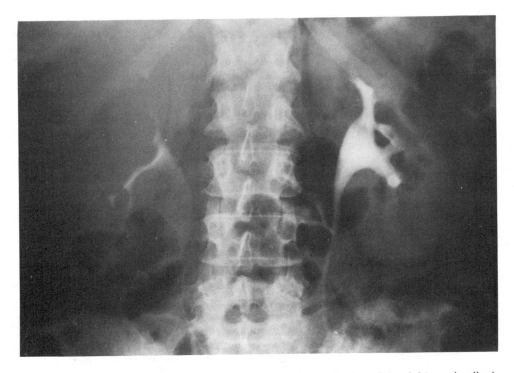

Figure 6–1. An excretory urogram showing incomplete visualization of the right renal collecting system and a suggestion of a mass lesion in the mid-right kidney and the right upper pole. This was an extensive adenocarcinoma involving the right kidney. The left kidney is normal.

ferential being a renal cyst vs. a renal malignancy. It is very helpful if nephrotomograms are obtained at the time that the excretory urogram is done because these studies will often help both to detect mass lesions within the kidney and to suggest whether these mass lesions are cystic or solid. Unquestionably, renal cysts are far more common than renal malignancies, but it is nevertheless extremely difficult, perhaps even foolhardy, to try to make a definitive distinction between cyst and malignancy based on the excretory urogram and the nephrotomograms alone.

Retrograde Ureteropyelogram. One very definite indication for this study is the presence of a nonfunctioning (nonvisualizing) kidney on excretory urography. At other times when the collecting system is seen but incompletely filled, retrograde ureteralpyelography may also be indicated.

Ultrasonography. After the excretory urogram has been done, and with or without a retrograde ureteropyelogram, if there is a suggestion of a mass lesion within the kidney ultrasonography is probably the next diagnostic step to be taken. Although this test is not definitive, that is, additional studies will still need to be done after it has been completed, it is most helpful in making a provisional distinction between a renal cyst and a solid renal lesion (renal carcinoma) by the absence or presence of internal echoes.

Renal Cyst Puncture and Cystography. If the ultrasound is quite conclusive that the lesion in the kidney is cystic, the next step is a percutaneous puncture of the cyst, with aspiration of the fluid within. A true cyst invariably has clear, straw-colored fluid in the aspirate, and a microscopic examination of this fluid will show virtually no fat therein. Aspiration of bloody or chocolate-colored fluid is highly suspicious of tumor, and this aspirate will usually have a considerable amount of fat within it. If the aspirate is clear and straw colored, so that a renal cyst is virtually certain, contrast media is injected through the needle that has punctured the cyst and x-rays are taken (Fig. 6–2). A smooth, clear outline of the cyst within the kidney as seen on an x-ray following injection of the contrast medium is fairly certain evi-

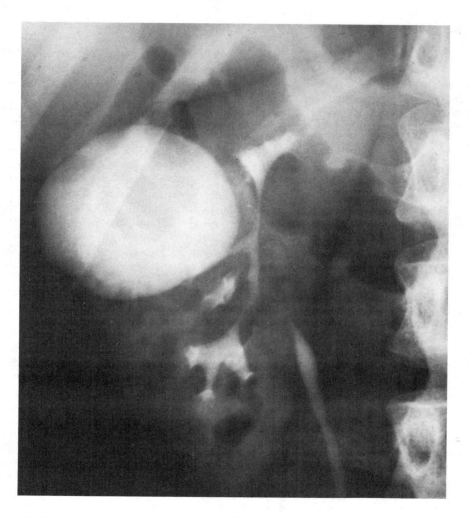

Figure 6-2. A renal cyst that was aspirated, after which contrast medium was injected into the cystic area that had just been aspirated. The smooth, clear outline of the cyst seen following injection of the contrast medium is fairly certain evidence that the mass lesion is indeed cystic.

dence that the mass lesion within the kidney is cystic and not a malignancy and the diagnostic workup can probably stop at this point.

CT Scans. If the ultrasound studies suggest internal echoes within the mass or a solid lesion (in other words when the ultrasound fails to confirm that the mass lesion is a renal cyst), the CT scan is probably the next diagnostic step to take and this is a much more definitive study. It is extremely helpful in diagnosing renal mass lesions because it can precisely determine the density of lesions and thus whether a renal mass is cystic or otherwise. Some physicians like to obtain a CT scan even in the presence of an ultrasound finding that is compatible with a renal cyst because the CT scan is the more definitive of the two studies. Whenever a mass lesion in the kidney is *not* cystic it must be considered to be a malignancy until proven otherwise (usually by surgery).

Renal Angiography. When all of the studies obtained thus far suggest a renal malignancy, renal arteriograms are helpful because they can delineate the blood supply to the involved kidney as well as the collateral circulation from the kidney that may result from the presence of some tumors. Although angiograms are certainly not a necessity in the workup of a patient with a renal mass lesion, they are often very helpful and the author personally prefers to obtain them prior to surgical intervention.

In patients where the CT scan is equivocal, angiograms are a virtual necessity because, by definition, they depict the vascularity of the affected kidney and usually very well demonstrate those findings that are associated with renal malignancies. The specific findings on the angiogram that are virtually pathognomonic of renal malignancies are "puddling" of the contrast medium within the kidney (Fig. 1–39) and an abnormal or "corkscrew" appearance of the small vessels feeding into the renal malignancy.

Used appropriately, the above diagnostic studies provide the clinician with close to a 99 percent accuracy regarding the diagnosis of a specific renal mass lesion.

Renal Scanning. Scanning generally does not provide any useful information regarding renal morphology and is neither helpful nor indicated in trying to differentiate renal cysts from renal tumors.

Laboratory Studies. Laboratory studies are important and play a definite role in the diagnostic methodology of renal cell carcinoma. As noted earlier, unexplained microscopic hematuria and certainly gross hematuria should be cause for further intensive investigation. Obviously, however, the absence of blood in the urine does not of itself overrule other findings that suggest the possibility of renal cell carcinoma. As many as 25 percent of patients with renal cell carcinoma may never have any blood in their urine during the course of the disease. Some elevation of urinary proteins is not uncommon with renal cell carcinoma; markedly elevated proteinuria may be associated with renal vein or vena cava obstruction caused by tumor thrombi. Lowered hemoglobin levels and resulting anemia may be found in between 25 and 50 percent of patients with renal cell carcinoma, but it is particularly interesting to note that polycythemia has been reported in as many as 5 percent of individuals with renal cell carcinoma. The kidney is known to have a role in the production of erythropoietin, and it is felt that this production is increased in some cases of renal cell carcinoma. Urinary cytology in cases of renal cell carcinoma is usually unrewarding inasmuch as malignant cells would only be expected to be present in the urine late in the course of the disease, after the tumor has broken into the collecting system of the kidney. Approximately 10 percent of patients with renal cell carcinoma have a hypercalcemia and it is thought that this is due to a parathormone-like substance elaborated by renal cell carcinoma. A very interesting phenomenon occurring with hypernephroma is hepatic dysfunction. Up to 40 percent of patients with hypernephroma may have laboratory tests indicating one or more of the following: increases in blood alkaline phosphatase activity, thymol turbidity, or prolonged prothrombin time, or decreases in globulin, albumin, or retention of bromsulphalein (BSP). In a large series of patients with such abnormalities of liver function and a definite diagnosis of hypernephroma, liver biopsies were done at the time of nephrectomy and nonspecific reactive hepatitis was found in some of these individuals. In no patient was metastatic disease found to be the cause of the abnormal laboratory values. With respect to these parameters of hepatic dysfunction, it is particularly important to realize that the presence of one or more abnormal tests of liver function does not indicate metastatic disease and therefore inoperability and incurability. Equally important is the observed fact over the last several years that the prognosis is very poor for those patients whose liver function tests failed to return to normal after nephrectomy or returned to normal and then became abnormal again.

Treatment.   The management of patients with renal cell carcinoma is basically surgical. Unless the patient is considered medically unable to survive a surgical procedure (radical nephrectomy) or unless the patient is known to have widespread and extensive metastatic disease such that life expectancy is brief, the treatment of choice is prompt and radical nephrectomy. Even in the presence of known metastases, if the patient is a good surgical risk it is probable that nephrectomy is still indicated. This is because as the disease progresses most patients with renal cell carcinoma develop flank mass, flank pain, or hematuria and there is an ever-present possibility of a significant bleed into the tumor itself that will produce considerable discomfort to the patient. It is also a clinical fact that some patients, following nephrectomy, seem to improve and to do better for a short period of time. For all of these reasons nephrectomy is probably indicated in most patients with renal cell carcinoma whether or not they have metastatic disease. Another reason that radical nephrectomy is the treatment of choice is that at the present time there are literally no other treatment modalities that can be expected to be of benefit to the patient. These tumors are not radiosensitive, and chemotherapy has not been found to be of any value. There are some studies suggesting that, in male patients, the use of intramuscular progesterone may be of some benefit, but the author feels that for the most part these are anecdotal experiences and not statistically valid. Immunotherapy may offer some hope for treating this malignancy in the future, but at present, there is certainly nothing definitive in this regard.

Survival Rate.   The 5-year survival rate for patients with hypernephroma depends, not surprisingly, on whether the tumor is completely confined within the kidney at the time of surgery. In those cases designated Stage 1 (tumor confined within the renal capsule), the 5-year survival is in the neighborhood of 70 to 80 percent following radical nephrectomy. If the renal capsule has been infiltrated and there has been perirenal tissue or adjacent nodal involvement, the 5-year survival rate drops to about 35 percent even when radical nephrectomy is carried out. If distant metastases are present, then the 5-year survival is about 5 percent regardless of therapy. It is particularly important to realize that renal cell carcinoma, absent for 5 years following nephrectomy, not infrequently recurs 10 and 15 years after treatment and for this reason constant surveillance for at least 15 years following nephrectomy is warranted. When local recurrences following nephrectomy are found in the retroperitoneum or even in the lungs and these are isolated, surgical removal is indicated.

Cancer of the Renal Collecting System

The second largest category of carcinoma of the kidney (after renal cell carcinoma), encompassing between 7 and 8 percent of all kidney cancers, is transitional cell epithelioma, or carcinoma, involving the renal collecting system. The etiology of this tumor is unknown but, as with bladder tumors, certain known carcinogens as well as the presence of chronic infection play a role in the etiology of a relatively small percentage of these tumors (see Cancer of the Bladder, above).

Symptoms and Signs. The symptoms produced by transitional cell epithelioma are those associated with the location of the tumor. Inasmuch as the cancer is growing within the collecting system, the likelihood is great that microscopic or gross hematuria will occur very early in the course of the disease. In fact, gross, painless hematuria is probably the most common symptom of this particular tumor and affects the vast majority of patients so afflicted. Additionally, about two thirds of these tumors produce an associated hydronephrosis because the location of the tumor tends to obstruct the ureteropelvic junction, bringing about the dilatation of the renal collecting system. If the hydronephrosis is large enough, a palpable mass may be noted by the patient or by the examining physician. If it is of sudden onset over a relatively short period of time, the hydronephrosis will produce definite costovertebral angle pain. If the hydronephrosis evolves over a period of weeks or months, there will in all likelihood not be any significant flank discomfort.

Diagnostic Methodology. Diagnosis of cancer of the renal collecting system is initiated by a high index of suspicion when an adult is found to have microscopic or gross hematuria. Excretory urography is the initial diagnostic step and the characteristic filling defect or negative shadow (Fig. 6–3) is often sufficient to warrant a provisional diagnosis of cancer of the renal collecting system.

The differential diagnosis of a visualized filling defect or negative shadow on the excretory urogram (in addition to cancer of the renal collecting system) is between nonopaque calculus and blood clot. If the details of the collecting system are not well seen on a high-dose excretory urogram or if there is a possibility that the defect is an artifact, cystoscopy and retrograde ureteropyelograms are helpful. In practice, this is almost always done inasmuch as cystoscopy is indicated in any individual with a suspected tumor of the collecting system because these tumors tend to spread both through the renal vein and by direct extension down the ureter and into the bladder, making cystoscopic evaluation of the bladder an absolute necessity. At the time of cystoscopy, urine can be collected for cytologic study directly from the side suspected of harboring the carcinoma. Unless the diagnosis of carcinoma can be made with certainty the usual procedure is to repeat the excretory urogram in 3 to 6 weeks so as to be more certain that the filling defect is a tumor and not a blood clot which would theoretically lyse in the intervening time period. Additionally, random specimens of voided urine may be collected for urinary

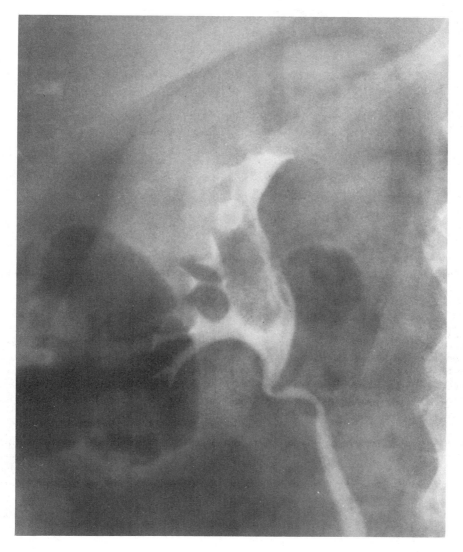

Figure 6-3. An excretory urogram showing a persistent filling defect in the right renal pelvis and infundibulum to the upper collecting system. Filling defects such as this are highly suggestive of transitional cell carcinoma.

cytology because, due to the location of the tumor on the urothelium of the kidney, there is a good chance of exfoliation of malignant cells, with subsequent recovery in the urine.

CT scanning can be quite helpful in the diagnosis of filling defects within the renal collecting system because of its unique ability to differentiate between different densities (i.e., tumor, stone, or blood clot). Selective renal angiography is not usually of any particular help unless it is felt that there may be tumor involvement of the renal parenchyma. In any case, angiography is sometimes employed when the issue is still obscure.

The recent development of ureteroscopes that are 10F and 11F in diameter often enables direct visualization of the filling defect within the kidney, but, obviously, this requires a general anesthetic. Through these ureteroscopes it is possible to obtain "brushings" of the tissue within the collecting system and this may also be helpful in making the diagnosis.

In general, when transitional cell carcinomas of the collecting system are suspected, laboratory tests are neither particularly helpful nor diagnostic, with two exceptions: (1) urinalysis that shows a persistent microscopic hematuria even if gross hematuria is not present, and (2) urine cytology that may be positive for tumor cells. The interpretation of urinary cytology, however, must be done by an experienced cytopathologist.

Treatment. Treatment of tumors of the renal collecting system is by nephrectomy, which need not be of the radical type, and total ureterectomy with removal of a cuff of bladder at the point where the ureter enters the bladder. As already noted, this is done because these tumors often tend to spread by direct extension down the ureter and into the bladder. In some cases where the collecting system tumor is extremely small and local excision shows it to be truly superficial, acceptable treatment may simply be removal of the tumor with a full thickness of collecting system wall with sparing of the kidney. This particular method for treating collecting system tumors is probably only truly justified in a patient with a solitary kidney, but there may be occasional instances where it is advisable in a patient with two kidneys. The long-term follow-up of a patient with cancer of the collecting system mandates frequent cystoscopic examinations as well as periodic and regular excretory urograms because these tumors, besides spreading by direct extension, are thought to be of multicentric origin. Thus the patient must be carefully observed for evidence of similar tumors arising in any other portions of the urothelium.

Survival Rate. The 5-year postnephrectomy survival rate of patients with tumors of the renal collecting system is not good and it depends on whether the tumor is papillary (85 percent) or invasive (15 percent) and how much invasion of the underlying muscle has occurred. Also, invasion of the renal vein is a grave prognostic indication. The best survival rate for patients with noninvasive tumors and no renal vein involvement appears to be around 50 to 60 percent and it decreases rapidly from there.

Wilms Tumor

Wilms tumor, considered to be the most common abdominal tumor of childhood and second to neuroblastoma if childhood and infancy are considered together, occurs almost exclusively in children under 5 years of age, although it has been reported in older children and adults (see Chapter 5).

Sarcomas of the Kidneys

Sarcomas are by far the least common of the four principal types of kidney cancer and fibrosarcoma is the most common of all the sarcomas. Sarcomas account for perhaps 3 percent of all kidney cancers, they are highly malignant, and the 5-year survival rate for patients is less than 10 percent. Treatment is radical nephrectomy.

CANCER OF THE TESTIS

Although testicular cancer accounts for less than 1 percent of all cancers in males of all age groups and no more than 0.2 percent of deaths from cancer in all males, it does remain the leading cause of death from cancer among men in the 25- to 34-year age bracket.

Testicular cancers comprise germinal cell tumors (over 97 percent) and nongerminal cell tumors (under 3 percent), the latter arising from the nongerminal elements of the testis, such as the interstitial cells, Sertoli cells, and the stroma. This text deals primarily with germinal cell tumors because they are by far the preponderant type. They can be divided into five histologic groupings:

1. Pure seminoma.
2. Embryonal cell carcinoma with or without seminoma.
3. Teratoma.
4. Teratoma, with embryonal cell carcinoma or choriocarcinoma and with or without seminoma.
5. Choriocarcinoma with or without embryonal cell carcinoma and with or without seminoma.

All of these tumors must be considered malignant.

The etiology of testicular tumors is not known but various intriguing carcinogenic factors have been suggested. It has long been felt that individuals with undescended testes have a 20- to 40-fold increased incidence of carcinoma as compared with a normally descended testis. Some studies have suggested a very high incidence of abnormal chromosomes in undescended testes when peripheral blood chromosome studies are normal, and it may be that these undescended testes are abnormal in some way that predisposes to carcinoma. It is also known that malignant testis tumors are considerably more common in an atrophic testis than in its normal contralateral mate. The relationship of testicular tumor to antecedent testis trauma has often been suggested, but this is extremely difficult to document because testis trauma of one degree or another is very common in young active males.

Symptoms and Signs

Although most testis tumors are first noticed as relatively painless swellings of the testis, it is important to recognize that the condition may be heralded in a more explosive manner by a coexisting acute inflammation of the testis or epididymis. Sudden bleeding into the testicular tumor may account for occurrences of acute and immediate pain. Hydroceles of inflammatory etiology have often been seen in association with testicular cancer. Such hydroceles can prevent adequate testicular palpation and lead to considerable delay in diagnosis and treatment.

Physical Findings

The paramount physical finding in a patient with testicular cancer is a hard and indurated area on the testis that is definitely firmer than the surrounding testicular tissue or the contralateral testis. This hard region may vary in size from a small nodule to involvement of the entire testis. Inasmuch as induration of the epididymis is extremely common and completely benign, it is essential that the examining physician be able to differentiate induration of the testis from that of the adjacent epididymis (see Chapter 1). This is best done with the patient in the dorsal recumbent position by palpating the testis and the epididymis between the fingers of both hands. The epididymis is normally clearly separate and distinguishable from the testis. Therefore, even when there is induration of this structure the normalcy of the adjacent testis should be easy to determine. When doubt exists about the normalcy of the testis or when the examining physician is reasonably certain that the testis is in fact considerably firmer than it should be, the patient should be referred to a urologist, without delay, for probable exploratory surgery.

It should be emphatically pointed out that testicular tumors do *not* spread to the inguinal lymph nodes except in most unusual circumstances, and therefore palpation of the inguinal area to determine possible spread of testicular tumors is invalid and potentially misleading.

Since it is not unusual for testis cancer to be masked by coexisting epididymitis or epididymoorchitis, it is incumbent upon the examining clinician making a diagnosis of epididymitis or epididymoorchitis to bear this fact in mind and to see the patient every 1 to 2 weeks for a 2- to 4-week period. At the end of this period if the testis itself has not returned to complete normalcy (i.e., if the orchitis has not totally subsided) the patient should probably be considered for exploratory surgery to rule out a carcinoma of the testis. On the other hand, the epididymis may take up to 3 months or longer to return to a normal state, and it is therefore again incumbent on the physician to be able to distinguish persistent induration of the epididymis from the adjacent testis, which hopefully has returned to normal. If there is doubt as to the normalcy of the testis, exploratory surgery can obviously be lifesaving. If the testis is normal and no cancer is present, the patient probably will be no worse off for having had surgical exploration.

Differential Diagnosis

The differential diagnosis of testicular carcinoma could, in a very broad manner of speaking, encompass all of those conditions leading to mass, edema, induration, and such within the scrotum. Such conditions include epididymitis, epididymoorchitis, orchitis, indirect inguinal hernia, torsion of the cord, torsion of the appendix testis or the appendix epididymis, varicocele, spermatocele, hydrocele of the cord or testis, lipoma of the cord, gumma of the testis, tuberculosis of the testis, granulomatous orchitis, and hematocele (see Chapter 11). In spite of the seemingly formidable nature of this list, it must be recalled that the differential diagnosis of testicular cancer is not a problem as long as the testis can be palpated and normalcy clearly determined. Strange areas of induration or tenderness elsewhere in the scrotum are almost invariably benign and it is only in the testis that cancer must be feared. If any intrascrotal condition inhibits normal palpation of the testis or if such testicular palpation leads to the conclusion that absolute normalcy cannot be ascertained, surgical exploration is warranted, particularly when the patient is in the 20- to 40-year age group.

Laboratory and X-Ray Studies

Any young male presenting with an intrascrotal mass in which the diagnosis of testis carcinoma is considered should have two blood tests done for the so-called testis tumor markers: a serum α-fetoprotein (AFP) and the β subunit of human chorionic gonadotropin (hCG). Approximately 85 to 90 percent of patients with a nonseminomatous testis tumor have an elevation of one or both of these tumor markers. Other studies that should be carried out if testis malignancy is suspected include excretory urograms, chest x-rays with tomograms, or, preferably, CT scans of the chest and abdomen; all of these studies are to see if any obvious metastases are present.

Initial Treatment

The testis in which carcinoma is suspected should be explored though an inguinal incision using a large rubber-shod clamp across the cord at the level of the internal ring in order to minimize dissemination of cancer cells during the mobilization of the testis. When both palpation and visual inspection of the testis lead to suspicion of testicular carcinoma, radical orchiectomy (removal of the testis with the entire cord up to the level of the internal inguinal ring) is carried out. Except in cases of a solitary testis, biopsy is not warranted because of the possibility of tumor dissemination and because of the fact that accurate visual inspection and palpation of the testis will rarely lead to the removal of a normal testis.

Follow-up therapy depends on the histologic type of tumor present. If the removed testis is a pure seminoma and if the tumor markers are negative, the treatment of choice is radiation therapy to the retroperitoneal, mediastinal, and left supraclavicular areas, with about 4000 rads administered over a 4-week period. However, if the human chorionic gonadotropin is elevated significantly, this may suggest the possibility of malignant elements other than seminoma being present. This is a very controversial area and if the decision is made to go with radiation therapy alone at this point, the patient should be very carefully monitored for 2 or 3 years following radiation therapy with serial hCG levels.

If the radical orchiectomy disclosed a nonseminomatous tumor, then the next step is probably a retroperitoneal lymphadenectomy and this is really done for staging purposes. Cancer of the testis spreads to the retroperitoneal lymph nodes, specifically the iliac, preaortic, and renal hilar nodes, and these nodes are removed en bloc and examined for any evidence of metastatic carcinoma. If there is no carcinoma found then the patient is followed every 3 months for 2 years and then every 6 months for another 2 years with serial tumor markers, tomograms, or CT scans of the chest and retroperitoneum. If any retroperitoneal nodes are involved with metastatic tumor, then chemotherapy is indicated (see below).

Definitive Treatment

The definitive treatment for nonseminomatous cancer of the testis is now chemotherapy, and this particular treatment for this particular disease represents one of the very real and very dramatic therapeutic breakthroughs of the past decade. It might fairly be said that the modern era of chemotherapy for testis cancer began in 1960, but it was not until 1974 when protocols using cis-platinum, vinblastine, and bleomycin were put together that the "modern" era of chemotherapy for testis cancer began. Various combinations of these chemotherapeutic agents have been used in protocols since 1974, and at present the combination chemotherapy consistently produces 70 percent complete remissions and a further 10 percent of patients can be rendered disease free following surgical excision of residual disease. The projected cure rate for patients with disseminated testis cancer is 70 percent, an absolutely remarkable improvement in comparison with the cure rate of less than 10 percent in the 1960s and an almost uniformly fatal outcome prior to that time. Of all the genitourinary tract malignancies, it is only cancer of the testis for which chemotherapy can be described as curative.

CANCER OF THE PENIS

Extremely uncommon, penile cancer is seen almost exclusively in uncircumcised males who practice poor personal hygiene. Penile cancer is invariably associated with chronic infection of the glans and the underside of the foreskin, and it is invariably seen in patients who rarely, if ever, fully retract the foreskin in order to carefully cleanse the glans, coronal sulcus, and undersurface of the foreskin.

The carcinomas are usually squamous cell in nature and may be ulcerating or fungating in appearance. It is extremely important that the examining physician retract the foreskin (or have the patient do it himself) of all uncircumcised patients for the purpose of examining the glans penis specifically for carcinoma. Biopsy of any suspicious lesion is virtually always warranted if a definitive diagnosis cannot be made otherwise. Penile cancer spreads by way of the inguinal lymph nodes, but it should be noted that the inguinal adenopathy frequently present in association with cancer of the penis is often inflammatory and not neoplastic.

Treatment

Treatment of penile cancer usually consists of partial amputation of the penis if the lesion is on the distal portion of the penis. If it is not possible to retain at least a 2-cm tumor-free margin proximal to the lesion following amputation and still leave a phallus that is suitable for voiding and intercourse, total penectomy is indicated. On occasion, radical penectomy with groin dissection and radiation is warranted. For further discussion and illustrations of this condition see Chapter 12.

REFERENCES

Carter WC III, Rous SN: Etiology of gross hematuria in 110 consecutive adult urology hospital admissions. Urology 18:342, 1981

Donohue JP: Tumors of the testis. In Kendall AR, Karafin L (eds), Urology. Philadelphia, Harper and Row, 1980, vol 2, chap 8

Durant JR: Chemotherapy of genitourinary tumors. In Kendall AR, Karafin L (eds), Urology. Philadelphia, Harper and Row, 1982, vol 2, chap 25

Lakey WH, Lieskovsky A: Tumors of the kidney. In Kendall AR, Karafin L (eds), Urology. Philadelphia, Harper and Row, 1981, vol 2, chap 6

Myers RP: Tumors of the renal pelvis, ureter and urinary bladder. In Kendall AR, Karafin L (eds), Urology. Philadelphia, Harper and Row, 1981, vol 2, chap 7

Nelson RP: New concepts in the staging and follow-up of bladder carcinoma. Urology 21:105, 1983

Paulson DF: Current concepts in the management of prostate adenocarcinoma. Surg Rounds 24–31, December 1983

Rous SN, Mallouh C: Prostatic carcinoma: The relationship between histologic grade and incidence of early metastases. J Urol 108:905, 1972

Rous SN: Squamous cell carcinoma of the bladder. J Urol 120:561, 1978

Symposium on Adenocarcinoma of the Prostate. Olsson C, Moderator. Contemp Surg 24:115, 1984

Turner WR Jr, Rous SN: The management of metastatic carcinoma of the prostate. J Carolina Med Assoc 73:415, 1977

7
Benign Prostatic Hyperplasia

EDUCATIONAL OBJECTIVES

1. List the symptoms associated with benign prostatic hyperplasia.
2. Discuss the reasons why hesitancy, frequency, nocturia, intermittency, hematuria, urgency, and foul-smelling urine may occur in benign prostatic hyperplasia.
3. Discuss the causes of stones in the bladder.
4. Discuss with a patient and his family the implications of surgery for prostatic hyperplasia and subsequent complications.
5. Determine if a patient is delirious postoperatively.
6. Discuss the management of a patient who is delirious postoperatively.
7. Discuss the anatomic relationships and the pathophysiology of BPH.
8. List the indications for the surgical treatment of BPH.

Benign prostatic hyperplasia (BPH) is the most common cause of bladder outlet obstruction in men. As determined by autopsy studies, more than 50 percent of men over 50 years of age and 75 percent of men beyond age 70 are affected by hyperplasia of the prostate. These figures, however, do not reflect the incidence of individuals requiring prostatic surgery to relieve symptomatic bladder outlet obstruction. Since similar pathologic processes produce symptoms of differing severity in different individuals, the physician becomes aware of a clinical problem only in those patients in whom the symptoms become distressing enough to warrant medical attention.

Inasmuch as the dog is the only animal with a prostate gland similar to that of man, all basic research to date on the etiology of benign prostatic hyperplasia has been done in dogs. Although it is risky to extrapolate human data from animal data, until recently, based on this dog research, the etiology of benign prostatic hyperplasia appeared to be the accumulation of dihydrotestosterone within the prostate gland. Still further investigation into this excess accumulation of dihydrotestosterone within the prostate gland, however, has disclosed that faulty controls had led to this conclusion. Accordingly, there is at this time virtually nothing that is known about the etiology of BPH.

What do we know of BPH clinically? It is a clinically observed fact, for example, that eunuchs do not develop BPH. It is also a clinical fact that BPH is unrelated to sexual activity or its absence inasmuch as it exists in celibate priests in the same degree as it does in the general public. Furthermore, BPH is probably unrelated

161

to antecedent sexual excesses, prolonged periods of abstinence, or impotence. Still further, the condition does not appear to be related to prostatic infection or venereal disease, and finally, it is additionally well known that the administration of estrogens will cause prostatic adenoma (BPH) to shrink, albeit with the production of many disagreeable side effects.

ANATOMY OF THE PROSTATE GLAND

Fundamental to a complete understanding of the pathophysiology and therefore the symptoms of BPH is a thorough comprehension of the normal and the pathologic anatomy of the structures involved.

Normal Anatomy

Graphically, the prostate gland may be conceived of as an apple with the core entirely removed. The hole thus produced through the center of the apple may be visualized as the prostatic urethra, which is contiguous with the bladder neck superiorly and the membranous urethra inferiorly. This relationship may be conceptualized by thinking of the core opening of the apple (on the stem side) in snug approximation to the bladder neck. The skin of the apple can be considered the true capsule of the prostate gland, with the pulp of the apple representing the gland itself, which consists of fibrous, muscular, and glandular elements. The entire prostate gland in a young, healthy adult weighs abut 20 g and is about the size of a large chestnut.

Pathologic Anatomy

In most men at about 40 years of age adenomatous tissue consisting of glandular, muscular, and fibrous components (histologically very similar to the true prostate tissue) begins to grow within the prostate gland. Invariably beginning just beneath the mucosa of the prostatic urethra, this growth develops in a circumferential pattern (periurethrally) that may be uniform but is more often irregular, with the principal adenomatous growth occurring in an upward direction from the floor of the prostatic urethra (the so-called middle lobe of the prostate gland) and in an inward direction from the lateral aspects of the prostate (the lateral prostatic lobes). The anterior lobe of the prostate plays a minor part in the obstructive adenomatous process and the posterior lobe is not involved at all.

As the adenomatous growth slowly continues to enlarge, generally over a period of years, it may do so in an outward direction (towards the true capsule of the gland, or the skin of the apple), thereby enlarging the entire prostate gland. This enlargement is palpable on digital rectal examination of the prostate as enlarged lateral lobes. The adenomatous growth may also enlarge in an inward direction so as to intrude on the lumen of the prostatic urethra; in this case, enlargement is *not* palpable on digital rectal examination of the prostate. It may also enlarge in *both* directions, which is usually what happens. As the adenomatous growth expands towards the periphery of the prostate gland, it compresses the true prostate tissue between the expanding adenoma itself and the true capsule of the gland (the skin of the apple). Between the expanding and outward growing adenoma and the true prostatic tissue is a cleavage plane known as the surgical capsule.

SURGICAL TREATMENT OF BPH

The principle of all prostatic surgery for benign prostatic hyperplasia, regardless of the approach, is to remove all of the tissue within the surgical capsule, leaving behind the true prostate tissue (which may be compressed into a thin rim of tissue) and the true capsule. When this is done, the normal mucosal lining of the prostatic urethra will be removed along with the adenoma; thus, in the immediate postoperative period the prostatic urethra is lined with the true prostatic tissue (Fig. 7–1). Over the next 3 to 4 months, epithelium from the vesical neck grows downward

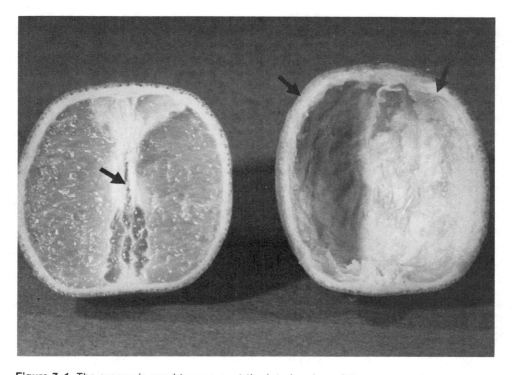

Figure 7-1. The orange is used to represent the interior view of the prostate. On the left the rind of the orange represents the true capsule of the prostate and the white part of the orange just inside the rind represents the compressed true prostatic tissue. The pulp of the orange represents the prostatic adenoma and the arrow points to the area where there should be a channel running up and down through which the urine passes. This channel is obliterated by the pulp of the orange, which represents the prostatic adenoma. The junction between the pulp of the orange (the prostatic adenoma) and the compressed true prostatic tissue (which is just inside the rind of the orange) is known as the surgical capsule which is really only a cleavage plane. The goal of the surgery is to remove all of the tissue within this cleavage plane, thereby leaving the prostate, or the orange, as it is seen in the figure on the right. This postoperative figure on the right represents the prostate following surgery for the removal of the benign adenomatous tissue (regardless of the surgical approach) and as can be seen the true capsule (*arrow* on the left of the postoperative orange), represented by the rind of the orange, is untouched. Just inside the true capsule is the compressed true prostatic tissue (*arrow* on the right side of the postoperative orange) and the rest of the prostatic fossa (or the orange) has been surgically removed, thereby leaving the prostatic fossa (immediately after surgery) lined by the true prostatic tissue.

to line the entire prostatic urethra once again. During this time, and as part of the normal healing process, there is a constant desquamation of white blood cells (pus cells). This is perfectly normal and the presence of these cells in the urine should not be construed as indicative of urinary tract infection. However, bacteria found in the urine may indeed signify infection.

The surgical procedure just described is termed an adenomaectomy, or, more accurately, an adenectomy, although it is generally referred to by most laymen and even physicians as a "prostatectomy." Because this surgery does *not* remove the true prostate gland, however, it is obvious that the possibility exists for regrowth of the prostatic adenoma, and in fact it does regrow enough to produce symptoms in about 10 percent of individuals who have had prostatic adenectomy. The chances that additional prostatic surgery will be necessary in any given patient are therefore related to the age of the patient (the younger the patient the longer he is expected to live and therefore the greater the chance of repeat surgery) and the thoroughness of the surgical removal of the adenoma. It should be called to the attention of the patient that inasmuch as the true prostate gland is not being removed and inasmuch as the true prostate gland is the normal and usual site for carcinoma of the prostate to arise, the patient who has had a prostatic adenectomy for BPH is no less at risk for cancer of the prostate than any other male and should therefore have annual digital rectal examinations of the prostate.

SYMPTOMS AND SIGNS

The symptoms and signs of BPH are nocturia, frequency, dysuria, hematuria (gross and microscopic), intermittency, hesitancy, weak urinary stream, terminal dribbling, overflow incontinence, and acute urinary retention. The physician must realize, however, that it is rare for any single patient to present with all of these symptoms and that meticulous questioning is often necessary to elicit *any* of them. Objective signs that may be present when obstructive BPH exists are bladder trabeculation, bladder infection, the presence of residual urine, hematuria, dilatation of the ureters or renal collecting systems, and elevation of blood urea nitrogen (BUN) or creatinine levels with or without the symptoms and signs of uremia, coma, and even death.

When periurethral adenomatous tissue grows in an inward direction (whether or not it additionally grows in a peripheral or outward direction), it tends to diminish the lumen of the prostatic urethra. The act of voiding is basically a function of detrusor muscle contraction on one side and resistance anywhere in the urethra on the other side. As the lumen of the prostatic urethra becomes smaller due to increasing encroachment of the periurethral adenoma the detrusor muscle must work harder against this increased resistance in order to initiate and complete the act of voiding. When detrusor muscle (or muscle anywhere in the body) must work against increased resistance, it undergoes a work hypertrophy. Significantly, the bladder trigone musculature is embryologically different from the rest of the bladder (it is of mesodermal origin whereas the rest of the bladder is of endodermal origin). The trigone is the most sensitive part of the bladder and the first to undergo work hypertrophy, and it is also the most dependent part of the bladder. Therefore, relatively small amounts of urine are detected by the hypertrophied and very sensitive trigone and perceived by the patient as a desire to void.

Nocturia
Because of the greatly increased irritability and sensitivity of the trigone secondary to its work hypertrophy, the desire to void becomes manifest when relatively small amounts of urine are present in the bladder, resulting in nocturia, (awakening during the night because of a need to void), which is the most frequent early symptom of bladder outlet obstruction. It is fair to ask why this trigonal hypertrophy that produces nocturia does not produce daytime frequency as well, inasmuch as the trigone is as much hypertrophied and irritable during the day as it is at night. Daytime frequency is not as early a symptom as nocturia simply because during waking hours an individual's mind is otherwise occupied so that the threshold for perceiving a minimal voiding urge is diminished and at times even ignored. Daytime frequency as a symptom of BPH, therefore, occurs considerably later than nocturia, and when it does occur, it is usually minimal and not bothersome enough to distress the patient. When highly distressing daytime frequency occurs, it is not caused by simple trigonal hypertrophy and increased irritability but usually by secondary bladder infection or a high level of residual urine, both of which are discussed subsequently.

Hesitancy
As the lumen of the prostatic urethra diminishes in size as a result of the inexorable inward growth of the periurethral adenoma, the detrusor muscle must work progressively harder to initiate voiding and to empty the bladder completely. Eventually, the obstruction of the prostatic urethra is such that the detrusor must contract with far more than its usual contractile strength in order to initiate the urinary stream, and several seconds may elapse before this very forceful contraction can be accomplished. Delay between attempting to initiate the flow of urine and the actual start of the flow is referred to as hesitancy. This is usually most noticeable during the first voiding of the morning because the bladder is usually fullest at this time and a bladder that is extremely full often has a muscular atony secondary to overdistention. When this atony is combined with the already present bladder outlet obstruction, there may be 15, 30, or more seconds of hesitancy.

Residual Urine
A bladder that can be and is emptied during the act of voiding, with or without intermittency, terminal dribbling, or any of the other symptoms associated with BPH, is said to be *compensated.* It should be obvious from much of the foregoing, however, that as the prostatic urethra becomes progressively more obstructed, the detrusor muscle eventually becomes unable to contract with sufficient force to empty the bladder, so that urine remains following the completion of voiding. This urine is called residual urine, and once it is present the bladder is considered to be *decompensated.* Note that the presence of residual urine immediately following voiding is never normal and the severity of the obstructive process may be gauged by the amount of residual urine remaining in the bladder following voiding. From the onset of bladder decompensation (as noted by the presence of residual urine), the symptoms of BPH frequently accelerate and become more unpleasant. The amount of residual urine inevitably increases over the months or years until anywhere from several ounces to a pint or a liter of urine is present in the bladder following voiding. The presence of any residual urine following voiding is an ominous finding because such urine is a good culture medium for bacteria, growth of which is promoted

and aided by a breakdown in the intrinsic bladder mucosa defense mechanism that has resulted from the acquired mucosal abnormalities (due to the trabeculation and perhaps even to the effect of the residual urine itself on the bladder mucosa).

Bacteria arrive in the bladder from foci in the urethra, where they frequently may be present but insignificant when the patient is in good health, from lymphatic spread from the gastrointestinal tract, or by hematogenous spread from a distant focus of infection. The significant point to recognize is that in the male a perfectly normal bladder with no residual urine is usually most resistant to the establishment of any bladder infection, even given the introduction of bacteria from the sources just noted. However, the bladder damaged by trabeculation and particularly the bladder with postvoiding residual urine is no longer able to ward off bacterial infection. Once bladder decompensation occurs, it is usually only a matter of time before acute bacterial cystitis follows.

Frequency and Urgency

With the onset of acute cystitis, the bladder mucosa becomes acutely inflamed, resulting in severe frequency, with the urge to void occurring as often as every 15 to 30 minutes. Acute inflammation in the region of the bladder neck and trigone also often produces the symptoms of urgency, wherein the desire to void is followed by the very strong need to void within a few seconds or a very few minutes. If voiding does not occur, there is often an involuntary loss of urine in varying amounts (urgency incontinence).

Foul-Smelling Urine

The majority of organisms capable of producing acute bladder infection are also capable of splitting urea, with a resulting release of ammonia. This ammonia release gives infected urine its characteristic offensive odor. The splitting of urea with the release of ammonia occurs in an alkaline pH and it should be noted that anytime the urine is strongly alkaline, the odor of ammonia may result. This ammonia odor is not always caused or accompanied by urinary tract infection but may result simply from a very high (alkaline) urinary pH.

Intermittency

As the obstructive process continues, and the bladder begins to decompensate (due to a buildup of residual urine), the detrusor contraction at the time of voiding empties the bladder as well as it can, but urine still remains following this contraction. It is then not unusual for a second and weaker contraction of the detrusor to occur after its refractory period has passed, and this represents an attempt by the detrusor to empty the bladder more completely. It is during this refractory period for the detrusor that there is no flow of urine and the start–stop–start of the urinary stream is known as intermittency.

Terminal Dribbling

When there is advanced bladder outlet obstruction and residual urine remains following voiding, the second and weaker detrusor contraction following the refractory period for the bladder muscle attempts to empty the bladder of remaining urine. If just a small amount of urine remains and the patient is unaware that he has not emptied his bladder, he will close his trousers thinking that micturition has ceased. The weak secondary detrusor contraction can then bring about a terminal dribbling after the patient has closed his trousers, resulting in small amounts of urine wetting the patient's clothing. Some patients learn to anticipate this and do not close their trousers until the secondary detrusor contraction has brought out the last bit of urine. Terminal dribbling and intermittency are therefore both related to incomplete bladder emptying and the bladder's attempt to compensate by means of a second contraction.

Bladder Stones

Recurrent urinary tract infection with persistent alkalinization of the urine because of the action of urea-splitting organisms forces calcium phosphate and magnesium ammonium phosphate crystals out of solution and allows them to precipitate in the very alkaline pH. If there is significant residual urine following voiding, these precipitated crystals remain in the bladder and gradually coalesce to form bladder calculi. The composition of these calculi is inevitably calcium phosphate, magnesium ammonium phosphate, or both, and the presence of bladder stones is valid evidence of bladder outlet obstruction and long-standing infection within the bladder. It is uncommon, however, for a kidney stone to pass into the bladder and remain as the nidus for further growth, resulting in bladder stone formation in the absence of urinary tract infection and outlet obstruction.

Although bladder stones often form when the bladder urine is infected and when a high level of residual urine is present, the physician must realize that conditions other than BPH may be etiologic. In males, any condition that produces urinary retention postvoiding can result in infection and stone formation, and urethral stricture and neurogenic bladder are two other not uncommon causes of stones. Bladder incrustations (known as alkaline encrusted cystitis) and calculus formation also can occur in female patients with chronic urinary tract infections that produce significant urinary alkalinity and precipitation of large amounts of calcium phosphate and magnesium ammonium phosphate crystals.

Hematuria

Superficial blood vessels supplying the prostatic urethra, the bladder neck, and the bladder all course in the submucosa. As the prostatic adenoma enlarges in its normal submucosal position these blood vessels are often greatly stretched, and not infrequently they rupture spontaneously, leading to microscopic hematuria, gross hematuria, and even frank (and frightening) hemorrhage (depending on the size of the vessel that ruptures). This hematuria is usually of a transient nature but is a common enough occurrence that, in men over 50, hematuria secondary to BPH is possibly more common than hematuria caused by anything else (bladder cancer and BPH are considered to be the two most common causes of microscopic and gross hematuria in men over 50 years). Hematuria may also occur as a result of acute cystitis, often a sequella to the decompensated bladder with residual urine; in these cases acute inflammation of the bladder mucosa and submucosa may result in the rupture of small submucosal blood vessels.

Overflow Incontinence, Acute Urine Retention and Renal Failure

Although frequency has already been discussed in relation to trigonal hypertrophy with increased irritability and in relation to acute cystitis secondary to residual bladder urine, there is another cause that must be understood because, although uncommon, it can be the first symptom of BPH. In these cases, an individual will deny or be truly unaware of any urinary tract symptoms but will come to the physician's office with the complaint of having to void every 10, 20, or 30 minutes with some involuntary loss of urine if an appropriate place for voiding is not promptly available. In these patients the buildup of residual urine has been silent but complete to the point where a pint or more of urine remains in the bladder at all times. As additional urine arrives in the bladder from the kidney, the "overflow urine" produces a sudden desire to void with involuntary leakage of urine if voiding does not occur. In a less severe situation, the patient might come to the physician's office with a more modest amount of residual urine and complain of a frequency of every 30 to 60 minutes or every 2 hours without any incontinence. This latter symptom occurs because the patient may be carrying 100 to 200 ml of residual urine at all times; thus it does not take very long between voidings for fresh urine arriving from the kidney to bring the bladder capacity up to the level where the patient has another urge to void.

Although the majority of patients with BPH do in fact present with the "classic" symptoms of nocturia, hesitancy, frequency, weak urinary stream, and so on, a significant minority are completely unaware of any such early symptoms and may well initially present with the pronounced frequency, urgency, urgency incontinence, or even frank incontinence just outlined above. It is probable that this minority of patients are genuinely unaware of the more typical and classic symptoms of BPH because their symptomatology has been present over such a long period of time that they truly have not recognized any change in the usual voiding pattern. Other patients may feel that a difficulty in voiding somehow reflects negatively on their overall genital performance and thus deny symptoms at all costs, often at the subconscious level. A still smaller minority with BPH apparently have no symptoms whatever of which they are aware and then are suddenly forced to go to a hospital emergency room because of acute urinary retention with a pint or a quart or more of urine in the bladder. Still others will present with a true overflow incontinence wherein the bladder capacity is at its maximum and additional urine coming down from the kidneys results in an involuntary and virtually continuous leakage of urine per the urethra. It is worth bearing in mind that when involuntary leakage of urine occurs in men it is far more commonly due to BPH and overflow than to any neurologic disease. Finally, there is a very small group of individuals in whom the classic symptoms of BPH have never manifested themselves sufficiently to warrant the patient's attention, but a progressive back pressure on the ureters from a severely decompensated bladder results in uremia, which then becomes the first finding. These patients characteristically present with nausea, vomiting, lethargy, or uremic frost and sometimes they are comatose when first seen by a physician.

PHYSICAL EXAMINATION

Physical examination of the genitourinary tract in any man should always include suprapubic percussion and palpation to identify a distended bladder that might be otherwise unsuspected. Suprapubic palpation should also be done to disclose any tenderness that might suggest bladder infection. Attempted palpation of the kidneys and percussion of the costovertebral angle should be carried out to detect unsuspected kidney enlargement (hydronephrosis) or otherwise asymptomatic kidney infection (see Chapter 1).

After the external genitals are examined for normalcy, the physician should gently introduce a well-lubricated index finger into the rectum and note the anal sphincter tone. During this procedure, the patient is best placed in the knee–chest position on a table or bent sharply at the waist in the standing position with the feet well apart and the toes pointed medially. It is most important that the glans penis be briskly squeezed while the examining finger is still in the rectum to detect the normal bulbocavernosus reflex, which should produce a contraction of the anal sphincter on the examining finger. The absence of this contraction may possibly be of no significance, but it may be a major clue in detecting a defective sacral reflex arc that may be contributing to a neurogenic bladder of the atonic type. The physician must constantly bear in mind that atonic bladders may simulate all of the symptoms of BPH and that any individual with this condition may also have an atonic bladder. Not surprisingly, if these two conditions coexist, the expected results of surgical intervention to remove the periurethral adenomatous growth will not be as good as if only BPH is present.

After careful examination of the rectal mucosa so as not to miss any rectal lesions, the prostate gland should be palpated carefully to determine anatomic landmarks, consistency, size, firmness, and the presence of any nodules. A prostate gland that is not enlarged should have an easily palpable median sulcus and two lateral sulci and it should be readily possible to pass the index finger up over the base of the gland (see Chapter 1). Enlargement of the prostate gland is designated as follows:

- *Grade I:* The gland is up to twice its normal size and may be considered as having from 20 to 25 g of adenomatous growth (above the normal 20-g weight of the gland).
- *Grade II:* The gland is two to three times its normal nonhypertrophied size, with an estimated 25 to 50 g of adenomatous growth. A gland this size may not demonstrate a median sulcus due to enlargement of one or both lateral lobes.
- *Grade III:* The gland is three to four times its normal size, with 50 to 75 g of adenomatous growth. Such a gland is perhaps the size of a lemon, and the physician's examining finger may just reach the base of the gland. The median sulcus will commonly be obliterated.
- *Grade IV:* The gland is more than four times its normal size, with over 75 g of adenomatous growth. Such a gland is at least the size of an orange and it is not possible for the physician's examining finger to even reach the base of the gland. One or both lateral sulci will frequently be obliterated by the large growth of the lateral lobes. Clinically, less than 5 to 10 percent of patients coming to surgery have Grade IV prostatic enlargement.

It is imperative that the physician realize that the size of the prostate gland on rectal palpation does not necessarily reflect prostatic encroachment on the lumen of the prostatic urethra. It must be emphasized that a high degree of obstruction of the bladder outlet may be produced by a middle lobe hyperplasia that is absolutely not palpable on digital rectal examination (the middle lobe cannot, under any circumstances, be palpated by a digital rectal examination of the prostate gland) and that palpation of enlarged lateral lobes of the prostate gland does not necessarily indicate that there is lateral lobe encroachment on the prostatic urethra commensurate with the degree of enlargement found on rectal examination.

Digital rectal examination is likely to cause the patient a great deal of anxiety. The physician can allay these fears by describing the procedure before it is carried out and by asking the patient to verbalize any concerns that he may have about it.

DIAGNOSTIC METHODOLOGY

Laboratory Findings

Although there are no specific tests that are used to diagnose benign prostatic hyperplasia, urine analysis and a urine culture should be done to determine if urinary tract infection exists. Tests of blood urea nitrogen and creatinine levels are indicated to determine the functional status of the upper urinary tracts.

X-Ray Studies

X-ray studies are not done in patients with BPH for the purpose of establishing or refuting the presumptive diagnosis, but rather to evaluate the upper urinary tracts, to rule out any dilatation of these tracts secondary to prostatic obstruction, and to get a rough idea from the postvoiding film of the quantity of residual urine that may be present (Fig. 7–2). An excretory cystogram may disclose a trabeculated bladder with or without a postvoid residual urine; it may also disclose a filling defect in the bladder caused by an enlarged middle lobe or enlarged lateral lobes, and these findings may help to confirm the presumptive diagnosis. It must be pointed out that the absence of any of these roentgenographic findings or the presence of a perfectly normal excretory urogram in no way speaks against the diagnosis of benign prostatic hyperplasia if other factors, such as clinical history (from the patient) and digital rectal exam, tend to confirm the diagnosis.

Cystourethroscopy

Endoscopic visualization (cystourethroscopy) of the bladder and urethra contribute vital information to confirm the presence or absence of bladder outlet obstruction as well as the specific type of obstruction if one is present. This information is of the utmost importance in determining whether any surgical intervention is indicated and, if so, in selecting the best surgical approach from the several that are commonly used.

In the patient whose symptoms suggest a bladder outlet obstruction or in whom the excretory cystogram phase of the excretory urogram discloses bladder trabeculation, significant residual urine, or an enlarged prostate gland, cystoscopic examination is absolutely necessary. The only question is whether it should be done on an outpatient or inpatient basis. Although cystoscopy can virtually always be carried out under local anesthesia without discomfort to the patient, the suspected presence of significant residual urine greatly increases the chance of acute bladder infection following the procedure. For this reason it is wisest for the patient to be hospitalized before cystoscopy is carried out and it is most advantageous to carry out the procedure immediately prior to contemplated prostatic surgery. In this manner, the preliminary cystoscopy and the actual prostatic surgery (assuming that the latter is in fact indicated) are done under the same anesthetic and in the same operating time. If suspected prostatic obstruction is confirmed cystoscopically, surgery can follow immediately; if it is not, the patient can leave the hospital that day or the next. In evaluating patients for BPH, it is generally the author's practice to cystoscope on an outpatient basis only those patients with relatively few symptoms in whom it is felt that surgery will *not* be needed. The purpose of cystoscopy in these cases is to confirm the preliminary decision not to carry out surgery, to measure the residual urine, and to establish a baseline for future reference.

Regardless of whether cystoscopy is performed on an inpatient or outpatient basis an 18F or 21F cystourethroscope is generally used, as it permits thorough

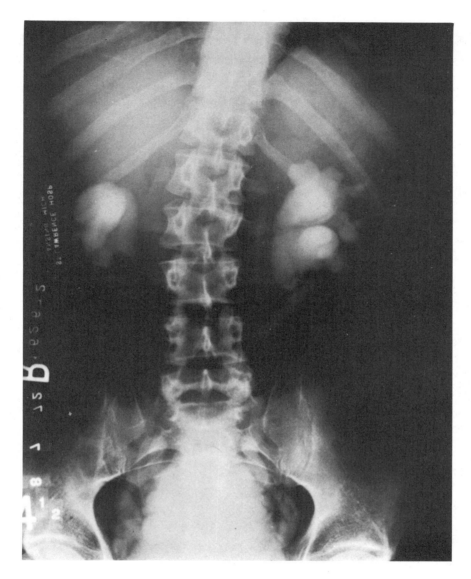

Figure 7-2. An excretory urogram. **A.** Considerable bilateral hydronephrosis and an enlarged and heavily trabeculated bladder in a 39-year-old male with significant bladder outlet obstruction secondary to prostatic hyperplasia.

evaluation of the interior of the bladder. Unsuspected bladder tumors may be diagnosed in this manner and the overall condition of the bladder mucosa can be thoroughly evaluated. The presence of bladder trabeculation, with or without cellules or diverticulae, offers objective evidence of bladder outlet obstruction. The already noted residual urine is a vital parameter of the bladder's ability to empty itself against an increased resistance, and this determination may be readily measured by having

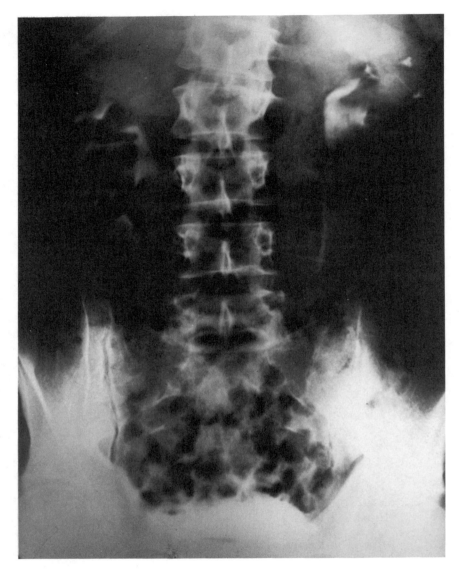

Figure 7-2B. The same patient 8 months after surgical relief of the outlet obstruction and the upper urinary tracts have returned to normal and the bladder is no longer distended.

the patient void immediately prior to cystourethroscopy. The amount of urine present in the bladder when the instrument is introduced offers an accurate measurement of residual urine.

Perhaps the most important thing to be determined by cystourethroscopy, however, is confirmation of the bladder outlet obstruction by direct observation of the prostatic urethra (recall that a neurogenic bladder and a urethral stricture can both simulate bladder outlet obstruction). The other important piece of knowledge to be gained from the urethroscopic evaluation is the type and extent of prostatic hyperplasia that is present. When this preoperative measurement is carefully determined, the specific surgical approach may be planned and carried out. Prostatic surgery, therefore, should not be carried out without the preliminary cystourethroscopic evaluation of the bladder and urethra to confirm the presence of bladder outlet obstruction, the best surgical approach, and the normalcy or abnormality of the bladder.

Urodynamic Studies

Extraordinarily sophisticated studies to measure pressures generated within the bladder during voiding, pressures within the prostatic urethra during voiding, urethral and anal sphincter activity during voiding, and voiding flow rates have been developed and perfected in the last 5 to 10 years. Most of these studies are best used in a research setting or for the purpose of evaluating voiding difficulties in patients whose symptoms are obscure and clearly not due to the normally encountered type of benign prostatic hyperplasia. An example of the type of patient in whom urodynamic studies might be helpful would include the patient with a neurogenic bladder of one sort or another. However, it is often helpful to measure a peak urine flow rate, and this can simply be done with a measured container and a stopwatch. A peak urine flow rate of over 20 ml/sec is normal (this varies with age) and under 10 ml/sec suggests a significant bladder outlet obstruction. In the range from 10 to 20 ml/sec there is probably a bladder outlet obstruction that exists, but how significant it is and whether or not surgery is indicated are dependent upon other findings in the diagnostic workup.

TREATMENT

Nonsurgical Treatment

For many years various estrogens have been used in an attempt to shrink the prostate gland, but the results have been far too variable and the side effects much too troublesome and unpleasant for these agents to become accepted. The general feeling of those individuals actively pursuing research in this field seems to be that there may someday be an appropriate agent to prevent BPH, but the discovery within the foreseeable future of a drug without any unpleasant side effects that can reverse already present BPH is not anticipated.

Surgical Treatment

Surgery remains the preferred method for the treatment of benign prostatic hyperplasia. Indications for surgical intervention include the following:

1. Symptoms of bladder outlet obstruction, such as nocturia, frequency, hesitancy, intermittency, weak urinary stream, and terminal dribbling. This group of symptoms constitutes what might be called the subjective indications for prostatic surgery. Ideally, there should also be objective evidence of outlet obstruction such as bladder trabeculation, residual urine, back pressure on the upper urinary tract as seen on excretory urography, and recurrent urinary tract infection. This last group of findings constitutes what could be called objective indications for prostatic surgery.
2. Evidence of bladder outlet obstruction determined by rectal palpation, excretory urography, and cystourethroscopy. Such evidence could consist of

bladder trabeculation or trigonal hypertrophy, residual urine, recurrent infection, or the like. Obviously, this group of indications would also come under the heading of objective indications.

3. Residual urine, with the larger the volume of residual urine the greater the need for surgery. Inasmuch as residual urine is a very late finding in the pathophysiology of BPH it is fallacious to say that surgical intervention is not necessary *until* residual urine is present. When it is present, surgical intervention is probably mandatory.

4. Recurrent urinary or prostatic infection that is secondary to bladder outlet obstruction.

5. Impaired renal function due to long-standing obstruction. Note that in these cases preliminary drainage by catheter may be indicated prior to surgery.

6. Hemorrhage from dilated blood vessels, a finding that is usually associated with a massive prostatic hyperplasia.

7. Acute urinary retention or overflow incontinence.

Transurethral, perineal, suprapubic, and retropubic approaches are common in prostatic surgery for benign hyperplasia. Each has its advantages and disadvantages.

The principal advantages of the *transurethral approach* are reduced hospitalization time and lower morbidity than with other surgical approaches. Patient mortality is between 1 and 2 percent, about the same as in other methods of prostatic surgery, with the mortality almost always resulting from a myocardial infarction or a pulmonary embolus. The transurethral approach is probably the procedure of choice in the majority of cases of BPH, but there is no question that it is by far the most difficult surgically; special equipment is necessary and a high degree of skill on the part of the urologist is mandatory because the risks of blood loss and urinary incontinence are real (although minimal, in skilled hands) and other unpleasant postoperative complications such as bladder neck contracture and urethral stricture are also possible. This operative approach is *not* indicated in patients with severe hip ankylosis that would preclude the lithotomy position and it would probably not be indicated in cases of massive adenoma (Grade 3 or 4 prostatic hyperplasia) unless the skill of the urologist is exceptional.

Perineal prostatectomy has a few advantages but they are mostly theoretical; It affords the most direct surgical approach to the prostate gland through a relatively avascular field; the incision provides for a physiologic dependent drainage of the operative wound. However, there are few or no practical advantages to this approach in the treatment of BPH. Some physicians feel that there is an increased incidence of impotence and incontinence following this perineal procedure, but this is probably not the case.

The prime advantages of the *suprapubic approach* are that it is relatively easy to do and very large adenomas are amenable to this approach. Also, a minimum of special equipment is needed. Moreover, it can be done without benefit of excellent relaxation or exposure. The primary disadvantage is the difficulty in controlling bleeding because the points of bleeding are not adequately visualized. There are few, if any, specific indications for this type of procedure except perhaps the absence of surgical assistants, a paucity of specialized surgical instruments, and the necessity to examine the interior of the bladder, which may not have been done previously for one reason or another. The procedure is contraindicated for known carcinoma of the prostate gland.

Retropubic prostatectomy is indicated, as is the suprapubic approach, when a massive adenoma is present. It is indicated, as in the suprapubic approach, in patients in whom ankylosis of the hips precludes the lithotomy position. It is contraindicated in the presence of carcinoma of the prostate gland. The advantages of the retropubic approach are that it permits ideal exposure of the prostatic bed and vesical neck and greatly facilitates precise control of bleeding. Its disadvantages are that special equipment is needed and the exposure can be very difficult in obese patients or in those with a narrow or deep pelvis.

Transurethral cryosurgery has had its advocates and achieved a very mild degree of popularity in the 1960s but there are frankly few, if any, indications for this form of surgery the complications of which far exceed its advantages.

It should be noted that for all of the surgical approaches noted above the incidence of incontinence runs about 1 percent. Although there is absolutely no physiologic reason for impotence to occur following any of these surgical procedures (except possibly the perineal approach) there are some patients that claim erectile dysfunction following surgery. It is the author's feeling that this could be greatly minimized if each patient is firmly told prior to surgery that he should anticipate an erectile state postoperatively comparable to what it was preoperatively.

PSYCHOLOGIC CONSIDERATIONS

From the technical point of view, surgery of the prostate gland is now highly refined and very successful. From the patient's point of view, however, it is just as fearful a procedure as it has ever been because the prostate gland and sexuality are inevitably intertwined in the minds of most men. The clinician who would reassure a patient about impending prostate surgery must first be fully conversant with the pathophysiology of the obstructive process of BPH, and at least have a passing familiarity with the operative procedures involved in treating this condition. It is of paramount importance that primary care physicians explain the operative procedure to the family and the patient, and also important that they elicit from the patient his expectations about how he will function, in a urologic and sexual sense, following surgery. Clinicians should question patients about the kinds of fears they have about being in the hospital, for example, the necessity of an indwelling catheter, and particularly any fears about change in sexual or other physiologic function following recovery from surgery. Once the clinician has allowed the patient to verbalize all of these anxieties, it is but a short step to reassure him by explanation based on an understanding of the clinical situation that his sexual function will not be altered following surgery, that his pain will be very minimal (unless he has open prostate surgery), and that the presence of an indwelling catheter will produce frequent sensations of having to void, but no true discomfort in most patients. The clinician must also explain carefully to the patient the role of the nursing staff in the postoperative period so that he may be reassured about being physically exposed to, and particularly about having his genitalia handled by, a female nurse should there be any necessity to irrigate the catheter, change the catheter, or so on.

POSTOPERATIVE DELIRIUM

Postoperative delirium can be an aftermath of any kind of surgery. It is perhaps more frequent after prostatic surgery, because the patients are often elderly. The physican should be alert to the possibility of delirium and, when visiting the patient after surgery, establish that he is oriented to time, place, person, and recent memory. This may be done by asking the patient to recall, for example, what he had for breakfast, who his last visitors were or various aspects of current events. The patient should also be asked to perform simple calculations such as serial subtraction of sevens. Signs and symptoms of delirium include manifest confusion, hostile behavior that did not previously exist, and lack of cooperation regarding his medical regimen, as evidenced by pulling on the catheter or by removal of intravenous needles. Also, deterioration in his levels of awareness and cooperativeness, particularly in the evening and night hours, and even extreme depression that was nonexistent before surgery may be signs of delirium. The clinician should be particularly careful to search for major organic causes and factors in postoperative delirium, such as electrolyte imbalance, elevated BUN level, dehydration, or congestive heart failure, in addition to the possibility of exacerbation of impaired mental function by drugs such as barbiturates, other sedatives, and Valium. Combatting delirium involves restoration of the normal physiologic functions of the patient and removal of noxious agents as well as general supportive measures such as leaving a light on in the patient's room at night, orienting the patient continually to time by placing a clock in the patient's room (the constant ticking of the clock can become a comfort to the confused patient), and limiting the number of staff who come into contact with the patient so that he is not constantly exposed to new faces. This last problem makes many elderly patients become delirious and confused. The rationale of the loudly ticking clock by the bedside is that it tends to serve as a constant presence to which the patient can become accustomed and upon which he can rely for continuity in the face of ever-changing hospital personnel.

REFERENCES

Brugh R, Rous SN: The incidence of bladder obstruction in male inguinal hernia patients over 50 years of age. Urology 10:550, 1977

Hinman F Jr (ed): Benign Prostatic Hypertrophy. New York, Springer, 1983

Rous SN: Urology in Primary Care. St. Louis, Mosby, 1976

Rous SN: Benign lesions of the prostate and vesical neck. In Kendall AR, Karafin L (eds), Urology. Philadelphia, Harper and Row, 1983, vol 2, chap 15

8
Stone Disease

EDUCATIONAL OBJECTIVES

1. List the most common metabolic causes of renal stone formation.
2. Discuss the relationship of obstruction and infection to stone formation.
3. List the common types of urinary tract stones.
4. Discuss the medical management of recurrent stone formation for calcium oxalate stones, calcium phosphate stones, and uric acid stones.
5. Discuss the management of the patient with a 5-mm stone in the ureter.
6. Discuss the management of the patient with a 1.5-cm stone in the ureter.
7. List the indications for surgical intervention when there is a stone (1) in the kidney, and (2) in the ureter.
8. List the symptoms of stones in the bladder.
9. List the steps to be taken in determining the etiology of stone formation in the patient with recurrent urolithiasis.

Medicine is a science in which spectacular breakthroughs in diagnosis and treatment occur with regularity. Stone disease of the urinary tract is almost as old as recorded history itself and very little change in either diagnosis or treatment of this common problem occurred through most of this recorded history. Within the past few years, however, the progress in diagnosis, medical management, and surgical management of stone disease has been so extraordinary that it may even be compared to the change in the management of infectious diseases after the introduction of antibiotics.

INCIDENCE

Although it is obviously difficult to give any figures regarding the precise incidence of urolithiasis, various studies from around the world suggest that from 6 to 15 percent of males and 3 to 5 percent of females are afflicted with this condition. The incidence of urolithiasis in males as compared to females is about 3:1. About 1 percent of hospital discharges in the United States indicate urolithiasis as the presenting problem or a secondary problem. It is safe to say that urolithiasis is a common problem and it is seemingly becoming even more common. There is also general agreement that the highest incidence of stone disease in the United States is found in the Southeast (the so-called stone belt), but the precise reason or reasons for this are not known.

In the United States the most common type of stone found in patients with urolithiasis is composed of calcium oxalate; approximately three quarters of the patients with stone disease have this type of stone. About 17 percent of patients have a mixed phosphate type of stone and about 7 percent to 8 percent of patients have uric acid lithiasis. In general, the disease is much more likely to occur in males than in females and this follows a ratio that is somewhere between 3:1 and 4:1. It is far more common in whites than in blacks by a ratio of somewhere between 7:1 and 10:1.

ETIOLOGY

Although a great deal of research has been done within the last several years with regard to the causative factors of urolithiasis, it has primarily centered around diagnostic approaches to lithiasis and to finding the best approach to stone prevention based on particular characteristics of the stone itself and of the urine produced by the individuals susceptible to stone formation. To date, what we do know is that urinary tract calculi are composed primarily of crystalline and organic substances, but the interrelationship of these two components as far as which of the two is the initiating factor in stone formation is still uncertain. Some researchers feel that the organic material in a stone, which is known as the matrix, plays only a very minor role in the inception or the organization of the stone and that it is simply trapped by the deposit of the inorganic crystals such as uric acid, calcium phosphate, or calcium oxalate. Others, probably the majority of those working in the field of urolithiasis, feel that the precipitation of inorganic salts (the crystalline material) is dependent on the presence of an organic matrix that consists of a large molecular mucopolysaccharide, such as uromucoid, upon which the inorganic crystals can precipitate. If indeed this latter theory, the so-called matrix theory, is correct, then one possible etiology of stone occurrence might be through increased urinary osmolarity (caused, for example by dehydration), resulting in a precipitation of uromucoid with deposition of calcium oxalate or calcium phosphate on this precipitated uromucoid. The complex thus formed would stick within the lumen of the renal tubules and, by the enzymatic action of sialic acid, the uromucoid would be converted to a permanently insoluble complex that would then become the nidus for a stone. It must be noted, however, that this theory is neither universally accepted nor thoroughly documented and may prove to be nothing more than a theory.

Without question, there are many other factors in urolithiasis that indeed play a major role in stone formation, regardless of what will ultimately prove to be the primary initiating factor. The pH of the urine, the osmolarity of the urine, the presence or absence of various inhibitors or promoters of crystallization in the urine, the concentration of ions such as calcium and oxalate in the urine, and the state of saturation of the urine are among the factors that are well known to be critical in stone formation.

THE ONE-TIME STONE FORMER

The author feels that the one-time stone former is in a rather different situation from the patient with recurrent lithiasis, as it is likely that the one-time stone former has no underlying metabolic abnormality or other disease process predisposing to stone formation. At least half of the one-time stone formers will probably not form another stone in the foreseeable future, if ever, and so the author does not feel it necessary to determine an etiology for the single episode. The principal goal in establishing an etiology for lithiasis is to then be able to put the patient on the correct prophylactic medication such that lithiasis will not recur. In the author's experience, it is not only unnecessary for half of the patients with a one-time episode of lithiasis to receive *any* prophylactic medication, but it seems to be extremely unlikely that there will be any patient compliance with a regimen of medication two, three, or even four times daily for an indefinite period when a patient has had only one episode of lithiasis. For these reasons, the author feels that the one-time stone former should be properly treated for the episode of lithiasis and a definite screening should be made for hyperparathyroid disease because this disease requires surgical therapy regardless of whether or not it has contributed to urolithiasis; however, further attempts at a full-scale metabolic workup are probably not indicated.

THE PATIENT WITH RECURRENT UROLITHIASIS

In addition to patients who have clinically had more than one episode of lithiasis, there is another group of patients that should also be included in the group of patients whom the author feels require a full metabolic workup. These are the patients that may be said to have metabolically active disease. Specifically this means that within the previous year, they have had any or all of the following: documented passage of gravel in the urine; documented growth of a preexisting stone within a kidney; and documented growth of a new stone within a kidney. Thus, patients with urolithiasis that is either metabolically active or clinically recurrent should be included in the group of patients undergoing full diagnostic workup for therapeutic purposes.

EVALUATION OF THE PATIENT
WITH RECURRENT UROLITHIASIS

The cornerstone for the evaluation of these patients rests with two or three serially repeated 24-hour urine collections for calcium, uric acid, oxalate, and creatinine clearance and three or four serum determinations of calcium, uric acid, creatinine, electrolytes, and phosphorus. The creatinine clearance study is for baseline purposes. The 24-hour urine for oxalate is an extremely important determination and is notoriously difficult to do with any degree of reproducibility and accuracy. The author has found that the oxalate decarboxalase enzymatic method is an excellent, if somewhat tedious method, and there is now at least one new enzymatic method that. is automated and equally excellent. In addition, a new "kit" has recently been marketed for the determination of urinary oxalate levels. This new kit is extremely accurate and yields highly reproducible results; it is made by Sigma Diagnostics of St. Louis, Missouri. The 24-hour urine for calcium should be collected in an acid medium at a ph of 2–3, and this may be done by using 20 millileters of bN HCl (Hydrochloric acid). Failure to do so will result in precipitation of calcium phosphate and even calcium oxalate crystals; this precipitated calcium cannot be driven back into solution if the acid is not added until *after* the precipitate has formed. This error in the technique of making the urine collection will result in extremely and falsely low 24-hour urinary calcium levels.

In referring to patients with recurrent urolithiasis the author specifically means those patients who have had more than one clinical episode of lithiasis as well as those patients who are felt to have metabolically active disease. This is the group in whom definitive therapy is indicated and therefore in whom a careful metabolic investigation is warranted so that specific therapy can be tailored to the specific etiology. Therapy means definitive drug therapy but it goes without saying that this should only be employed when a patient with recurrent lithiasis is either unable to ingest sufficient fluids to keep his urine volume at three or more liters daily or this therapy proves not to be effective.

In trying to evaluate the patient with recurrent urolithiasis it is helpful to realize that there are many etiologies for this problem, with approximately the following breakdown:

1. "Idiopathic" lithiasis— ± 70 percent of patients
2. Tubular or enzymatic disorders— ± 1 percent of patients
3. Primary hyperparathyroidism— ± 5 percent of patients
4. Other primary disorders, such as hypercalcemic states (besides hyperparathyroidism), uric acid lithiasis, and gastroenterologic disorders ± 20 percent

All patients in the "idiopathic" renal lithiasis category are normocalcemic by definition. First let us look carefully at the "idiopathic" category, which is really not idiopathic at all, and which may be divided into two broad groups of patients: those with *hypercalciuria* (more than 300 mg of calcium per 24 hours of urine in men and 275 mg per 24 hours in women) and those with *normocalciuria*.

Those patients with *hypercalciuria* are then subdivided into patients who are renal tubular "leakers" and patients who are "hyperabsorbers" (from the gut). The renal tubular "leakers" fail to reabsorb much of the calcium that is presented to the renal tubules and the hyperabsorbers absorb abnormally large amounts of calcium from the gut even when normal amounts of calcium are ingested. There are numerous protocols that have been devised so that the clinician can separate the hypercalciuric patient who is a renal tubular "leaker" from the hypercalciuric patient who is a hyperabsorber. One of the simpler methods used is to keep the patient on his or her regular diet followed by an overnight fast for about 14 hours, after which a 2-hour urine collection between 7 and 9 A.M. is taken. If there is less than 20 mg of calcium in this specimen, it is probable that the patient is a hyperabsorber, because fasting a patient who is a hyperabsorber will reduce the amount of calcium in the urine. If the 2-hour urine specimen, however, discloses more than 20 mg of calcium in the urine, then the study should be repeated and the fasting period lengthened. Persistent presence of more than 20 mg of calcium in the 2-hour urine specimen after a prolonged fast strongly suggests that the patient is a renal tubular "leaker."

It must be emphasized that the patient should be on a normal diet (for that individual) immediately prior to the fasting period if the study is to be meaningful, but it should be noted that some hypercalciuric patients will require a high calcium diet if it is suspected that these patients are hypercalciuric because they periodically go on calcium intake "binges." The basic rule of thumb, however, is to try to have them stay on a diet that is as close as possible to their regular diet both during the 24-hour collection period, when the decision will be made as to whether they are hypercalciuric or normocalciuric, until the overnight fast and the 2-hour collection period, when the attempt will be made to differentiate the hyperabsorbers from the renal tubular leakers. In the author's experience the renal tubular leakers outnumber the hyperabsorbers by a ratio of at least 3 to 1.

The other broad category of patient fitting under the heading of "idiopathic" is the *normocalcemic, normocalciuric patient,* and these patients represent about 50 to 60 percent of the patients in the "idiopathic" category. The usual reason for the normocalcemic, normocalciuric form of urolithiasis is probably a defect of one or more of the urinary inhibitors of crystallization, of which some of the better known ones are magnesium, citrate, pyrophosphate, RNA-like substances, heparin-like substances, and glycosaminoglycans (GAGS). Other known causes of normocalcemic, normocalciuric "idiopathic" urolithiasis are hyperuricosuria, in which the increased number of uric acid crystals seems to bring about an increased precipitation of calcium oxalate crystals, a secondary hyperoxaluria usually due to dietary factors such as the ingestion of large amounts of iced tea, and an increased urinary alkalinity that is fairly persistent in the region of pH 6.5 to 7.0 and that leads to precipitation of calcium phosphate crystals with resulting calcium phosphate lithiasis.

Renal Tubular Syndromes and Enzyme Disorders

In this category are very uncommon conditions such as cystinuria, renal tubular acidosis, and primary hyperoxaluria. Cystinuria may be identified by the presence of hexagonal crystals in the urine, and by positive nitroprusside tests; renal tubular acidosis in its complete form may be suspected if the patient has a persistent hyperchloremic acidosis, which, unfortunately, is not present in its incomplete form. This condition may be suspected if the pH of the *second* voided morning specimen after an overnight fast is not less than 5.5. Confirmation may then be obtained by testing the patient with an ammonium chloride load that will (if positive and the patient has renal tubular acidosis) fail to acidify the urine below 5.8. Based on this test, a diagnosis of type I renal tubular acidosis may be made. Primary hyperoxaluria, a condition usually found in children, may be diagnosed if the 24-hour urinary oxalate level is over 40 mg. It may be differentiated from a hyperoxaluria that is secondary due to dietary excesses by carefully obtaining a dietary history and also by measuring the plasm glycolate. If this level is elevated above 0.3 mmol/l, a constant value in adults and children that is not affected by renal failure, the diagnosis of primary hyperoxaluria may be made; if it is less than 0.3 mmol/l, a diagnosis of secondary or dietary hyperoxaluria may be made.

Hypercalcemic States

That produce hypercalcemia and a secondary hypercalciuria can be responsible for recurrent urolithiasis in numerous ways. Undoubtedly the most common is through primary hyperparathyroidism, which the author feels is best diagnosed by an elevated serum calcium level. Other conditions leading to a hypercalcemia are prolonged immobilization, milk alkali syndrome, sarcoidosis, hypervitaminosis D, neoplasms, excessive steroid use, or Cushing syndrome and hyperthyroidism.

Uric Acid Lithiasis

Comprises between 5 and 10 percent of calculi in this country and most often the lithiasis is idiopathic in that there is no associated gout and the patient has normal blood and urine uric acid levels. The condition may be suspected by the fact that the urine pH is usually less than 5.5.

Gastrointestinal Disorders:

Ileostomies and protracted diarrhea states will lead to excess loss of water and bicarbonate, with a resulting low urine volume and a pH near 5. Uric acid lithiasis will frequently result with these conditions. Additionally, the so-called short bowel syndrome and conditions such as small bowel bypass for obesity, small bowel resections, primary small bowel disease, etc. will often lead to an excess of fatty acids in the gut and these tend to bind the calcium that is in the gut, thereby leaving the intestinal oxalate free to become absorbed in sufficient quantities to lead to a secondary hyperoxaluria and a resulting calcium oxalate lithiasis. As a general rule, the large intestine must be intact in order for this secondary hyperoxaluria with resulting calcium oxalate lithiasis to occur.

It is almost always possible to uncover the proper etiology of recurrent lithiasis, but it takes persistence, a definite protocol of procedures to be followed, and particularly an excellent laboratory that is able to do highly accurate and reproducible 24-hour urine determinations. Inasmuch as the vast majority of recurrent urolithiasis (about 75 percent in the United States) is calcium oxalate, it would not be unwise for the clinician to concentrate on this type of lithiasis and become thoroughly familiar with the metabolic steps outlined above to determine the precise etiologies for its different forms. It is also absolutely mandatory that a very precise stone analysis be carried out, and the author feels that this can best be done by using a crystallographic technique of x-ray diffraction that will elucidate any stone nidus that is present and will also give specific percentages of stone ingredients.

Therapy for each of the various etiologic types of lithiasis is very specific. Inasmuch as each has its definite drawbacks and complicating side effects, it is imperative that the clinician establish the precise etiology for the recurrent urolithiasis so that appropriate, and not "shotgun," therapy may be used.

OBSTRUCTION AND INFECTION

Until a few years ago, obstruction and infection were felt to be the most common causes of recurrent urolithiasis, but this is no longer the case. Unquestionably, these entities still play a role, either contributory or primary, but this role is not nearly as great as was formerly thought. Obviously, the kidney damaged by infection may be predisposed to lithiasis. For the most part, however, these stones are the so-called infected stones and consist of magnesium ammonium phosphate or "triple" phosphate, as it is sometimes called. They form in a highly alkaline pH that results from the urea-splitting action of certain organisms, with *Proteus* being the most notorious offender. However, virtually any organism capable of causing infection in the urinary tract can split urea and produce highly alkaline urine if present in a virulent enough form and in large enough numbers. The other way, perhaps theoretical, in which infection can lead to urolithiasis is if the infection produces areas of mucosal damage or alteration of the renal pyramids or the renal papillae on which organic matrix material and crystalline material can precipitate to become the nidus of a renal stone. The author feels that this type of situation is probably much more theoretical than real, but it certainly may occasionally be a factor in urolithiasis.

Obstruction anywhere in the urinary tract can obviously lead to a slowing of the urine flow within the kidney. This may contribute to stone formation because a sharply decreased urine flow rate may permit organic matrix and crystalline material to precipitate out of solution and adhere to the urothelium.

In summary, there is no question that infection and obstruction can play a role in urolithiasis; however, the role is indeed a small one in terms of the overall picture. Perhaps the most important point for the clinician to realize when talking about the role of infection and urinary tract calculi is that it is extraordinarily difficult to treat a kidney infection successfully when there is a coexisting renal calculus. Removal of the calculus must be accomplished before successful sterilization of the kidney can be carried out.

BLADDER CALCULI

If obstruction or infection is an uncommon cause of upper urinary tract calculi, it certainly represents the most common cause of bladder calculi. Although a stone in the bladder may sometimes originate in the kidney, pass into the bladder, and then remain and grow after reaching the bladder, the vast majority of bladder calculi are secondary to bladder outlet obstruction, a condition that inevitably leads to the presence of residual urine. This, in turn, usually becomes infected unless the bladder outlet obstruction is relieved surgically. The infected urine, which is alkaline, in turn leads to the precipitation of crystals and ultimately to stone formation. Once bladder infection has occurred, antibiotic usage can only treat the specific infection; a recurrence of the infection is inevitable unless the bladder outlet obstruction is removed. Stones in the bladder secondary to bladder outlet obstruction and infection are usually either magnesium ammonium phosphate or calcium phosphate. Because the patient is unable to empty his or her bladder during voiding, the initial crystalline deposits are not washed out with the urine but remain behind and serve as a nidus onto which more crystals adhere, until ultimately one or more calculi form in the bladder.

Bladder outlet obstruction and infection need not coexist in order for bladder calculi to form. Infection alone may lead to a crystalline precipitation of sufficient magnitude to permit encrustation and the formation of small calculi; however, the presence of significant postvoiding residual urine contributes heavily to the formation of bladder calculi and, in the majority of patients, infection and obstruction do occur together. As mentioned above, efforts to remove the calculi or to cure the infection without also relieving the obstruction will only result in a recurrence of both.

Any condition that causes a decompensated bladder with postvoiding residual urine can and usually does lead to infection and calculus formation. In addition to benign prostatic hyperplasia, chronic urethral strictures, congenital bladder obstruction, neurogenic bladder, urethral valves, and meatal stenosis are other pathologic entities that may contribute to infection and bladder stone formation. In the absence of any lower urinary tract disease, such as bladder outlet obstruction, small calculi reaching the bladder from points of origin in the kidney are usually voided spontaneously. Nevertheless, it is justifiable to carry out a metabolic workup, even if only for screening purposes, when any patient has bladder calculi even if these calculi are initially thought to arise in the bladder. More than one patient has presented with bladder calculi that appeared to be of bladder origin but were ultimately proven to have resulted from parathyroid adenomas.

DIAGNOSTIC METHODOLOGY FOR THE PATIENT THOUGHT TO HAVE UROLITHIASIS

History

Patients who have had prior episodes of urolithiasis are often able to identify their symptoms as those of renal colic; however, for the first-time stone patient, the history may have many variables. Classically, there is an acute onset of severe flank, upper abdominal, lower abdominal, or groin pain, with the location of the pain depending on the location of the stone. If the calculus is obstructing the drainage from the kidney and causing a hydronephrosis that results in an outward pressure against a fairly rigid renal capsule, the pain will be predominantly in the flank or costovertebral angle. As the stone moves down the ureter, the pain tends to become more anterior, is characteristically colicky in nature, and is often extremely severe. The reason for the severity of the pain is poorly understood but it may possibly be due to ureteral anoxia secondary to the pressure of the stone on the ureteral wall. As the stone passes down the ureter and if the kidney remains acutely obstructed, pain will be present in the flank as well as anteriorly. However, if the downward movement of the stone relieves the obstruction to the drainage of the kidney, there will be little or no flank pain and all of the discomfort will be anterior. As the calculus gets into the lower third of the ureter, and particularly as it approaches and enters the intramural ureter, there are usually accompanying symptoms of urgency, frequency, suprapubic pressure, and pain referred into the testes or labia majora. There is almost always microscopic hematuria and there may be some gross hematuria accompanying the downward progress of a stone *unless* the stone is completely occluding the ureter so that blood from the proximal ureteral trauma cannot pass the stone and reach the bladder.

Physical Examination

Physical examination of the patient who is passing a ureteral stone classically reveals a patient in acute pain and discomfort. When the pain is in the upper or lower abdomen, differentiation from intraabdominal pathology must be made. There is usually abdominal guarding and tenderness and there often may be rebound tenderness as well because the posterior peritoneum is lying directly over the ureter, with peritonitis possibly resulting from direct contact with an inflamed ureter. In the differential diagnosis of ureteral colic one must often consider virtually all of the intraabdominal and intrapelvic conditions that can cause severe inflammation and pain.

It is worth noting that if the stone is in a renal calyx there are usually no symptoms whatever and certainly no findings on physical examination. If the calculus is floating free within the renal pelvis, there may be no symptoms at all or they may be intermittent pain and discomfort, usually in the flank, when the stone drops down to the point that it obstructs the ureteropelvic junction and produces a transient hydronephrosis.

Urinalysis

Analysis of the urine sediment of patients with stone disease typically shows several to many red blood cells per high power field with or without accompanying white blood cells. Several crystals may also be seen in the urinary sediment and are helpful in reaching a diagnosis inasmuch as their presence in normal urinary sediment is uncommon. The urine should also be cultured when the patient is seen because if urinary tract infection is present, it may significantly change the management of the patient with urolithiasis.

Roentgoengraphic Studies

Definitive diagnosis of stone disease is usually made with an infusion excretory urogram. Not infrequently, the osmotic diuresis produced by the injection of the contrast medium is sufficient to bring about spontaneous passage of a small calculus. Urograms usually disclose dilatation of the ureter and the renal collecting system above the point of the calculus, although this finding is dependent on the size of the stone and the degree of obstruction present (Fig. 8–1). It is also possible that a small stone might be radiolucent or have already passed into the bladder by the

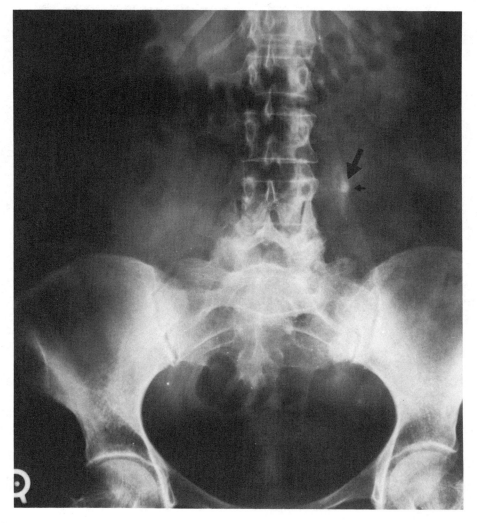

Figure 8–1. A. Plain film showing a stone in the midportion of the left ureter (*arrow*).

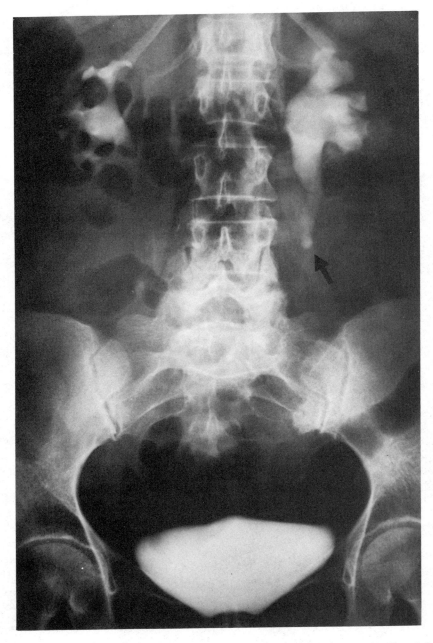

Figure 8–1. B. An excretory urogram in the same patient showing a significant hydro-ureteronephrosis above and down to the level of the stone (*arrow*).

time the urograms are done. Typically, calcium oxalate and calcium phosphate stones are radiopaque, whereas uric acid stones are frequently radiolucent and not visible on x-rays although there may be sufficient calcium within the stone to allow for some radiopacity. Cystine stones are less dense than calcium oxalate or calcium phosphate stones, but they are clearly visible when found in the adult; in children they are usually radiolucent. Although most urinary tract calculi are visible on the excretory urograms, some calculi, as just noted, are not. In these special situations, retrograde ureteropyelograms, with or without air contrast studies, may be helpful in the identification and localization of calculi.

It is the author's feeling that excretory urograms should be performed in virtually all patients suspected of having symptomatic urinary tract calculi unless there is a valid reason to circumvent this. A known severe allergy to contrast medium, for example, is certainly a bona fide reason not to perform excretory urography. Also, if a patient has a prior history of renal/ureteral calculi and is able to tell the physician that his or her present and previous symptoms are the same, there is probably no overriding need to obtain urograms. For the vast majority of patients, however, there are two primary reasons for obtaining the excretory urograms. First, it is used to document the provisional diagnosis of calculus disease. This is particularly important in the face of a totally normal excretory urogram, particularly if there is no microscopic hematuria. A diligent search must be made for other causes that could be producing the patient's severe pain because some of these causes are genuine surgical emergencies (i.e., leaking aneurysms) that must be addressed and investigated. The other overriding reason that excretory urograms should be done in patients suspected of having calculus disease is because the management of the patient often depends on the results of these studies. A small calculus that is not causing any obstruction to kidney drainage, for example, can often be observed indefinitely to see if it will pass spontaneously. However, the same small calculus (or any calculus for that matter) that is causing a moderate to severe hydronephrosis cannot be observed indefinitely and some sort of surgical intervention may well be indicated. It is extremely difficult to determine the degree of obstruction above a calculus (and to simultaneously document the diagnosis of a calculus) without an excretory urogram.

MANAGEMENT OF THE PATIENT WITH A DOCUMENTED URINARY TRACT CALCULUS

Indications for hospitalization of the patient with calculus disease include severe pain that is only temporarily relieved by narcotics; inability to hold down oral fluids because of nausea or vomiting; an elevated temperature such that infection above the obstructing calculus is suspected; and a moderate or high-grade obstruction above the calculus in a patient felt to be too unreliable to return as requested for follow-up. When the patient is hospitalized, the urine should be cultured if this has not already been done and each voiding for a 24- to 48-hour period checked for pH since that often gives a good hint as to the type of stone present. A pH that is fairly constant around 5.5 or lower suggests a uric acid or a cystine stone. A pH that is consistently higher (more alkaline than 7) should lead the physician to suspect a magnesium ammonium phosphate stone, which is invariably associated with urinary tract infection. A pH in the range of 6.5 to 7 might indicate a calcium phosphate stone, but these stones, and also calcium oxalate stones are often associated with a highly variable pH. The author does not suggest that all of these pH determinations be done in the hospital laboratory because this would be quite costly, but rather that they be done at the nurses station using nitrazine paper or some other type of pH indicator. Examination of the urine sediment when the patient is hospitalized can be most helpful particularly if hexagonal crystals of cystine are seen because this is almost always indicative of cystinuria and cystine lithiasis. Other crystals seen in the urine may or may not be helpful indicators in determining the type of stones present. The patient should be well hydrated when hospitalized, and this is best done with intravenous fluid if the patient is not able to tolerate an oral intake of at least 3000 ml daily and preferably even more. The objective is to induce a sufficient diuresis so that the passage of the stone is mechanically assisted; in willing patients, the author encourages a high intake of beer for this purpose. Probably the most important thing that is done for the hospitalized patient, however, is to keep him or her dosed with sufficient narcotics to make the pain tolerable because the pain is about as severe as any pain can possibly be and it has often been said to be "worse than childbirth." Also, while the patient is hospitalized, serial blood calciums are very important to search for possible hyperparathyroid etiology for the lithiasis. This is done even on the very first episode of lithiasis because hyperparathyroid disease warrants surgical correction on its own merits and quite unrelated to its role in urolithiasis. Serum phosphorus determinations and uric acid determinations should be made and blood protein determinations are also important inasmuch as calcium is bound to these proteins for the most part and it is only the free calcium that contributes to stone formation. Abnormally low protein levels in the presence of normal serum calcium levels could therefore mean that an abnormally large amount of free (unbound) calcium is available to contribute to stone formation. Therefore, the determination of hyperparathyroidism is best made by detecting an elevated blood calcium level on at least one occasion in the presence of normal blood proteins. This is a very difficult disease to document, and serial serum calciums are indicated in lithiasis patients. Blood chloride and bicarbonate levels should also be obtained as a rough screen for the complete form of renal tubular acidosis, which usually shows an elevated blood chloride level with a decrease in the CO_2 level (a hyperchloremic acidosis).

For the patient initially seen in the emergency room or the physician's office and in whom the diagnosis of urinary tract calculus has been documented, treatment in the patient's home setting is possible if there is minimal or no obstruction to the urinary tract above the stone, if there is no infection in the urinary tract, if the patient is well enough to take fluids by mouth, and, particularly, if the patient's pain has subsided enough after the initial dose of narcotics so that injectable narcotics are not required on a repetitive basis. Oral pain medication is simply not adequate for patients suffering from renal colic. Obviously, the patient who is not hospitalized cannot readily have the repeat urine analyses, pH checks, or the various blood studies that have been mentioned, although the blood studies, at least, can be done on an outpatient basis once the patient has become asymptomatic.

As already suggested, definitive management of the patient with a urinary tract calculus is dependent in large measure on the location of the calculus, the presence or absence of infection above the calculus, the degree of obstruction above the calculus, and the size of the calculus as seen on excretory urograms. Spontaneous passage is far preferable for the patient than cystoscopic manipulation or any other procedure to remove the stone provided that there is a reasonable expectation of such passage and provided that kidney damage or sepsis does not result prior to such spontaneous passage.

As a general rule, a stone that measures (on x-ray film) 5 mm or less in its greatest diameter has an excellent chance of spontaneous passage and it is often justifiable to wait for weeks or even months for this to occur, except under the following circumstances:

1. If there is a high-grade obstruction behind the stone that persists for more than a very few days, the fear of resulting permanent renal damage militates strongly against any delay while waiting for spontaneous passage.
2. If there is evidence of diminishing renal function, regardless of the severity of the hydronephosis. This diminishing renal function may be determined by excretory urography or renal scanning.
3. If there is infection behind the stone, as determined by a febrile course or by bacteriuria, the possibility of a potentially dangerous closed space infection within the kidney exists and spontaneous passage cannot usually be awaited.
4. If the pain is so severe that the patient must take narcotics continually for several days or longer and is unable to resume his or her usual occupation while awaiting spontaneous passage, manipulative or surgical intervention is certainly warranted.

Generally speaking, the vast majority of stones 5 mm or less in their greatest diameter will, and should be allowed to, pass spontaneously. Stones between 5 mm and 1 cm in their greatest diameter may pass spontaneously but often do not and in such cases the physician's clinical judgment and the patient's clinical course will determine the preferred mode of treatment. Stones that are over 1 cm in size will, in all likelihood, not be able to pass spontaneously and are probably too large to be extracted cystoscopically. Such stones are preferentially removed by open surgical procedures. The caveat to be observed here is that the patients who have passed many stones previously are frequently able to tell the physician that they *know* some of their spontaneously passed stones were larger than 1 cm and in these instances it would behoove the physician to give the patient an adequate clinical trial at spontaneous passage before surgical intervention is undertaken.

A general rule is that blind cystoscopic manipulation and extraction of the stone by means of a stone basket inserted into the ureter from the bladder is only attempted when the stone is less than 1 cm and is in the lower third of the ureter. Within the very recent past, however, direct vision ureteroscopy has become quite successful and is becoming more commonplace as a means of removing stones from the middle and upper portion of the ureters. Because it is done under direct vision the chances of ureteral trauma are minimized. Even with ureteroscopy, however, it is doubtful whether stones much bigger than 1 cm can be extracted from below through the ureter because of the risk of a traumatic ureteral stricture occurring and tearing or perforating the ureter. However, the use of ultrasound shock waves directly applied to the stone via the ureteroscope can successfully cause a fragmentation of the stone, and the pieces can then be extracted through the ureteroscope.

When a stone is present within the collecting system of the kidney, the question always arises regarding the justification and the indications for surgical intervention. The stone that is in a minor calyx in the presence of sterile urine can probably be left alone and it is most unlikely that such a stone will cause the patient any symptoms at all. A stone that is present in association with infected urine, however, will surely grow and should preferentially be removed surgically. A stone within the renal pelvis that is thought to be too large to pass into the bladder spontaneously should also be removed surgically inasmuch as there is a great risk that a stone of this size might suddenly drop into a position in which it would partially or completely obstruct the ureteropelvic junction. In general, the indications for surgical intervention for intrarenal calculi are concurrent infection, a stone in a position where there is a high risk of obstruction of the ureteropelvic junction, a stone that is large enough to produce a decrease in renal function, or a stone that is producing pain or significant obstruction to all or part of the kidney. In the last analysis decisions regarding management of stones in the urinary tract require a great deal of specialized knowledge and appropriate urologic consultation should always be obtained.

In the past couple of years, the percutaneous approach to stones in the kidney has gone far towards replacing "open" or traditional surgical approaches. With this new and exciting method, a small tract about the size of a fountain pen in diameter is developed (under anesthesia) from the skin into the collecting system of the kidney and a probe is introduced through an endoscope that is in the tract. The probe is placed in direct contact with the stone(s) in the kidney and the ultrasound waves are sent through the probe and shatter the stone(s). The stone fragments are then sucked back out through the endoscopic instrument by means of a small "vacuum cleaner" device.

An even newer instrument, developed in Germany, can shatter kidney stones (which then pass down the ureter) using shock waves focused on the stones from *outside* the body. The technique is entirely noninvasive. The equipment required for this at present is extraordinarily costly but many individuals, and companies, are working at new and cheaper modifications of this instrument. In the next decade, it is likely that most hospitals will have some form of extracorporeal device to shatter and destroy renal stones.

EXAMINATION OF THE RECOVERED STONE

In treating the patient with recurrent urinary tract lithiasis, it is of utmost importance that the stone be recovered and a proper analysis carried out. It is imperative that the physician know what the nidus of the stone is, because it may be quite different from the outer layers and it is one of the keys to the etiology of that particular stone. For example, it is not at all uncommon to have a uric acid nidus with a great deal of calcium oxalate laid down around it. There are virtually no hospitals in the United States currently doing adequate stone analyses and when a conventional hospital laboratory sends a report based on analysis of a stone it lists those elements present in the stone but does not identify a nidus nor does it indicate the percentages of each component present in the stone. Such a totally worthless report only serves to hinder the efforts of the clinician to create a prophylactic regimen for the patient. The technique of examining the nidus of the stone and reporting all of the various elements of it on a weight-percentage basis is highly complex and requires expensive equipment for the crystallographic analysis of the stone. The Louis Herring Company in Orlando, Florida, and Calculab, Inc. in Richmond, Virginia, do an outstanding job of stone analysis and their work is done at an extremely modest cost. The stone is shipped to the laboratory in a special mailing container provided by that laboratory and a report is usually in the hands of the clinician within 1 week to 10 days.

MEDICAL MANAGEMENT OF PATIENTS WITH RECURRENT UROLITHIASIS

Medical management must be precisely tailored to the etiology of the lithiasis. This in turn depends upon a meticulous workup involving serum and 24-hour urine studies, as discussed earlier in this chapter, and upon a proper analysis of the stone. It cannot be reiterated too often that the cornerstone of therapy for virtually all urinary tract calculi is a fluid intake that is large enough to produce at least 3 liters or urine daily. Besides a measurement of urine output to determine if, in fact, 3 liters of urine is being made, an alternate means of determining the adequacy of urine volume is to make certain that the urine is colorless at all times. When the patient is not able to comply with this or when compliance is good but the patient continues to form stones then one of the medical therapies outlined below is indicated.

1. When the patient is *normocalcemic* and *normocalciuric*, the treatment of choice is the long-term use of oral phosphates. The author prefers to use Neutra-Phos (Willen Company, Baltimore) in powder form. This is dissolved in water and given three or four times daily to a dosage of 1½ to 2 g daily in three or four divided doses. When administered orally, Neutra-Phos significantly raises the pyrophosphate and citrate level in the urine and actually brings about an approximately 80 percent decrease in calcium oxalate crystal formation in the urine. This therapy is highly effective, resulting in a cessation or significant reduction in stone formation in better than 90 percent of patients who are normocalcemic, normocalciuric, normouricosurvic, and normooxalovic. They form recurrent calcium oxalate (or, rarely, calcium phosphate) stones because of a defect of one or more urinary inhibitors of crystallization. Neutra-Phos directly addresses this underlying problem by increasing the urinary levels of two of the most potent inhibitors of crystallization, pyrophosphate and citrate. Although Neutra-Phos may occasionally be efficacious in the normocalcemic, hypercalciuric patient, the rationale for its success in these cases is obscure. Neutra-Phos should not be used in patients with renal insufficiency or in patients in whom infection or obstruction accompany the lithiasis because it may result in additional stone formation in these cases due to phosphate precipitation. Magnesium oxide may also be used in the normocalcemic, normocalciuric type of idiopathic calcium oxalate lithiasis, and its obvious rationale is the strong role of magnesium as another known inhibitor of crystal formation. The dosage is 100 mg three times per day and it does not generally produce the drastic gastrointestinal side effects that magnesium hydroxide produces.

2. For the *normocalcemic, hypercalciuric* patient who is a renal tubule "leaker," oral thiazides are the drugs of choice in a usual dosage of 50 mg twice per day. The author prefers to use Hydro-DIURIL for this purpose but there is probably not too much difference among the thiazides. Thiazides act on the distal tubule or collecting duct and decrease the urinary calcium excretion by about 50 percent. This effect may be blocked by a high sodium intake and this should be carefully measured (by means of a 24-hour urine sodium) if it appears that thiazides are not producing the desired therapeutic effect. Thiazides generally do not lower the calcium level in the normocalciuric patient, however, so they are not generally indi-

cated in normocalcemic, normocalciuric stone formers. The side effects of thiazides can be quite unpleasant and include significant weakness, fatigue, and somnolence, along with impaired glucose tolerance and an elevated serum uric acid. As many as 10 to 20 percent of patients placed on thiazide treatment discontinue the therapy because of these side effects. Although it must be emphasized that thiazides are only indicated and logical in the normocalcemic, hypercalciuric patient, it very occasionally is therapeutic, for unknown reasons, in the normocalcemic, normocalciuric patient in whom Neutra-Phos has not been successful or in whom urinary tract infection precludes the use of Neutra-Phos.

3. For the *normocalcemic, hypercalciuric* patient who is a hyperabsorber, cellulose phosphate is a helpful agent. It tends to bind the calcium in the gut, thereby minimizing its absorption. However, in doing this, free oxalate is left unbound and its absorption significantly raises urinary oxalate levels. Cellulose phosphate also tends to decrease the urinary magnesium level and these two factors are major causes of urolithiasis. Therefore, if and when cellulose phosphate is used, a low oxalate diet and supplemental oral magnesium are mandatory. In the author's experience, hyperabsorbers from the gut are not common and the author prefers to treat these patients by sharply limiting their calcium intake to 200 mg/day, thereby making this specific category of stone former (the hyperabsorber) the only type of lithiasis patient in whom severe restriction of dietary calcium is recommended. For those hyperabsorbers who cannot comply with a decreased calcium intake or in whom this decreased intake does not produce the desired results, oral thiazides are used because these patients are, in fact, hypercalciuric.

The reason the author is so meticulous about separating the normocalciuric from the hypercalciuric patient and further subdividing the hypercalciuric patient into the renal tubular "leaker" and the "hyperabsorber" is because each abnormality has its own optimum form of therapy based upon the etiology of the stone and therapeutic success is unlikely *unless* the therapy is tailored to the problem. Moreover, the side effects of thiazides, at least, can be less than pleasant, thereby reinforcing the wisdom of using it *only* when it is specifically indicated.

For the patient with recurrent calcium oxalate lithiasis based upon the diagnosis of primary hyperoxaluria, the treatment of choice is oral Pyridoxine, and 6 to 8 months of therapy or longer may be necessary before the full therapeutic effect has been realized. Neutra-Phos is sometimes added to the Pyridoxine regimen and may be beneficial. For the patient who is a calcium oxalate stone former due to a secondary (dietary) hyperoxaluria, the elimination of as much oxalate as possible from the diet is usually therapeutic. In the author's experience iced tea is the biggest single dietary cause of secondary hyperoxaluria.

4. For the *calcium phosphate* stone former whose metabolic workup may be normal or in whom there may be an elevated urinary phosphorus level, urinary acidification to a pH below 6.2 may be helpful in minimizing the precipitation of calcium phosphate crystals. If this therapy alone is not successful, oral phosphates (Neutra-Phos) can be added to the therapeutic regimen if the patient is normocalciuric or thiazides may be used if the patient is hypercalciuric.

5. For the *uric acid* stone former, in whom the metabolic workup is usually normal, the therapy of choice (in addition to hydration) is alkalinization of the urine to a pH of 6.5. This increases the solubility of the uric acid tenfold and this alkalinization may be accomplished with sodium bicarbonate or with polycitra or bicitra. Sometimes, Allopurinol, 300 mg daily in three divided doses, is the treatment of choice, and this is particularly true if the urinary pH is normal (thereby indicating that alkalinization therapy will probably not be successful) or if clinical gout is present or if alkalinization is not adequate for any reason. Allopurinol therapy may be stopped after the stones have been dissolved unless clinical gout is present.

6. For the patient with *cystine* stones, hydration is certainly the most important step in therapy because 3 liters or more of urine produced each day will usually keep all the cystine in solution and prevent or minimize stone formation. Alkalinization to a pH of 6.5 does not greatly increase the solubility of cystine, but it *is* significantly increased if alkalinization can be pushed to a pH of 8.0. If this cannot be accomplished, then penicillamine is the treatment of choice, but occasional side effects with this type of therapy can be serious (agranulocytosis and the nephrotic syndrome) and require cessation of therapy.

7. For the magnesium ammonium phosphate (struvite) stone former (these are usually staghorn calculi), the etiology is chronic infection with urea-splitting organisms (usually Proteus) leading to a highly alkaline ph with resulting crystalline precipitation. Therapy is directed at surgical removal of the stone and the use of a new drug, Acetohydroxamic acid (Lithostat), which inhibits the bacterial enzyme urease, thereby decreasing urinary ammonia and alkalinity, which in turn facilitates treatment of the underlying proteus in infection and minimizes the likelihood of stone regrowth.

REFERENCES

Carter WC III, Halushka PV, Jones D, Roof B, Rous SN, Spector M: Indomethacin lowers urinary calcium excretion in normal volunteers and normocalciuric stone-formers. In Smith LH, Robertson W, Finlayson B (eds), Urolithiasis, Clinical and Basic Research. New York, Plenum, 1981, pp 723–725

Greene LF, Rous SN: Manipulative treatment of ureteral calculi. GP 141–148, March, 1963

Rous SN: Urology in Primary Care. St. Louis, Mosby, 1976

Rous SN, Turner WR: Retrospective study of 95 patients with staghorn calculus disease. J Urol 118:902, 1977

Rous SN: A review of 171 consecutive patients with urinary lithiasis. J Urol 126:376, 1981

Smith LH: Urolithiasis. In Earley LE, Gottschalk CW (eds), Strauss and Welt's Diseases of the Kidney, 3rd ed. Boston, Little, Brown, 1979, vol 2, chap 21

Spector M, Garden NM, Rous SN: Ultrastructural features of human urinary calculi. In Fleisch H, Robertson WG, Smith LH, Vahlensieck W (eds), Urolithiasis Research. New York, Plenum, 1976, pp 355–359

Spector M, Garden NM, Rous SN: Ultrastructure and pathogenesis of human urinary calculi. Br J Urol 50:12, 1978

9
Renal and Adrenal Hypertension and Related Adrenal Problems

EDUCATIONAL OBJECTIVES

1. Discuss the mechanism by which a narrowed renal artery may produce hypertension.
2. Discuss the actions of cortisol.
3. Discuss the steps taken to determine if hypertension is of adrenal origin.
4. Describe the mechanism of action of aldosterone.
5. List the symptoms associated with failure of the adrenal cortex.
6. Discuss the relationship of the adrenal glands to hypertension.
7. List the symptoms of pheochromocytoma.

HYPERTENSION

Cardiovascular disease with or without hypertension is the leading cause of adult death in the United States. Hypertension, so often related to cardiovascular disease either as an etiology or a result, affects an estimated 10 percent of the entire population and has an even higher incidence in adults. Hypertension in the adult is defined as blood pressure higher than 140/90; with regard to its clinical significance, however, a blood pressure of 160/90 in a 60-year-old is not nearly as distressing as blood pressure of 160/100 in a 30-year-old. Although "essential hypertension" is the etiologic category in the vast majority of cases, it is possible that as many as 5 percent of hypertensive individuals suffer from this clinical condition as a result of potentially curable disease within the renal arteries. It is also possible that many patients with so-called essential hypertension have as yet unexplained or incompletely comprehended underlying disease mechanisms within the kidney or the renal vessels.

RENAL MECHANISMS OF HYPERTENSION

The connection between the kidney and cardiovascular disease has been known since the 1920s as a result of the observations of the English physician, Richard Bright. In the 1930s the research of the American pathologist, Harry Goldblatt, elucidated at least one connection between the kidney and hypertension by demonstrating that blood pressure elevation occurred in the experimental animal when one or both main renal arteries were diminished in caliber by the placement of an arterial clamp across the artery. Additional investigations by Goldblatt and others determined that if a renal artery was constricted, the kidney supplied by that artery responded by releasing a substance into the general circulation by way of the renal vein and this substance initiated a series of events that ultimately led to the development of hypertension. The substance released by the kidney was subsequently identified as renin, a material that had been serendipitously identified and forgotten 35 years earlier. Goldblatt's studies set off a furious chain reaction of basic research, which continues to this day, that soon showed that renin was *not* the cause of blood pressure elevation, but was a proteolytic enzyme stored and probably manufactured in the juxtaglomerular cells located within the walls of the afferent arterioles of the glomeruli. It was found that renin has no vasoconstrictive or pressor properties in itself but does act on a renin substrate known as angiotensinogen, which is manufactured in the liver and is normally present in circulating blood. The action of renin on this substrate yields a decapeptide fragment called angiotensin I, a weak vasoconstrictor. During its circulation through the lungs, however, the angiotensin I is acted on by a converting enzyme to produce an octapeptide, angiotensin II, an extremely potent vasoconstrictive pressor substance responsible for hypertension. It acts directly on the smooth muscle of the arterial walls, resulting in contraction of these vessels, an increase in their peripheral resistance, and blood pressure elevation. Circulating within the blood are various angiotensinases, which split angiotensin II into inactive fragments and thereby serve to keep blood pressure in balance.

RENAL ARTERY NARROWING

There are three mechanisms by which a functional narrowing within the main renal artery or one of its branches can bring about excess renin release, ultimately resulting in hypertension. First, and probably foremost, a decreased mean pressure at the level of the glomerular afferent arteriole will probably change the tension on the wall of that afferent arteriole and stimulate an excess renin release. A decreased mean pressure such as this can result distal to a stenosis of the renal artery, occurring from fibromuscular hyperplasia, atherosclerotic plaques, intimal hyperplasia, or any of several other vascular lesions. An effective decrease of mean pressure at the level of the afferent arteriole can also result from a proximal arteriovenous fistula or a renal arterial aneurysm.

A second mechanism by which excess renin release is thought to be triggered is based on the amount of sodium (or chloride) delivered to the macula densa, specialized cells of the distal convoluted tubule that are anatomically in close proximity to the juxtaglomerular cells of the afferent arteriolar walls. When the delivery of sodium is decreased, renin production is increased. This decrease in the amount of sodium is felt to be secondary to local factors such as renal arterial constriction or generalized factors such as a reduced extracellular fluid volume, as might be found with dehydration or hemorrhage.

Another mechanism that is thought to effect excess renin release is stimulation of the β-adrenergic (sympathetic) nerve fibers to the kidney.

Under these various stimuli, and possibly others yet to be determined, renin stored in the juxtaglomerular cells is released into the bloodstream through the renal vein, at which point the chain of events already noted is begun.

In addition to the mechanisms by which renal artery narrowing can bring about renin release with resulting hypertension, it should be pointed out that various intra renal disease processes, which perhaps alter the blood flow to given areas of the kidney by means of pressure ischemia, can also stimulate the renin–angiotensin mechanism. Examples of this group of diseases are renal cysts, renal tumors, or hydronephrosis, any of which may produce pressure on adjacent renal tissue, or renal infarction, in which some renal tissue is still viable but ischemic.

Anatomic narrowing of the renal arteries is not uncommon, being present in as many as 50 percent of some autopsy series. It must be emphasized, however, that the presence of anatomic narrowing of the renal arteries does not necessarily mean that hypertension will result, and, more important, it is not necessarily the etiologic factor when hypertension *is* present. In order for hypertension to result from a decreased mean pressure, it is generally felt that there must be at least a 50 percent reduction in the lumen of the affected artery, but it is also a fact that all renal arteries that are narrowed by 50 percent do *not* result in hypertension.

How, then, can the physician determine if the patient is hypertensive because of some observable renal arterial narrowing as seen on selective renal angiography (see Fig. 1–38)? Probably the most accurate means to make this determination is by comparing the renal vein renin levels from both the affected and the contralateral sides by direct catheterization of the renal vein; this procedure is most conveniently done at the same time as the selective renal angiography and the renin activity is measured by means of bioassays or radioimmunoassays. This activity is expressed in terms of nanograms of angiotensin I per milliliter of plasma per hour. Although rarely used because the renin activity determinations are so much more diagnostic, split renal function tests are another means of determining whether or not renal arterial narrowing is causing hypertension. This rather sophisticated procedure in which various parameters of the function of *each* kidney are determined and then compared is based on the knowledge that ischemic kidneys will behave in a different manner than their normal mates when challenged by certain substances requiring tubular secretion and reabsorption.

RENAL ADRENAL MECHANISMS OF HYPERTENSION: RENIN–ANGIOTENSIN–ALDOSTERONE AXIS

In addition to the vasoconstrictive action on the smooth muscle of the arteriolar wall, angiotensin II and to a lesser degree angiotensin I are known to act directly on the adrenal cortex to stimulate the production of aldosterone. Other stimuli to the production of aldosterone are hyponatremia, hyperkalemia, and adrenocorticotropic hormone (ACTH). The physiologic functioning of the renin–angiotensin–aldosterone axis may be conceptualized by visualizing a diminished filling of the arteriolar tree, such as might result from a sudden change to an upright posture, a low-salt diet, dehydration, or blood loss. This will be sensed by receptors in the wall of the afferent glomerular arteriole; in response, excess renin will be released into the circulation. The angiotensin II that is ultimately produced may possibly act locally within the kidney to decrease glomerular filtration; it may act peripherally to cause arteriolar constriction; and it will also reach the adrenal cortex, where it stimulates the production of aldosterone. This hormone in turn enhances sodium reabsorption in the renal tubules, with a resulting increase in plasma volume and reexpansion of the arteriolar tree; this reexpansion is the signal within the juxtaglomerular apparatus for the cessation of renin secretion. Angiotensin II is thus seen to act in two manners: direct vasoconstricting action on the arteriolar tree, which serves to raise the blood pressure; and action in stimulating the production of aldosterone, which in turn acts on the distal renal tubule to promote the reabsorption of sodium and water, further raising the blood pressure. Both of these mechanisms work most efficiently in the normal maintenance of body homeostasis, but under abnormal conditions, such as a pathologic narrowing of the renal artery, they can work together to perpetuate blood pressure elevation. It must be stressed that in cases of renal artery narrowing causing excess renin release, it is clearly the action of angiotensin II on the arteriolar system that contributes the most to the initial blood pressure elevation. However, the etiology of the perpetuation or continuation of hypertension is obscure and, whereas the angiotensin–aldosterone mechanism is undoubtedly an important factor, the direct pressor effect of angiotensin II in the arteriolar system probably is not.

It is known that autonomously secreting aldosterone tumors can also raise blood pressure by direct action on the distal renal tubule to cause excess reabsorption of sodium and water. How may the clinician differentiate so-called primary aldosteronism, where there is an autonomous aldosterone-producing tumor or a diffuse hyperplasia within the adrenal gland, from secondary aldosteronism, in which it is excess renin production that is responsible for the excess aldosterone by way of the angiotensin system? In primary aldosteronism, the resulting increase in plasma volume actually suppresses the secretion of renin; therefore, demonstration of suppressed renin levels in the presence of elevated aldosterone levels has become an important diagnostic test for primary aldosteronism. This may actually be demonstrated using the Lasix stimulation test while the patient is on a regular diet. Forty mg of Lasix is administered at 2:00 P.M., 6:00 P.M., and again at 6:00 A.M., and 4 hours after this third dose of Lasix the renin activity is measured. A suppressed renin activity level, which would be compatible with a diagnosis of primary aldosteronism, would be less than 2 ng/ml/hr.

TREATMENT OF HYPERTENSION CAUSED BY RENAL ARTERIAL LESIONS

After a diagnosis of hypertension caused by renal artery disease has been accurately and properly made, treatment may involve long-term antihypertensive medications or corrective surgery in some cases. This corrective surgery may involve revascularization of the kidney by means of a bypass graft or reconstruction of the arterial lesion by means of a patch graft; where the arterial lesion is intrarenal and in an inaccessible place, nephrectomy may be indicated. An analysis of the results of surgical treatment in large series of patients shows that about two thirds may be cured or significantly improved; one third of such operations must be considered failures. When the renal arterial lesion is a fibromuscular lesion, however, approximately 80 percent of patients may be cured or significantly improved, compared with improvement in just over 60 percent of patients with unilateral atherosclerosis. When bilateral renal arterial disease exists, the improvement rate is somewhat over 50 percent. The key to good surgical results involves meticulously performed preoperative diagnostic studies, with heavy emphasis on the relative renin activity levels found in each renal vein. Equally important for successful surgery is that the contralateral or uninvolved kidney be normal or virtually normal. When these determinations are properly carried out and where the operation is anatomically successful (no postoperative arterial thrombosis) as many as 80 percent of patients may be significantly helped by surgery. The general thinking among physicians in this field is that patients with atherosclerotic lesions in the renal arteries are not ideal candidates for corrective surgery, inasmuch as this is usually a generalized systemic condition involving many arteries, often including the contralateral renal artery. It is therefore quite probable that patients with this sort of problem do better on a long-term antihypertensive medical regimen. It is interesting to note that in the very recent past, some medical centers have been treating renal arterial narrowing selectively with transluminal angioplasty, which is a nonsurgical (although invasive) technique of dilating renal arterial narrowing using balloon catheters that have been inserted into the arterial system percutaneously. These results, in very selected cases, appear to be promising, but long-term follow-up is as yet unknown.

ADRENAL MECHANISMS

In addition to primary and secondary aldosteronism, the adrenal gland can have at least two other known pathologic entities leading to and directly productive of hypertension, one involving the cortex and one the medulla. In Cushing's syndrome (adrenal hyperplasia) there is hyperfunction of all of the elements of the adrenal cortex; in pheochromocytoma, epinephrine and norephinephrine are produced by a tumor of the adrenal medulla.

Cushing's Syndrome (Adrenal Hyperplasia, Adrenal Adenoma, or Adrenal Carcinoma)

In addition to hyperaldosteronism, the second of the three known adrenal mechanisms for producing hypertension in Cushing's syndrome, or Cushing's disease (these terms may, for our purposes, be used interchangeably). As originally described, Cushing's disease referred to a basophilic adenoma or a chromophobe tumor of the pituitary gland that led to an excess production of ACTH, with resultant adrenal overproduction of glucocorticoids and sex hormones. As it is now commonly used, Cushing's disease or Cushing's syndrome may also refer to primary adrenal pathology producing the same excess hormonal production just noted. This adrenal condition is histologically most often an adrenal adenoma although it may be an adrenal hyperplasia or even an adrenal carcinoma. The other group of hormones resulting from normal adrenal steroidogenesis, mineralocorticoids, is only secondarily under the control of the pituitary gland (it is under the primary control of angiotensin), and therefore excess production of mineralocorticoid is not a usual feature of Cushing's syndrome.

About one third of the patients suffering from Cushing's syndrome have hypertension because of the mineralocorticoid effect of the glucocorticoid cortisol, which is produced in great excess. The mineralocorticoid effect of the excess cortisol serves to cause sodium and fluid retention, with resulting hypertension, but it should be realized that hypertension associated with Cushing's syndrome is not a result of excess production of mineralocortocoid itself.

Cushing's syndrome, with its excess of cortisol production, is manifested clinically by the classic findings of moon facies, prominent supraclavicular fat pads, so-called buffalo humps of the neck and upper back, truncal obesity and thin extremities, abdominal striae, and easy bruisability. Associated mood and personality changes are not uncommon, and frank psychoses sometimes develop. Additional findings are thinning of the scalp hair, acne, facial plethora, and increased body and facial hair, all of which result from the increased androgen production that usually accompanies Cushing's syndrome.

Cardiovascular and renal involvement from this condition may include cardiomegaly and congestive heart failure secondary to hypertension when it is present, and there may be definite electrocardiographic changes such as lengthening of the Q-T interval as hypokalemia develops. Other effects of this condition seen in the peripheral blood may be eosinopenia, lymphocytopenia, shortened coagulation time, and increases in platelet count, sedimentation rate, polymorphonuclear leukocytes, red cells, hematocrit, hemoglobin, and total blood volume. Increased gluconeogenesis may additionally occur secondary to the excess production of cortisol, and the anti-insulin effect of this steroid may result in the production of so-called steroid diabetes in patients with Cushing's syndrome.

Pheochromocytoma

The third of the known pathologic conditions of the adrenal gland causing hypertension is pheochromocytoma. Unlike the above two conditions, pheochromocytoma is a disease of the adrenal medulla, which is quite distinct from the adrenal cortex, the anatomic portion of the gland involved in aldosteronism and Cushing's syndrome.

The adrenal cortex originates from the mesonephric blastema and is mesodermal in origin; the adrenal medulla originates from the neural crest and is ectodermal in origin. The adrenal medulla arises in common with the sympathetic chain, the ganglia, and the celiac plexus. Cells from these structures migrate in utero to enter the anlage of the developing adrenal cortex and form the adrenal gland. These migrating cells eventually develop into two distinct types—ganglion cells and chromaffin cells. Chromaffin cells produce the adrenal medullary hormones. The two types of tumors of this cell line are pheochromocytoma and paraganglioma. Ganglion cells differentiate into a different tumor group, one of which is the lethal neuroblastoma. All of the cells of the adrenal medulla arise in common with the sympathetic chain, the ganglia, and the celiac plexus, which helps to explain the fact that these chromaffin tumors (pheochromocytomas) can arise not only within the adrenal medulla but anywhere along the sympathetic chain and ganglia. The vast majority of these tumors do arise within the adrenal medulla, but they have been reported in other places along the sympathetic chain and in places as distant as the urinary bladder. Pheochromocytomas are relatively rare catecholamine (epinephrine and norepinephrine) secreting tumors that typically are seen clinically with episodic or persistent hypertension that may be associated with flushing, sweating, tachycardia, arrhythmias, fever, glycosuria, headache, palpitation, nervousness, and tremor. The variability in clinical symptomatology is based on whether the catecholamine release is constant or intermittent and also on which vasopressor substance is actually released. An acute hypertensive episode may be precipitated by exercise, external pressure on the tumor, anesthetic, surgery, or monoamine oxidase inhibitor drugs.

The diagnosis of this condition can be confirmed by elevated urine levels of catecholamines or elevations of vanillylmandelic acid (VMA) and metanephrines, both of which are metabolites of catecholamines. In the face of definitive and diagnostic chemical studies indicating the presence of pheochromocytoma, various radioisotopic scanning and roentgenographic techniques such as adrenal venography are used to localize the tumor and surgical removal is then carried out.

Relationships Yet Unknown Between the Adrenal Gland and Hypertension

The known adrenal causes of hypertension—aldosteronism, Cushing's syndrome, and pheochromocytoma—together probably account for less than 10 percent of all cases of hypertension. There are some endocrinologists who firmly feel that there are at least as many additional hypertensive patients who have as yet unknown and undescribed adrenal lesions that are etiologic in their hypertension. The mechanisms of such adrenal hypertension are not worked out and may be considered to be nothing more than hypotheses at this time; nevertheless, when one considers the enormous spectrum of action of adrenal hormones and the complex biosynthesis in their manufacture, it does not seem at all unlikely or farfetched to presume that there may indeed be unknown substances produced by the adrenal gland that will ultimately be found to have an etiologic or related role in the production of or maintenance of hypertension.

DIAGNOSIS AND MANAGEMENT OF ADRENAL HYPERTENSION

What approach should the physician take to determine if known and demonstrable adrenal abnormalities are etiologic in the production of hypertension in a patient? The specific entities that would have to be considered are primary aldosteronism, Cushing syndrome, pheochromocytoma, and perhaps in the interest of completeness, secondary aldosteronism related to abnormalities of the renin–angiotensin mechanism.

Primary aldosteronism can be diagnosed by determinations of plasma renin activity and by testing 24-hour urine specimens for aldosterone levels. In primary aldosteronism, the plasma renin activity should be decreased (see above) and the urine aldosterone level increased. The additional finding of hypokalemia is helpful but not necessary. Primary aldosteronism must be differentiated from secondary aldosteronism, which may occur in several clinical situations, one of which is renovascular hypertension, in which the aldosterone elevations are secondary to excess production of angiotensin. In individuals with such secondary aldosteronism, renin activity will be significantly increased and should be measured directly from blood samples obtained from the renal veins. The vast majority of primary aldosteronism results from a secreting adenoma of the adrenal gland. Definitive diagnosis of this lesion depends on sophisticated roentgoengraphic and isotope scanning techniques, and definitive therapy requires surgical removel of the adenoma. In a small percentage of cases of primary aldosteronism, the condition is caused by a diffuse adrenal hyperplasia; surgical intervention in these cases is usually not beneficial.

Cushing's syndrome, the second of the known adrenal etiologies of hypertension, brings about excess cortisol production and leads to numerous symptoms that should make the clinician suspect this entity. Although Cushing's syndrome has occurred in association with other conditions that are neither of pituitary or adrenal origin, the vast majority of patients with this disease do suffer from pathologic pituitary or adrenal conditions, usually the latter. In those rare cases of Cushing's syndrome without adrenal or pituitary gland involvement, it is most likely that cancer of organs such as the lung, pancreas, and colon exists and presumably causes elaboration of polypeptides with ACTH-like activity, thereby producing Cushing's syndrome.

As already noted, the diagnosis of Cushing's syndrome should be suspected by the clinician when the characteristic findings of cortisol and androgen excess are present (see below). The early features of Cushing's syndrome may include weakness, emotionalism, menstrual problems, obesity, mild hypertension, and glucose intolerance.

Definitive diagnosis of *Cushing's syndrome* is preferentially made by means of the dexamethasone suppression test, in which this steroid is administered over a 4-day period in increasing dosages. In cases of adrenal hyperplasia, a high dose of dexamethasone will cause suppression of the urinary metabolite of cortisol, 17-hydroxycorticosterone. High doses of dexamethasone do not suppress the urinary metabolite of cortisol when an adrenal adenoma or carcinoma is present.

In patients with *pheochromocytoma*, 50 percent may exhibit paroxysmal hypertension with episodes of flushing or pallor, headache, palpitations, excessive perspiration, tremors, arrhythmias, and tachycardia; the other 50 percent may demonstrate only hypertension. If this condition is suspected, the diagnosis may be confirmed by 24-hour urine collections tested for vanillylmandelic acid (VMA), metanephrine, and catecholamine levels. Localization of pheochromocytoma may be difficult because it may be more than a single lesion and it can occur anywhere along the sympathetic chain and ganglia. Radioisotopic scanning techniques and adrenal venography are necessary, and sampling of vena cava blood for catecholamines at different levels of the cava is of particular importance. Treatment of pheochromocytoma, once isolated, is surgical removal of the lesion. This must be done under rigid and appropriate surgical monitoring to prevent catastrophic blood pressure fluctuations during the procedure.

CORTISOL: NORMAL AND ABNORMAL ACTIONS

All adrenal steroid hormones, including cortisol, come from the adrenal cortex and are derived from cholesterol, which is abundant in the adrenal gland. All normal adrenal steroidogenesis deriving from cholesterol results in three hormone types— glucocorticoids, sex hormones, and mineralocorticoids. The glucocorticoids, of which cortisol may be considered the prototype, are produced largely in the two inner zones of the adrenal gland, the zona fasciculata and the zona reticularis. Cortisol is by far the most abundant and the most active of the glucocorticoids, and one of its most important actions is *gluconeogenesis*. This process is fundamentally catabolic. There is a deamination of amino acids making up the protein, with resultant nitrogen loss and increased formation of glucose with a rise in both liver glycogen and blood glucose levels. The rise in glucose levels of the blood may temporarily be counterbalanced by an increase in insulin output, which may or may not be sufficient to prevent glycosuria. However, if cortisol is present in excess (as it is in Cushing's syndrome) or if it is administered exogenously for prolonged periods, the β cells of the pancreas may become exhausted and steroid diabetes ensues.

Although a normal action of cortisol is not primarily directed at protein catabolism, it must be realized that cortisol excess will in fact lead to an abnormal breakdown of protein, resulting in muscle weakness and wasting and loss of bone matrix. This in turn leads to resorption of calcium, with increased excretion of calcium in the urine and possible stone formation in the urinary tract. In addition, calcium absorption from the gut is impaired in the presence of cortisol excess, because of cortisol antagonism to vitamin D. As in the case of glucose, total fat is increased at the expense of protein in the presence of excess cortisol. This is deposited in a characteristic distribution limited to the head and trunk, bringing about the well-known findings of Cushing syndrome.

Cortisol acts to enhance water diuresis. This is probably due mostly to glomerular filtration and to a lesser extent to its antagonistic action toward antidiuretic hormone, which affects water resorption at the tubule level. Glucocorticoids (cortisol) also protect target tissue against the ill effects of antigen–antibody complexes, and cortisol serves to maintain normal bone marrow and skeletal structure as well as stability of the central nervous system. The presence of an excess or a deficiency of cortisol commonly leads to psychiatric disturbances.

It is of interest that cortisol serves to reduce the number of circulating lymphocytes and eosinophils. This effect is not due to suppression of the bone marrow but to increased sequestration in the lungs and spleen and increased destruction in the blood. The overall white blood cell count, however, is significantly raised by cortisol administration, as are the number of erythrocytes and thrombocytes. On occasion, hypotensive states that are unresponsive to pressor agents will yield to permissive amounts of cortisol, apparently because of the cortisol effect of sensitization of the arteriole walls to the actions of catecholamines.

Cortisol and other glucocorticoids additionally serve to decrease inflammatory responses and fibrosis and, to some extent, inhibit reparative and fibrotic changes. Thus these hormones tend to abolish the manifestations of disease without antagonizing the causative agents directly.

In summary, then, the main actions of cortisol are homeostasis, gluconeogenesis from protein catabolism, action on water metabolism to increase diuresis, sensitization of the arterioles to the action of catecholamines, antiinflammatory effect, maintenance of the normal bone marrow and skeleton, and stabilization of the central nervous system. Excess cortisol (as in Cushing's syndrome) leads to a negative nitrogen balance, cessation of growth, muscle wasting, thinning of the skin, osteoporosis, reduction in lymphoid tissue, and an increase of gastric secretion of acid and peptin. Variation of cortisol levels may be found in different conditions, running the full spectrum from Addison's disease (virtually absent), to adrenal insufficiency, myxedema, or anterior pituitary gland insufficiency (low normal), to the first trimester of pregnancy, virilism, or severe hypertension (mild elevation), to thyrotoxicosis (moderate elevation), to Cushing's syndrome due to adrenal hyperplasia (moderate to marked increase), and finally to Cushing's syndrome due to adrenal adenoma or adenocarcinoma (marked increase).

ADRENAL FAILURE

Failure of the adrenal cortex, also known as acute adrenal insufficiency and as Addison's disease, is life threatening in a patient whose physiologic requirements for glucocorticoid and mineralocorticoid steroid hormones exceeds the available supply. Acute adrenal insufficiency is generally characterized by one or more of the following signs and symptoms: hypotension, nausea and vomiting, severe weakness, hyperthermia, hypoglycemia, hyponatremia, and hyperkalemia. In addition, the intravascular volume depletion secondary to mineralocorticoid deficiency may cause severe hemoconcentration, with an elevated hematocrit level and prerenal azotemia.

The diagnosis of acute adrenal insufficiency is necessarily empirical because there is generally not sufficient time to confirm the clinical impression. This diagnosis should be suspected in any patient with shock of uncertain etiology or who is in a rapidly deteriorating clinical situation without obvious cause. Before treatment is initiated blood samples should be obtained for a complete blood cell count (CBC) with differential, electrolyte determinations, blood glucose and urea nitrogen levels, and, particularly, plasma cortisol levels. It must be realized that a normal plasma cortisol level in the context of a severe clinical stress situation must be considered as inappropriately low and is therefore suggestive of adrenal insufficiency.

Acute adrenal insufficiency may occur in patients with long-standing chronic adrenal insufficiency or in those who are having long-term anticoagulant therapy, with resulting adrenal hemorrhage, or long-term nonspecific use of corticosteroid therapy. It can result from anterior pituitary thrombosis and hemorrhage during pregnancy, it may be secondary to extreme clinical stress, particularly surgical, and it may occur with overwhelming sepsis. Finally, it may be tuberculous or idiopathic in etiology.

Therapy of acute adrenal insufficiency primarily involves the replacement of glucocorticoid intravenously; a total dose of 200 mg of hydrocortisone over the initial 24-hour period is usually adequate. Following stabilization, glucocorticoid therapy may be continued with oral administration of hydrocortisone or cortisone acetate. Mineralocorticoid therapy is not necessary during the acute adrenal crisis because the large dose of replacement glucocorticoid in the first 24 hours will provide sufficient mineralocorticoid activity. However, as the total glucocorticoid dose is reduced below 75 mg per 24 hours, supplementary mineralocorticoids such as desoxicorticosterone acetate or fludrocortisone acetate are indicated.

Rapid correction of fluid and electrolyte abnormality should be carried out intravenously, using 1 liter of 5 percent dextrose in normal saline during the first 1 to 2 hours. Specific therapy is usually not required for hyperkalemia because serum potassium levels will return to normal following rapid hydration with saline and treatment with glucocorticoids. A serum potassium level above 6.5 mEq/l, however, will usually require some sodium bicarbonate given intravenously until the potassium level is lowered and any cardiac arrhythmias are corrected. Hypoglycemia, another finding with acute adrenal insufficiency, should be corrected early in the therapy by infusing saline solution containing glucose. Occasionally, vasopressor agents may be necessary if the blood pressure does not respond properly to rapid hydration with physiologic saline solution and the prompt administration of glucocorticoid.

REFERENCES

Herwig KR: The adrenal gland. In Kendall AR, Karafin L (eds), Urology. Philadelphia, Harper and Row, 1981, vol 1, chap 12

Nelson RP, Evins SC, Turner WR, Rittenberg G, Brackett NC, Hughson M, Rous SN: Asymptomatic hypovascular renal mass in a hypertensive patient. A clinicopathological conference. J Urol 121: 665, 1979

Novick AC: Renovascular hypertension. In Kendall AR, Karafin L (eds), Urology. Philadelphia, Harper and Row, 1983, vol 1, chap 11

Rous SN: Urology in Primary Care. St. Louis, Mosby, 1976

10
Genitourinary Tract Trauma

EDUCATIONAL OBJECTIVES

1. State the anatomic and pathologic differences between intraperitoneal and extraperitoneal bladder rupture.
2. Discuss the diagnosis and the management of blunt and of penetrating trauma to the kidney.
3. List the indications for excretory urography and for renal angiography in blunt and in penetrating renal trauma.
4. Discuss the symptoms, the diagnosis, and the management of trauma to the urethra and to the bladder.

RENAL TRAUMA

Injuries to the kidney are not uncommon. Despite being well protected by the ribs, vertebral bodies, heavy lumbar muscles, viscera, and posterior peritoneum, the kidneys are very mobile and relatively friable and thus are liable to parenchymal trauma. Motor vehicle accidents, for example, result in a rapid deceleration, causing excessive movement of the kidney with resultant stretching of the renal hilar vessels, and this in turn may lead to major vascular trauma. In various collected series of patient trauma, injury to some part of the genitourinary tract occurs in 2 percent to 3 percent of all of these cases and injury to the kidney occurs in 1 percent to 2 percent of the overall number. Something under 10 percent of all patients seen for abdominal trauma resulting from either blunt or penetrating injuries are found to have a renal injury as well. Of particular importance to the clinician dealing with children is the observation that when comparatively minor blunt trauma causes major renal damage, the strong likelihood of underlying renal abnormality must be considered. It must be kept in mind that conditions such as ureteropelvic junction obstruction with hydronephrosis, polycystic kidney, and even Wilms tumor predispose the kidney to traumatic injury.

For purposes of both etiology and treatment, renal trauma is classified as either of the blunt type or the penetrating type.

Blunt Renal Trauma

Blunt renal trauma accounts for approximately 70 to 80 percent of all renal injuries and is usually the result of motor vehicle accidents, falls, or participation in contact sports. In view of these etiologies, it is not surprising that males are affected four times as often as females and that the peak ages of risk are at the third and fourth decades of life. The right and left kidneys are involved about equally. Hematuria, gross or microscopic, is the single most common sign of renal injury and is present in about 90 percent of the cases of renal injury. Unfortunately, the degree of hematuria does not necessarily correlate with the degree of renal injury and, in some cases, severe renal injury can exist without *any* hematuria being present. Its absence, therefore, does not rule out severe renal trauma, and without question an excretory urogram, preferably an infusion study, should be done in all patients with the history or physical findings of significant abdominal, chest, or retroperitoneal trauma with or without grosss or microscopic hematuria. If the patient is in shock from multiple injuries, a large bolus (150 ml) of contrast medium may be injected by push technique into the intravenous lines while the patient is being resuscitated. This often gives very adequate visualization of the kidneys once the blood pressure has come back to the point where renal perfusion can occur. Ideally, nephrotomograms should be done along with the excretory urogram, although this is not always possible in the severely ill patient. The excretory urogram (with or without nephrotomograms) seeks to establish the presence or absence of both kidneys, to define the renal outlines clearly, and ideally to outline the collecting systems of the kidneys and the ureters as well. The nephrographic phase of the excretory urogram may demonstrate cortical lacerations or poor parenchymal perfusion from injured arteries. Excretory urography combined with nephrotomography can adequately stage the vast majority of blunt renal injuries. When the excretory urograms do not provide sufficient information to allow for proper management of the patient, CT scans of the kidney are very helpful and provide very good definition of parenchymal lacerations, a clear demonstration of any urinary extravasation, an outline of nonviable tissue, and a definition of the extent and size of any perirenal hematoma that may be present. CT scans are particularly good in distinguishing the minor injuries of superficial parenchymal laceration from the major injuries of the kidney such as deep lacerations and lacerations with extravasation. These CT scans, or, alternatively, selective renal angiograms, are indicated in any patient with suspected renal trauma, with or without hematuria, if the excretory urogram discloses delayed, partial, or absence of visualization of the kidney. If there are associated injuries to the main renal artery or a devascularization of the majority of the renal parenchyma, renal exploration and repair are indicated. However, the vast majority of patients with blunt renal trauma can be treated conservatively and, overall, well under 10 percent of these patients with blunt renal injury, with or without hematuria, actually require surgical intervention. Conservative management, however, requires that the patient with blunt renal trauma be very carefully monitored as regards vital signs, hemoglobin and hematocrit, and any indication of increasing flank ecchymoses or fullness, either of which might indicate increasing retroperitoneal hemorrhage. It should be noted that flank fullness, a sign of possible continued bleeding in the retroperitoneum, should be searched for visually and by direct palpation of the flank. If the patient's clinical course seems to suggest continued bleeding, then selective renal angiography or CT scanning should be carried out even if the findings of the excretory urograms were unremarkable. Well over 90 percent of patients with blunt renal trauma respond with a full recovery to conservative (nonoperative) therapy. The time of hospitalization, of course, varies with the severity of the renal injury and may only be a few days or may be as long as 2 to 4 weeks. Those few types of blunt renal injury that require operative intervention include vascular injuries, expanding or pulsatile hematomas, and urinary extravasation. All in all, considerably fewer than 10 percent of patients having a blunt injury to the kidney will require surgical exploration. Within 3 months of the time of injury, it is a good idea to obtain a follow-up excretory urogram to make sure of the normalcy of the presumably recovered kidney.

Penetrating Renal Trauma

Penetrating trauma literally anywhere in the torso from the upper chest area to the perineum should suggest the possibility of renal injury. This type of trauma is the type produced by a knife or other penetrating object or a bullet of either high or low velocity. Because the path that a knife or particularly a bullet follows is totally unpredictable, renal injuries must be suspected and searched for even when the point of entry is in the lower abdomen or in the region of the chest. It must be assumed that the position of the patient at the time of injury as well as the actual trajectory of the penetrating object are totally unknown; thus the location of traumatized organs need not be in anatomic proximity to the visible external wound. Penetrating trauma comprises about one quarter of all renal injuries and about 10 percent of penetrating injuries to the abdomen involve the kidneys.

It is important to realize that between 90 and 100 percent of patients with penetrating trauma to the kidney caused by gunshot wounds have associated injuries to one or more intraperitoneal organs and about 70 to 75 percent of patients with knife wounds of the kidney have similar associated injuries. For this reason, if no other, surgical exploration is mandatory. Ideal management would provide for preoperative infusion urograms and possibly selective renal angiograms. Evaluation of the status of the contralateral uninjured kidney by means of an infusion urogram provides important and useful knowledge before any contemplated surgery on the traumatized kidney and selective renal angiograms undoubtedly offer the most definitive evaluation of the status of the renal parenchyma and vasculature. Some authors prefer the CT scan for an overall evaluation of the renal injury and it is probable that these two modalities (angiograms and CT scans) are equally excellent. Nonvisualization of an injured kidney should prompt immediate arteriography since this is the best diagnostic study to differentiate the major causes of a nonvisualized kidney which are arterial thrombosis, avulsion of the renal artery and vein, severe contusion to the renal vessels, and complete absence of a kidney.

It cannot be stressed strongly enough that it is not unusual to find no discernible abnormalities on excretory urography of a kidney that has suffered penetrating injury. In some large series of patients with penetrating wounds of the kidney, preoperative excretory urograms were normal in 20 percent of traumatized kidneys that had lacerations or fractures severe enough to require surgical repair. Although the urogram is mandatory in any case of penetrating renal trauma that is diagnosed or suspected, selective renal angiography is also mandatory and is the definitive diagnostic procedure. Penetrating injuries to the kidney will undoubtedly cause microscopic or gross hematuria unless there is a complete separation of the ureter from the kidney or the ureter is completely occluded. It must therefore be reemphasized that the absence of blood in the urine is not conclusive proof that a given penetrating (or blunt) injury does not involve the kidney.

Based on the infusion urograms and particularly on the selective renal angiograms, a given renal injury may be categorized as slight (minor) or severe (major). Minor injuries such as parenchymal contusions can usually be treated conservatively without any renal exploration, and renal angiography in these cases will show essentially normal kidneys. In view of the fact that most of these patients will have a laparotomy anyway because of the high probability of an associated intraperitoneal injury, the urologist should be available to examine the retroperitoneal space, see if any perirenal hematoma exists, and decide at the time of the surgery if any renal exploration or treatment is needed. Unquestionably, severe renal lacerations and complete fractures will be clearly seen on renal angiography (Fig. 10–1) prior to surgery and the urologist must decide at the operating table, based on the angiograms and the clinical picture in front of him or her, whether or not to open Gerota's fascia in order to explore and repair the kidney itself. Certainly an expanding hematoma, a pulsatile hematoma, or an extravasation of urine mandate definitive exploration and treatment, and each situation must be individualized at the time of surgery. The most severe form of renal trauma is sometimes referred to as a complete fracture, maceration, or shattering of the kidney, which is fragmented and partly or completely detached from the hilus. Severe hemorrhage is the usual result and these patients are generally in shock when first seen and have gross hematuria (unless the ureter has been completely avulsed from the kidney). It is not at all unusual for these individuals to exsanguinate before any steps can be taken to save them.

With a penetrating wound to the kidney, the transabdominal approach is mandatory both to explore and repair any intraabdominal damage and to secure the renal artery and vein before Gerota's fascia is opened. If these vessels are not secured, massive bleeding will occur, leaving nephrectomy as the only means of stopping the gross hemorrhage. When the vessels are properly secured before Gerota's fascia is opened, it is possible to leisurely debride and repair the areas of laceration, including the collecting system if the laceration extends into it. If the trauma is in the upper or lower pole of the kidney, a partial nephrectomy may be the treatment of choice. When a complete shattering of the kidney has occurred, a complete nephrectomy is a feasible treatment choice.

Separate mention should be made of those penetrating injuries to the kidney caused by high-velocity bullets. Experience has shown that renal injury from these missiles may appear to be small and discreet, but in fact the blast effect is so great that renal tissue 1 or even 2 cm away from the actual path of the trajectory is ultimately devitalized. In these wounds extensive and wide debridement is necessary for successful treatment.

In summarizing the diagnostic workup and treatment of a penetrating injury to the kidney, it may be said that all of these injuries should be explored surgically and should receive appropriate repair as needed unless the patient's general condition from associated injuries is such that renal surgery is contraindicated. If selective renal angiography and excretory urograms show no evidence of renal damage when there is a known penetrating wound without any hematuria, it is probably not necessary to explore the kidney itself during the course of the laparotomy. However, the kidney should certainly be carefully examined at the time of laparotomy (by inspection and palpation but without opening the retroperitoneum) with additional steps determined in the operating room. When hematuria *is* present it is even more important to at least explore the kidney manually during laparotomy, at which time the need for any additional steps can be determined.

TRAUMA TO THE URETER

Blunt ureteral trauma is extraordinarily uncommon and penetrating trauma involving the ureter is rare. Diagnosis in either case is by excretory urography and surgical exploration is necessary if there is any extravasation of urine. The specific type of repair effected at surgery would depend on the type and extent of the injury.

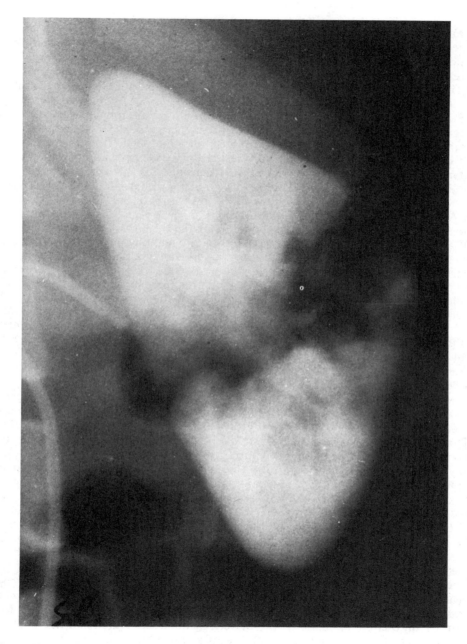

Figure 10-1. A selective left renal angiogram showing a severe fracture or laceration almost completely through the center of the kidney. Selective renal angiograms are particularly valuable in determining the extent of trauma suffered by the kidney.

TRAUMA TO THE BLADDER AND URETHRA

Traumatic injuries to the bladder occur most often from external force and are not uncommonly associated with pelvic fractures. Approximately 15 percent of all pelvic fractures are, in fact, associated with concomitant injuries to the bladder, the urethra, or both. The exact anatomic location of a tear in the bladder wall will determine if it is intra- or extraperitoneal, depending on whether the perforation is above or below the peritoneal reflexion that comes down on the anterior surface of the bladder. When the bladder is empty, it is almost entirely an extraperitoneal organ; it is only when the bladder is filled that large portions of it become intraperitoneal. Most bladder ruptures that result from pelvic fractures are caused by fragments of pelvic bone penetrating the bladder and are usually extraperitoneal in nature. Intraperitoneal bladder rupture is considerably less common and usually occurs only when the bladder is distended, making it more liable to rupture as a result of force exerted on it by a blow to the lower part of the abdomen that is not necessarily related to any pelvic fracture. In practice, an automobile-related injury in an individual with a distended bladder following the ingestion of a large amount of alcohol is a fairly common cause of intraperitoneal bladder rupture. Although these intraperitoneal bladder ruptures are far less common than the extraperitoneal variety, they are infinitely more severe because of the risk of chemical peritonitis from sterile bladder urine or bacterial peritonitis from urine that might possibly be infected. Of equal importance is the fact that the bursting force of an intraperitoneal rupture may also cause trauma to and perforation of the small intestine.

Many patients are unable to void following rupture of the bladder, either intra- or extraperitoneal, but when voiding does occur, hematuria is almost always present. Whenever a low abdominal or blunt penetrating injury is present or whenever there is a fracture of the bony pelvis, urine should be obtained promptly on the arrival of the patient in the emergency room. The urine is best obtained by spontaneous voiding or, if this is not possible, by catheterization. An absolute exception to this statement is that catheterization must definitely *not* be done if a bloody urethral discharge is noted or even if gross blood is present at the urethral meatus. These findings are strongly suggestive of urethral injury, and a retrograde urethrogram using 15 or 20 ml of contrast medium should be carried out before any catheter is inserted in the urethra because a catheter may convert a partial urethral tear into a complete disruption of the urethra and may furthermore introduce infection into the periurethral tissues. If the urethrogram discloses a partial or complete urethral disruption, catheterization of the urethra should not be attempted. Assuming an intact urethra or a normal urethrogram, a catheter may be placed into the bladder, which is then filled with 250 or 300 ml of contrast medium. X-rays are then taken to look for any evidence of extravasation with the medium present in the bladder and after it has been evacuated through the catheter. The evacuation film is very important because some areas of extravasation are concealed when the bladder is full of contrast medium. Should extravasation of contrast medium outside of the bladder be found on x-ray, the diagnosis of bladder rupture may safely be made. If the pattern of the extravasated contrast medium appears to be directly upward so that it seems to mix with the abdominal contents, there is probably an intraperitoneal rupture. If the extravasation appears to remain within the bony pelvis and extend laterally on either side of the bladder, the rupture is most likely extraperitoneal (Fig. 10–2). The clinician should realize that it

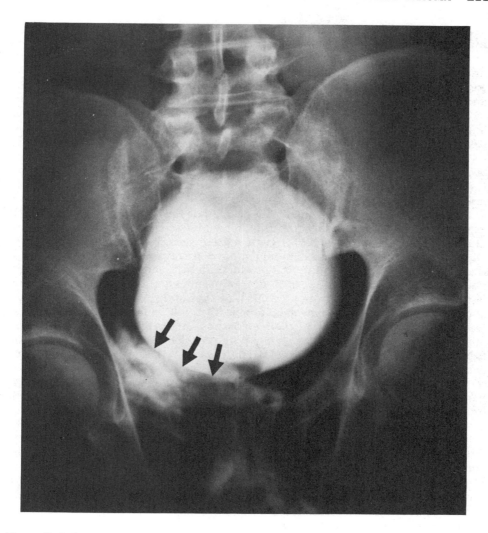

Figure 10-2. A retrograde cystourethrogram depicting an extraperitoneal rupture of the bladder secondary to an automobile accident. Note that the extravasation of the contrast medium is inferior to the bladder and also appears to be confined within the bony pelvis (*arrows* point to the extravasation).

is not rare to have *both* types of rupture. Intraperitoneal ruptures mandate prompt surgical intervention as soon as the patient's general condition permits in order to repair the bladder laceration, inspect the bowel for injury, and drain the peritoneal cavity of urine as best as possible. Extraperitoneal ruptures, depending on the physical findings, the degree of extravasation, and the patient's general condition, may be repaired surgically but in some cases may be treated by catheter drainage for 1 or 2 weeks providing that no infection occurs secondary to the extravasated urine and that the patient's general condition is not deteriorating. It is obvious that in both types of bladder rupture, associated nonurologic injuries must be managed appropriately, either in conjunction with the urologic treatment or even at times precluding immediate urologic treatment.

Urethral injuries, as noted above, are best suspected by a bloody urethral discharge or by blood seen at the urethral meatus. These injuries are relatively uncommon and occur almost always in men, usually associated with pelvic fractures and straddle type injuries. When the injury is to the posterior urethra (the prostatic or membranous portions of the urethra) the urethra is often sheared off just proximal to the urogenital diaphragm and the prostate is displaced superiorly by the developing hematoma in the periprostatic and perivesical spaces. Patients with these severe posterior urethral injuries are unable to urinate and, as already noted, blood at the urethral meatus is the single most important sign of this injury. Once this is seen or once urethral injury is suspected for any other reason, prompt retrograde urethrography is necessary to establish the diagnosis. In cases where the disruption of the posterior urethra is complete, the retrograde urethrogram shows the site of extravasation, which is usually at the prostatomembranous junction where free egress of contrast material into the periurethral space is seen. If urethral injury involves an incomplete urethral disruption, only minimal extravasation is seen and some of the contrast material passes into the prostatic urethra and then into the bladder. With complete disruption of the prostatomembranous urethra, digital examination of the prostate gland usually discloses marked superior displacement of the prostate and the area where the prostate should be is filled with a large pelvic hematoma. Obviously, partial disruption of the membranous urethra is not accompanied by any displacement of the prostate gland. With complete disruption of the prostatic urethra (this is more common than partial disruption), the long-range, postrepair complications of urethral stricture, impotence and incontinence, are considerable; the best results in a long-term sense are probably those achieved by the simple placement of a urethral catheter with a secondary repair of the disrupted urethra several months later.

Injuries to the bulbous and pendulous urethra may be secondary to self-instrumentation or iatrogenic instrumentation or even to straddle injuries. A severe straddle injury resulting in laceration of part of the urethral wall may allow extravasation of urine that may extend into the scrotum, along the penile shaft, up to the abdominal wall, and be limited only by the boundaries of Colles fascia. In these patients there is usually a history of a fall or of self-instrumentation; urethral bleeding is also present. As with the posterior urethral disruption, bleeding from the urethra or blood noted at the urethral meatus should trigger a retrograde urethrogram to demonstrate the extent and the location of the injury. The urethra should not be catheterized unless there is no evidence of extravasation seen on the retrograde urethrogram. When there is no extravasation seen on retrograde urethrogram studies, the patient is allowed to void after urethrography, and if the voiding occurs in a normal fashion, there is generally no additional treatment that is necessary. If extravasation is noted on the x-ray studies, it is probably best to divert the urine temporarily with a small suprapubic cystostomy tube that will allow the urethra to heal in a week or so. With more extensive injuries, diversion of the urine for 2 to 4 weeks usually allows for adequate healing; it should be recognized, however, that stricture formation is always a possible complication at the site of injury. Where there has been a severe laceration with pronounced extravasation, surgical drainage of the areas in which the extravasation has occurred is indicated and this may involve the perineum, the scrotum, and even the lower abdomen. Urinary diversion via suprapubic cystostomy is indicated while healing occurs.

TRAUMA TO THE PENIS

Tears of the tunica albuginea of the penis can occur during particularly traumatic sexual intercourse. This usually results in a certain degree of penile pain and, usually, hematoma formation as well. The resulting penile deformity can usually be successfully corrected surgically. Other penile injuries can occur as a result of self-mutilation or by overzealously applying constricting rings to the base of the penis in an attempt to achieve, maintain, or prolong erections, and this can result in gangrene or urethral injury. Avulsion of the penile skin can occur secondary to injury from different types of machinery, most often farm-type equipment. Penile injuries may be accompanied by urethral injuries and retrograde urethrograms should be performed to be certain that the latter has not occurred.

TRAUMA TO THE SCROTUM

The most common cause of scrotal injury is that caused by various types of machinery, and these injuries may lead to partial or total avulsion of the scrotal skin or to minor scrotal lacerations. As a general rule, the testes are spared in these types of scrotal injuries, but it is incumbent upon the clinician to determine the status of the testes at the time that the patient is seen.

TRAUMA TO THE TESTIS

One or both testes are most often damaged from blunt trauma and this is usually accompanied by severe pain. Nausea and vomiting usually occurs because of the sympathetic innervation to the testes and the crossover of these sympathetic pathways with those of the gastroenterologic (GI) tract. A hematoma may surround the testis following injury and the clinician will have to decide whether or not the condition warrants surgical exploration and repair or conservative therapy.

REFERENCES

McAninch JW: Trauma to the kidneys and ureter. Infect Surg 33–45, October 1982
McAninch JW: The injured kidney. In Stamey, TA (ed), 1983 Monographs in Urology. Princeton, NJ, Custom Publishing Services, 1983
Riehle RA Jr, Pierce JM Jr: Trauma to the lower urinary tract and genitals. In Kendall AR, Karafin L (eds), Urology. Philadelphia, Harper and Row, 1982, vol 2, chap 4
Sagalowsky AI, McConnell JD, Peters, PC: Renal trauma requiring surgery: An analysis of 185 cases. J Trauma 23:128, 1983

11
Intrascrotal Problems

EDUCATIONAL OBJECTIVES

1. Discuss the diagnosis and the treatment of torsion of the spermatic cord.
2. Discuss the differential diagnosis of torsion of the spermatic cord and acute epididymis and epididymoorchitis.
3. List the symptoms of torsion of the spermatic cord.
4. Discuss the causes and the treatment of hydrocele.
5. Describe the findings and management of torsion of the appendix testis and the appendix epididymis.
6. Palpate a scrotal mass and correctly identify: a hematocele, a hydrocele, a spermatocele, epididymitis, epididymoorchitis, torsion of the spermatic cord, testis carcinoma, and inguinoscrotal hernia.
7. List the early symptoms, physical findings and differential diagnosis of testis cancer.

PALPATORY FINDINGS

For the most part, urology is a reasonably straightforward discipline and its comprehension is based on the application of acquired knowledge. However, identification and correct diagnosis of the many intrascrotal pathologic conditions that can befall men are perhaps the exception to this generality. No phase of urology lends itself to more misunderstanding and misdiagnosis than the palpatory identification of the many and varied intrascrotal lesions. This chapter is intended to clarify for the medical student the pathogenesis, clinical and palpatory findings, and treatment of the more common abnormalities that occur within the scrotal sac (Fig. 11–1). From the point of view of an overall perspective, this chapter will help the medical student to identify torsion of the spermatic cord (a surgical emergency) and carcinoma of the testis (a life-threatening condition) and to differentiate these conditions from all of the other intrascrotal conditions that commonly occur. These many other conditions, though not serious in and of themselves, are distinct entities and warrant proper understanding and recognition.

TORSION OF THE SPERMATIC CORD

In terms of the extreme urgency of early and correct diagnosis and prompt therapy, no intrascrotal condition is more important than torsion of the spermatic cord.

First described in 1840, torsion of the spermatic cord occurs in about 1 of every 500 patients admitted to hospitals because of urologic problems, or about 1 in 5000 to 6000 general hospital admissions. In a moderate-size hospital, about three pa-

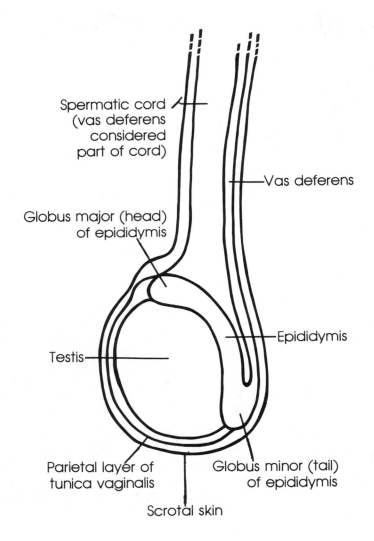

Figure 11-1. Normal intrascrotal contents. Note the insertion of the parietal layer of the tunica vaginalis upon the head of the epididymis.

tients with testicular torsion are seen per year. Undoubtedly, the true incidence of this condition is far greater than these modest figures would indicate, because probably at least two or three times as many cases are misdiagnosed or are not diagnosed at all and therefore are not seen in hospitals. The vast majority (over 90 percent) of patients with torsion of the spermatic cord are afflicted within the first two decades of life. There are two distinct age groups in which testicular torsion has its maximum incidence: infants in the first year of life (extravaginal torsion, Fig. 11–2) and boys in the years of puberty (intravaginal torsion, Fig. 11–3). Incidents of testicular torsion after the age of 25 are most uncommon although it has been reported in all age groups. Torsion must, therefore, be included in the differential diagnosis of any condition in which a patient of any age has intrascrotal pain with or without obvious edema or distortion of the intrascrotal contents.

Intra- and Extravaginal Torsion

Torsion of the spermatic cord can take one of two distinct forms. The more common is intravaginal torsion, so designated because the cord, and therefore the testicle, twists within the tunica vaginalis. During normal in utero descent of the testis the processus vaginalis, a true outpocketing of the peritoneum, is carried along with the descending testis. This processus vaginalis is usually obliterated following testicular descent, leaving intact only the portion of the tunica surrounding the testis. In the normal individual, the visceral layer of the tunica closely invests the testis and the epididymis, and the parietal layer normally inserts superiorly on the globus major (head) of the epididymis. There is usually also a stabilizing attachment of the epididymis to the posterolateral scrotal wall, and the testis is in very close proximity to the stable epididymis. Both of these serve to prevent any excessive testicular mobility.

In some individuals, the parietal layer of the tunica vaginalis inserts higher up on the spermatic cord rather than on the superior portion of the epididymis and thereby permits a great deal of mobility of the testis and epididymis *within* this layer of the tunica vaginalis. Additionally, those individuals with little or no anchoring of the epididymis to the scrotal wall or with an abnormally long attachment between the epididymis and the testis (mesorchium) will have a great deal more testicular mobility than normal. Thus, the combination of the high insertion of the tunica on the spermatic cord and an abnormally long mesorchium or a failure of attachment of the epididymis to the posterolateral scrotal wall predisposes an individual to intravaginal torsion. (This condition is sometimes called a "bell clapper" deformity; the testis may be visualized as the clapper of a bell, freely mobile within the tunica vaginalis.) In patients with intravaginal torsion, spasmodic contracture of the spiraling fibers of the cremasteric musculature can produce an abrupt twisting of the spermatic cord and the testis. The direction of this twisting, which is determined by the alignment of the cremasteric fibers, is usually clockwise on the left and counterclockwise on the right, but this is only a general rule of thumb and by no means invariable. The mechanism that triggers the cremasteric spasm is not known; therefore it is not known why torsion occurs. Although in many patients it is related to strenuous physical activity, in almost as many others it can occur when the patient is sleeping, sitting down, or in some other inactive situation.

Extravaginal torsion of the spermatic cord is far less common and is seen virtually exclusively in the neonatal period and the first year of life. In this condition, the anatomy is normal in that the tunica vaginalis does not have an abnormally high insertion and the mesorchium is normal in length. However, it has been ob-

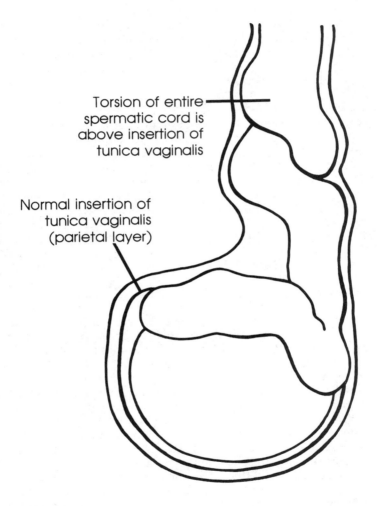

Figure 11-2. Extravaginal torsion of the spermatic cord occurs almost exclusively within the first year of life. The entire cord structure rotates extravaginally at the level of the spermatic cord *above* the insertion of the parietal portion of the tunica vaginalis.

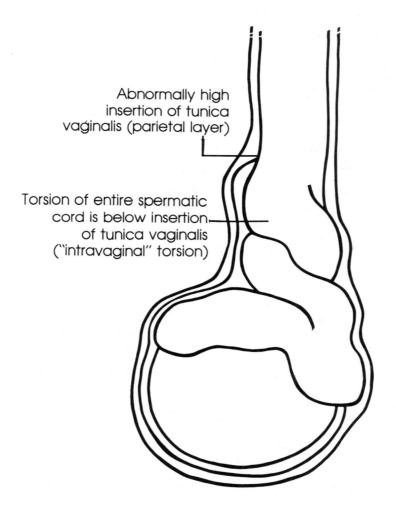

Abnormally high
insertion of tunica
vaginalis (parietal layer)

Torsion of entire spermatic
cord is below insertion
of tunica vaginalis
("intravaginal" torsion)

Figure 11-3. Intravaginal torsion of the spermatic cord occurs with peak incidence during puberty. Predisposing factors to this type of torsion are an abnormally high insertion of the parietal layer of the tunica vaginalis on the spermatic cord and an abnormally great testicular mobility because of an elongated mesorchium. These abnormalities permit intravaginal torsion although the factors actually inciting it are unknown.

served that in all neonates the attachment of the epididymis to the scrotal wall is extremely tenuous and weak, thereby permitting extensive mobility of the testis and spermatic cord. In this type of torsion, the entire cord structure rotates extravaginally, that is, the rotation occurs at the level of the spermatic cord above the insertion of the parietal portion of the tunica vaginalis on the globus major (head) of the epididymis. The inciting cause of extravaginal torsion is not known.

Clinical Findings—Extravaginal Torsion

Extravaginal torsion occurs almost exclusively in the neonatal period, and there are usually no symptoms or complaints to herald its onset both because the torsion frequently occurs in utero and also because it is apparently not as painful to the neonate as one might think. Diagnosis is based on frequent observation and examination of the scrotal contents—by the obstetrician at the time of birth, and then by the pediatrician and by the mother. If torsion is present it can usually be determined by an alert physician skilled in palpation of the scrotum in newborns. Diagnostic findings are an erythematous and edematous scrotum or hemiscrotum and a firm intrascrotal mass that is four or five times the normal testicle size for a neonate. Extravaginal torsion should be suspected in those infants with a scrotal mass in which transillumination is not possible and in which the normal testis cannot be felt adequately enough to rule out this condition. Because extravaginal torsion may occur in utero, its time of occurrence in relation to its time of discovery is the key factor in whether salvage of the testis is possible. Chances of testis salvage are greater in the neonate than in the older infant in whom torsion may have been present for weeks or months before discovery. In any case, the clinician must be constantly alert to this condition throughout the infant's first several months of life

History and Clinical Findings—Intravaginal Torsion

The greatest incidence of intravaginal torsion occurs in pubescence. However, it should be stressed that although torsion of the testis is extremely rare beyond the second decade of life or perhaps the mid-twenties, it must always be considered in a differential diagnosis of intrascrotal pain in older patients.

Some reviews of the literature suggest that torsion occurs more commonly on the left side; other reports indicate approximately equal incidence in the two testes. If indeed the left testis is involved more frequently, it may be because the left spermatic cord is longer than the right and thus, theoretically at least, is more susceptible to intravaginal torsion.

Probably the most prevalent first symptom of the patient with intravaginal torsion of the spermatic cord is moderate to severe pain of an abrupt onset. This is followed by an exquisite tenderness in the involved testis. Both the pain and the tenderness are generally localized to the testis or within the scrotum on the affected side; however, although uncommon, in some patients the pain may be referred along the course of the spermatic cord to the groin or the lower abdomen. On rare occasions intravaginal torsion has been misdiagnosed as appendicitis; therefore, the clinician should always examine the testes in patients with low abdominal pain. An extremely helpful and important finding in these patients would be a past history of severe intermittent testicular pain with spontaneous remission after a few minutes. This is of immeasurable help in establishing the diagnosis, as it indicates that in the past the patient has had some partial testicular torsion with spontaneous detorsion. In addition to pain, nausea and vomiting are relatively common findings, and although these are secondary to the severe pain they are nonspecific and simply represent crossovers of sympathetic innervation between the testes and the gastroenterologic (GI) tract. Urinary tract symptoms are almost universally absent. Results of urinalysis are virtually always within normal limits and examinations of the prostate gland and prostatic fluid show no unusual findings. White blood cell and differential cell counts are usually normal. Fever is striking by its absence and a temperature elevation above 100°F is extremely uncommon. In addition to the history of an abrupt onset of pain, the physical examination is most helpful in establishing the diagnosis. Physical findings depend on the elapsed time since the onset of symptoms. With intravaginal torsion there is initially an obstruction to the venous return, causing engorgement and edema of the testis. As the torsion continues, the arterial supply to the testis is compromised and ultimately leads to infarction and death of the testis. It is generally felt that without therapy irreversible destruction of the testis will occur between 5 and 12 hours after the onset of acute testicular pain; hence the need for haste in arriving at a diagnosis and proceeding with treatment. Within the first hour or two after the onset of symptoms, palpation of the involved testis is usually most rewarding because it may be possible to differentiate the epididymis from the testis and palpate a relatively normal epididymis in the presence of an exquisitely tender and edematous testis. If the torsion is 180 degrees, the epididymis may be palpated in the anterior position, thereby confirming the diagnosis. In those patients in whom the torsion is 360 or even 720 degrees, the epididymis is usually in its normal posterior relationship to the testis but it is generally not in its normal alignment with the testis, tending to be more diagonally placed posterior to the testis. On careful palpation of the cord above the testis, it is virtually always possible to establish that the cord is twisted and therefore thickened beyond its normal anatomic dimensions, and this impression is confirmed by comparing it with the cord on the contralateral side. A thickened spermatic cord should alert the clinician to the most likely diagnosis of torsion. Also, elevation of the testis characteristically increases the pain because such elevation, with the patient in the supine position, is tantamount to a virtual pulling motion on the cord. This elevation, or pulling motion, can help to differentiate the condition from acute epididymitis, which is the condition with which torsion is most commonly confused. Elevation of the hemiscrotum, with the patient in the supine position, tends to relieve the pain in the patient with epididymitis or epididymoorchitis because it removes the weight from the affected structure. The testis involved with a torsion of the spermatic cord is usually seen to be elevated and retracted within the scrotum, a not unexpected finding in view of the fact that twisting of the cord serves to shorten it. There is prompt and early edema of the scrotum on the involved side, usually extending only to the midline, raphé, and up as far as the twist in the cord. There may also be fixation of the skin to the underlying structures. These findings are helpful in establishing the diagnosis, but it must be stressed that, like so many other diagnostic findings, they are not infallible.

Treatment of Intra- and Extravaginal Torsion of the Testis

Inasmuch as it has been well documented, both clinically and experimentally, that infarction of the testis occurs if a normal blood supply is not restored in 5 to 12 hours after the onset of acute symptoms, therapy must be instituted virtually immediately after a diagnosis, or even a strong suspicion of intravaginal torsion, has been made. Prompt surgical exploration with detorsion through a scrotal incision is required if the testis is to be saved. Whether salvage is possible can be determined at the time of surgery by detorsing the testis, applying warm compresses, and observing it for 20 to 30 minutes to see if the blue–black testis returns to a normal color. It should be noted that even in those cases where it is felt that the testis might not be viable enough for spermatogenesis, it is very possible that Leydig cell production of testosterone may continue, and some urologists feel that these testes should be removed only if they are frankly gangrenous. If the testis is not removed, it should be sutured in two to three locations to the inside of the scrotum so that future torsion cannot occur. It is equally important to perform the same suturing of the contralateral testis to the scrotal wall because the congenital anatomic abnormalities that permit torsion usually are present bilaterally. In general, surgical exploration is indicated in virtually all patients when their age, history, and physical findings suggest the possibility of torsion. There is virtually no harm done in exploring a testis in which torsion is not found; there is a virtual guarantee of testicular infarction and atrophy if the testis in which torsion has occurred is not explored and detorsed.

The same treatment is indicated in extravaginal torsion, a condition that is virtually exclusive to the neonate. Inasmuch as this type of torsion is very likely to have been present for more than a few hours by the time of discovery, the salvage rate following surgery is extremely low and orchiectomy is usually carried out. Regardless, the presence of a firm, nontransilluminating scrotal mass in the neonate mandates prompt surgical exploration for those few individuals that may have a salvageable testis.

Differential Diagnosis

Although many intrascrotal abnormalities must theoretically be included in the differential diagnosis of torsion of the spermatic cord, acute epididymitis and epididymoorchitis are the major conditions from which torsion must be differentiated.

Accurate differential diagnosis of these conditions is based on the patient's age and history, the physical findings, and examination of the urine and prostatic fluid. Acute epididymitis rarely occurs in patients under 15 or 16 years of age, and the etiology of this condition when it does occur in this young age group is most commonly an antecedent or concurrent urethritis. Therefore, whenever it is possible to obtain a history of sexual activity, regardless of how young the patient might be, the possibility of epididymitis must be considered. A recent history of scrotal trauma may be helpful inasmuch as this may have produced a traumatic epididymitis. It must also be remembered that epididymitis can be a result of a blood-borne infection from a distant focus such as an infection of the skin, teeth, ears, or throat. When an absence of sexual activity can be established with some degree of certainty, the diagnosis of epididymitis warrants a careful search for an underlying focus of infection somewhere else in the body, and this must include a culture of the urine and examination of the prostatic secretions.

The onset of epididymitis typically is relatively mild and slow. From a few hours to a day or two will elapse between the onset of a vague testicular or low abdominal discomfort and the full-blown exquisite testicular pain that is characteristic of acute epididymitis and that is easily confused with testicular torsion. If there is an antecedent history of urethritis or urinary tract infection, the diagnosis of epididymitis is facilitated. Examination of the urine of these individuals not infrequently discloses pyuria and possible bacteriuria, and it is particularly important to obtain prostatic secretions for examination because they are occasionally loaded with pus cells, suggesting the possibility of prostatic infection.

Physical examination of the patient in the early stages of acute epididymitis discloses the same exquisite intrascrotal tenderness found with torsion; however, the tenderness is limited to the epididymis, which may be somewhat enlarged or even indurated (depending upon how early in the pathologic process the physical examination is done), and the adjacent testis will usually be normal (Fig. 11–4). Physical examination of the patient in the early stages of torsion of the spermatic cord usually discloses that the tender epididymis and testis are equally tender (since both are affected by the vascular compromise occurring with torsion of the cord) and additionally the epididymis may be palpated anterior to the testis or perhaps on either side of the testis or even in its usual posterior relationship to the testis but somewhat transverse in its lie. The big difference in the early stages of the patient with epididymitis compared to the patient with torsion of the cord is that the epididymitis patient will have all of his physical findings localized to the epididymis whereas the patient with torsion will have virtually all of his intrascrotal contents on the affected side abnormal as far as tenderness, pain, swelling, and the usual anatomic relationships. In the patient with torsion, the spermatic cord above the testis is usually thickened (as compared with the contralateral side) because there is a twist in the cord. In the patient with epididymitis, the cord in the affected testis usually feels about the same as the contralateral one. The problem in the differential diagnosis of torsion of the spermatic cord and epididymitis or epididymoorchitis is that patients are most often seen at least a few hours after the onset of symptoms and both of these disease processes change as regards physical findings to the degree that it is often not possible to differentiate one entity from the other. Within hours after the onset of torsion of the spermatic cord (or even less time depending upon the degree of torsion present) the entire intrascrotal contents on the affected side present the palpatory findings of one solitary, swollen, very tender mass, and it is not possible to differentiate testis from epididymis or even to determine the relationship of these structures to each other. Similarly, a significant percentage of patients with epididymitis progress to epididymoorchitis (Fig. 11–5), at which point the intrascrotal contents have the palpatory sensation of one very tender, firm, enlarged intrascrotal mass, and the two entites are similar enough as far as physical findings to make an accurate differentiation impossible. In each condition, the intrascrotal contents are usually significantly enlarged and can be somewhere between the size of a golf ball and a lemon. The thickening of the cord above the testis on the affected side is a constant with torsion, but this finding alone is often not enough to make a diagnosis with any degree of certainty.

At this point, great reliance must be placed on the patient's age, the history of the disease as given by the patient, and, to a lesser extent, findings within the urine and prostatic fluid. It is noteworthy that many patients with acute epididymitis and epididymoorchitis tend to have a low-grade temperature elevation whereas most patients with spermatic cord torsion are afebrile. In attempting to differentiate epididymitis/epididymoorchitis from torsion of the spermatic cord, it is helpful to remember that epididymitis/epididymoorchitis is an inflammatory process in which there is an increased blood supply to the affected testis and epididymis and torsion of the spermatic cord is a process in which there is a decreased blood supply to the testis and epididymis. Therefore, the use of the Doppler stethoscope, which detects increases or decreases of blood flow to a given area, or scrotal scanning using Tc—99m—DTPA, which also measures blood flow to a given area, may be helpful diagnostic techniques. It is the author's firm opinion, however, that these studies are only worthwhile if they confirm the clinician's own diagnostic impressions and

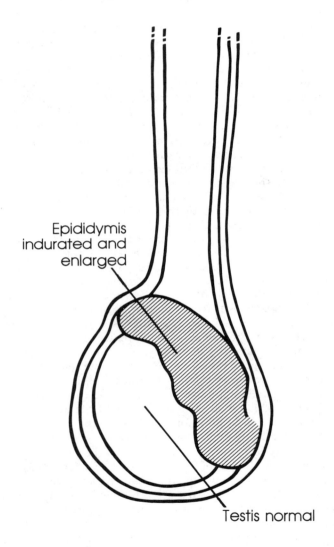

Epididymis
indurated and
enlarged

Testis normal

Figure 11–4. Epididymitis, a condition marked by inflammation, induration, and edema of the epididymis. In the early stages of the disease and in some patients, the adjacent testis remains normal.

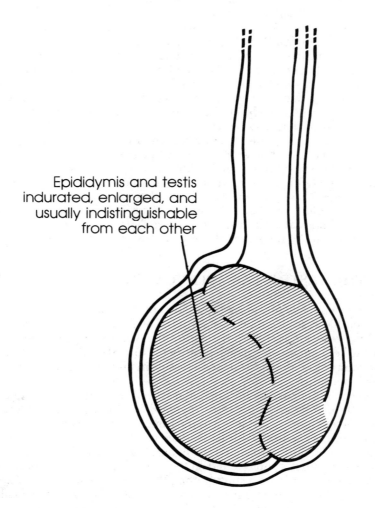

Epididymis and testis
indurated, enlarged, and
usually indistinguishable
from each other

Figure 11-5. Epididymoorchitis is a very common progression for epididymitis. The testis secondarily becomes enlarged and inflamed, producing an intrascrotal mass in which it is extremely difficult to differentiate the epididymis from the testis.

that, in the last analysis, surgical exploration of the scrotum is mandatory unless the clinician feels quite certain that the patient has epididymitis/epididymoorchitis and *not* torsion of the spermatic cord.

A pure orchitis, invariably of viral etiology, may also be confused with torsion, although it is relatively far less common than epididymitis or epididymoorchitis. There is sometimes an antecedent history of viral infection (such as mumps) elsewhere in the body. The onset of orchitis is gradual over a period of hours or a day or two and is a key in differentiating this condition from torsion. On examination, the cord will feel normal, with no suggestion of the thickening that accompanies torsion and the epididymitis will also be palpably normal.

A strangulated, or incarcerated, indirect inguinal hernia may sometimes be confused with torsion of the spermatic cord or epididymitis, although the differential diagnosis is really much simpler and reasonably straightforward. The patient is usually aware of the fact that he may have such an indirect hernia. Presence of a loop of bowel strangulated at the level of the external or internal ring produces nausea, vomiting, and pain that may be referred to the scrotal region but is more commonly abdominal. In these patients, examination of the intrascrotal contents reveals a normal testis and a normal epididymis and palpation of these structures does not produce any discomfort. Additionally, bowel sounds over the scrotum may be heard from the herniated loop of bowel (unless an ileus exists), and x-ray examination of the scrotum usually reveals the classic pattern of small intestinal gas within the scrotum. Palapation of the cord above the testis in these patients usually discloses the presence of normal cord structures, although a marked thickening will be present that is produced by the strangulated or incarcerated piece of intestine.

TORSION OF THE TESTICULAR APPENDAGES

Torsion of a testicular appendage was first described in the literature in 1922, and since then well over 300 cases have been reported. The frequency of this clinical entity, however, must be considered to be many times greater than the reported cases, inasmuch as the diagnosis is extremely difficult to make on a clinical basis alone and misdiagnosis or no diagnosis does not result in any particular complication or significant morbidity.

Anatomists describe four testicular appendages, but only two are of clinical significance (Fig. 11–6). The appendix testis (hydatid of Morgagni) is a constant finding in over 90 percent of men. Attached to the tunica albuginea on the anterior aspect of the upper pole of the testis, this appendage is a remnant of the müllerian duct. The appendix epididymis (also called the hydatid of Morgagni) is a remnant of the wolffian collecting tubules and is found on the globus major of the epididymis, usually anteriorly, and is a far less constant finding than the appendix testis. These vestigial structures are histologically similar, are composed of gelatinous and vascular connective tissue, and range in size from 0.1 to 1.0 cm in diameter. They are generally pedunculated and oval and may spontaneously twist for reasons poorly known. Torsion of the appendix testis is far more common than torsion of the appendix epididymis because a longer stalk is usually present with the former.

Clinical Findings
Mild to severe pain is present in patients who have a sudden twisting of one of the testicular appendages. The pain is of sudden onset, as with torsion of the spermatic

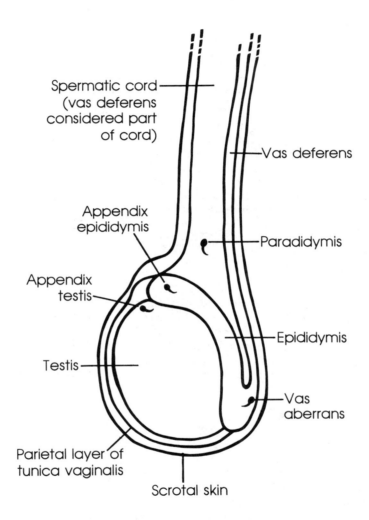

Spermatic cord
(vas deferens
considered part
of cord)

Vas deferens

Appendix
epididymis

Paradidymis

Appendix
testis

Epididymis

Testis

Vas
aberrans

Parietal layer of
tunica vaginalis

Scrotal skin

Figure 11-6. Torsion of the testicular appendages. This illustration points out all four appendages, but, in clinical practice, only the appendix testis (primarily) and the appendix epididymis (secondarily) undergo torsion and produce the clinical symptoms of infarction of the appendage which can simulate torsion of the spermatic cord.

cord, but may actually be localized to the specific twisted appendage. Physical examination may disclose a point of tenderness that helps to confirm the diagnosis. Unfortunately, in up to half the patients with torsion of a testicular appendage, a hydrocele will develop secondarily and obscure the localized findings, so the clinician cannot be certain if there is torsion of the testicular appendage or of the entire cord. In those cases where localization of the pain is possible, careful transillumination of the scrotum may reveal a dark blue or black body in the area of the appendage that represents the infarcted appendage and that will serve to confirm the diagnosis. Where the pain is diffuse throughout the testis or where a hydrocele obscures the physical findings, accurate diagnosis is not possible.

Treatment of Torsion of the Testicular Appendages

If accurate diagnosis is possible, that is, if the clinician is certain that torsion of one of the testicular appendages is present (and not torsion of the entire spermatic cord), symptomatic treatment by means of pain killers and bed rest is indicated. The pain may be expected to cease spontaneously in about 1 week when infarction and strophy of the appendage are complete or in less time if spontaneous detorsion takes place. It must be emphasized, however, that if accurate diagnosis is *not* possible, and if the possibility of torsion of the spermatic cord exists surgical exploration is mandatory. At the time of surgery, the testicular appendage may be simply removed. It is not necessary to remove the testicular appendage from the contralateral testis.

HYDROCELE

The most common cause of a mass lesion within the scrotum is a hydrocele, which is an accumulation of fluid between the visceral and parietal layers of the tunica vaginalis (Fig. 11–7). If the tunica vaginalis inserts very high on the spermatic cord instead of at the normal position on the globus major of the epididymis (see the section on intravaginal torsion of the spermatic cord), the collection of fluid will surround the cord as well as the testis and produce a hydrocele of both the testis and the cord.

Congenital Hydrocele

A hydrocele of the cord alone may result from a persistence of peritoneal fluid within one or more unobliterated segments of the peritoneal processus vaginalis. This constitutes a congenital form of hydrocele. As the testicle descends in utero—a descent that is sometimes delayed until the first few weeks after birth—the processus vaginalis is pushed ahead of it, causing an outpouching of the peritoneum. The processus vaginalis is usually obliterated by the time of birth. If it is not, however, it offers an open communication with the peritoneal cavity through which small amounts of fluid can run into and out of the tunica vaginalis (the former processus vaginalis) and produce a communicating hydrocele. This is another type of congenital hydrocele. When the child is crying or otherwise straining or active, the hydrocele forms in the tunica vaginalis; when the child is relaxed and lying down, the fluid runs back into the peritoneal cavity. Such communicating hydroceles are almost always accompanied by an indirect inguinal hernial sac and surgery is warranted to ligate the hernial sac because it will not resolve spontaneously. Occasionally, a small amount of fluid is trapped within the tunica vaginalis just before the

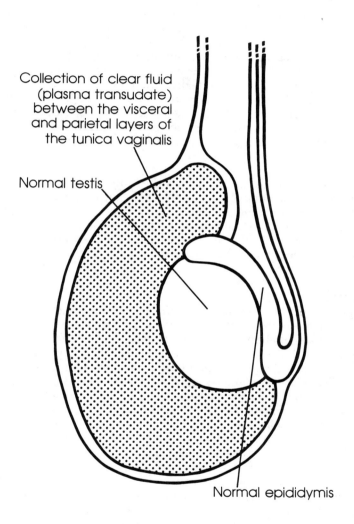

Collection of clear fluid
(plasma transudate)
between the visceral
and parietal layers of
the tunica vaginalis

Normal testis

Normal epididymis

Figure 11-7. Hydrocele, an accumulation of clear fluid between the visceral and parietal layers of the tunica vaginalis.

obliteration of the processus vaginalis and a testicular, noncommunicating hydrocele will be noted in the newborn child. This is yet another type of congenital hydrocele and most of these will commonly resorb within the first year of life; therefore, no specific treatment is indicated for at least this period of time.

Etiology of Noncongenital Hydroceles

The visceral and parietal layers of the tunica vaginalis are secreting membranes, and a small amount of plasma transudate is continually produced (secreted) by these membranes and reasbsorbed through lymphatic channels. Hydroceles result when a lymphatic obstruction causes a decrease in reabsorption of the fluid that is produced or by any mechanism that results in an increased production of fluid by the secreting membranes of the tunica vaginalis. The etiology of lymphatic obstruction, when it is the basis for a hydrocele, is poorly understood and usually not easy to diagnose. It is not at all uncommon among older patients for local extension from a primary prostatic or bladder carcinoma to result in lymphatic obstruction and hydrocele formation. However, when so-called spontaneous hydroceles occur in younger patients, the reason for the decrease in lymphatic resorption is not always apparent.

Hydroceles also result from an increase in fluid production, and this is a relatively common phenomenon. Injury to the testis, for instance, often causes an increase in transudate production, with resulting hydrocele. Infectious or traumatic epididymitis does the same, and it must not be forgotten that carcinoma of the testis can lead to a secondary hydrocele. In many of these cases, spontaneous resorption of the hydrocele may occur when the underlying process that stimulated the excess fluid production is resolved.

Physical Findings

On visual inspection of the scrotum, it is usually apparent that one side is larger than the other. Palpation of the affected hemiscrotum usually produces a sense of fluctuation and it may be relatively firm or soft depending upon the tension within the hydrocele. The outlines of the mass are usually smooth. The primary diagnostic step is to transilluminate the mass with a bright flashlight in a darkened room. A true hydrocele filled with the characteristic clear, straw-colored fluid readily transilluminates the light. Failure of transillumination may be due to a thickened tunica vaginalis secondary to chronic infection or the scrotal mass in question may not be a hydrocele at all. Hydroceles may be confined to the tunica surrounding the testis, or, as noted earlier, may also involve the distal portion of the cord, depending on the location of the insertion of the tunica vaginalis on the cord. Uncommonly, congenital hydroceles may also affect the cord alone.

Palpation of the testis within a hydrocele may be relatively easy if there is a minimum amount of fluid present, but it may be virtually impossible in the presence of a large collection of fluid. (Hydroceles range in size from only a little larger than the testis itself to the size of a cantaloupe or even larger). The general palpatory findings on examining the patient with a hydrocele are of a very thin rubber collecting device filled with fluid, which is unmistakable. Hydrocele is quite characteristic and should not be confused with any other intrascrotal lesion. It is important to palpate the cord above the level of the insertion of the tunica vaginalis, and in these cases a perfectly normal cord should be present. This helps to make a differential diagnosis from a large scrotal hernia, which on occasion may also be transilluminated. The presence of a large scrotal hernia can often be confirmed by bowel sounds within the scrotum, typical small bowel gas on x-ray films, and finally by actually reducing the scrotal mass by pushing it into the abdominal cavity while the patient is in the recumbent position. With most moderate or large hydroceles, it is not possible to palpate either the testis or the epididymis and it is incumbent upon the physician to be certain that a tumor of the testis is not responsible for the hydrocele. In these circumstances, when no etiology is apparent for the hydrocele and where spontaneous resolution does not occur within a few days, needle aspiration of the hydrocele fluid is permissible for the purpose of meticulous palpation of the underlying testis. As noted, the reason for palpating through the hydrocele is to feel the testis and epididymis in order to be certain that the hydrocele formation is not secondary to a cancer of the testis.

Treatment of Hydrocele

Some hydroceles, such as traumatic hydroceles in children, resorb spontaneously within 1 week to 1 month. In such cases, expectant and conservative treatment is indicated. In older age groups, the hydrocele may well resorb spontaneously if it has resulted from an overproduction of fluid by the secreting membranes of the tunica vaginalis such as one might find secondary to acute epididymitis. In the majority of adults with hydrocele, however, the etiology is that of an imbalance between fluid production and resorption and the hydroceles do not disappear spontaneously. In such cases, needle aspiration of the hydrocele does not constitute adequate therapy because the hydrocele will inevitably recur. Proper and adequate therapy involves surgical exploration of the scrotum, with resection and removal of most of the parietal layer of the tunica vaginalis so that a secreting membrane is removed, thus preventing a recurrence of the hydrocele.

INGUINOSCROTAL HERNIA

An inguinoscrotal hernia is an indirect hernial sac (although it may also represent a direct hernia) protruding through the inguinal canal, the external inguinal ring and down into the scrotum; it is seen as a mass within the scrotum. Diagnosis is based on palpable thickening along the entire course of the spermatic cord, due to pressure of the hernial sac and its contents (Fig. 11–8). This is true whether the hernia consists of omentum or bowel or both. Auscultation over the scrotum should reveal bowel sounds if a piece of small intestine has herniated into the scrotum unless there is an ileus. An x-ray film of the scrotum usually reveals a typical pattern of small bowel gas within the scrotum. Transillumination of the bowel may be possible, although not with the usual clarity that is seen with a hydrocele. If the hernia is reducible, as it usually is in the absence of any patient discomfort, it may be pushed back up through the external ring and the inguinal canal and into the peritoneal cavity. If it is not reducible, it must be considered to be incarcerated and surgical intervention should be seriously considered unless reduction can be accomplished. If the hernia is strangulated (with impairment of blood supply to the segment of bowel), the patient will have symptoms and findings compatible with intestinal obstruction, and the mass will be extremely tender. Finally, it is usually possible to palpate an entirely normal testis and epididymis within the scrotum in the presence of a scrotal hernia.

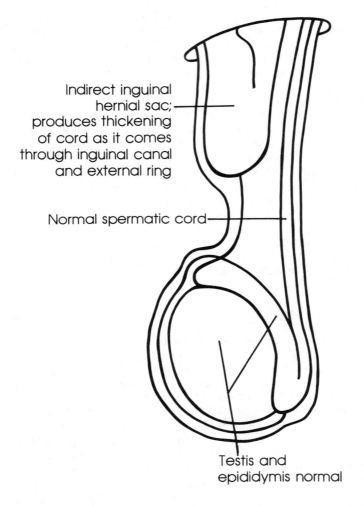

Indirect inguinal hernial sac; produces thickening of cord as it comes through inguinal canal and external ring

Normal spermatic cord

Testis and epididymis normal

Figure 11-8. Inguinoscrotal hernia, a scrotal mass produced by an indirect hernia sac protruding through the inguinal canal, the external inguinal ring, and down into the scrotum. There may or may not be intraabdominal contents such as intestine or omentum within the hernial sac. This type of hernia can also be of the direct variety.

SPERMATOCELE

A spermatocele is a retention cyst of the head of the epididymis or of an aberrant tubule or tubules of the rete testis (Fig. 11-9). It may occasionally be possible to transilluminate it. The critical point in the diagnosis of a spermatocele is the ability to palpate it quite distinctly from the testis, and this can be done easily because it lies outside the tunica vaginalis. The examining physician must be certain that it is in no way part of the testis itself because a lesion such as a spermatocele, were it a part of the testis itself, would be suspicious for cancer of the testis. On palpation, the spermatocele is firm, uniformly spherical in shape, and generally nontender. Spermatoceles are usually about the size of a marble and they are quite innocuous. No specific therapy is indicated. On occasion, however, these spermatoceles may become either large enough or sufficiently tender to warrant surgical removal on the basis of patient discomfort. Spermatoceles can only be definitely differentiated from epididymal cysts based upon the presence of spermatozoa in the aspirated spermatocele. In practice, however, this is not done because there is no need to make this differential diagnosis with any degree of certainty.

VARICOCELE

Varicocele is a redundancy and a dilatation of the veins within the scrotum and involves the internal and external spermatic and vasal veins (Fig. 11-10). It probably exists in 10 to 15 percent of men. The etiology is probably an incompetency of the valves within the internal spermatic vein or a congenital absence of these valves. To accommodate the resulting increased retrograding of blood down the internal spermatic vein, the other veins of the testicular circulation become greatly distended and redundant. Varicocele is much more common on the left side, probably because the left internal spermatic vein drains into the renal vein at a virtual right angle, whereas the right internal spermatic vein drains into the vena cava at a much smaller angle. Also, the left renal vein is anatomically prone to compression between the aorta and the superior mesenteric artery, and this can increase the pressure within that vein and thence into the internal spermatic vein.

The sudden appearance of varicoceles on either side must alert the clinician to the very slight possibility that they are caused by a tumor mass that is causing retroperitoneal obstruction to the internal spermatic vein. Varicoceles on the left side additionally should alert the clinician to the possibility of renal vein obstruction due to renal tumor. For these reasons excretory urography is probably indicated in any case of varicocele with sudden onset. There may be no symptoms of varicocele, or there may be a vague sense of intrascrotal heaviness or aching after the individual has been in an upright position for prolonged periods. Varicoceles have been implicated in the reduction of sperm motility and maturation and resulting infertility. This is probably because the large number of dilated and redundant veins within the scrotum result in a greatly increased blood flow within the scrotum, and this in turn tends to raise the scrotal temperature sufficiently to exert a deleterious effect on fertility.

Palpatory findings within the scrotum are very characteristic and consist of feeling a "bag of worms" when the patient is upright. The dilated and redundant veins collapse and are not palpable when the patient is recumbent.

No treatment is indicated unless the patient's discomfort warrants it, or if im-

234

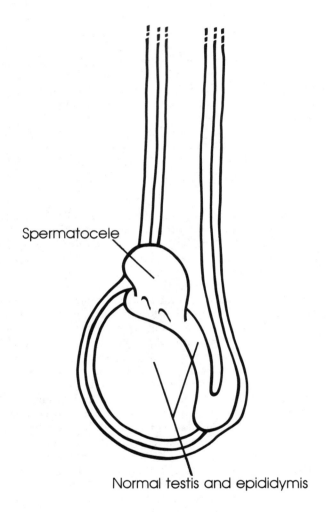

Spermatocele

Normal testis and epididymis

Figure 11-9. Spermatocele, a retention cyst of the head of the epididymis or of an aberrant tubule or tubules of the rete testis. It lies outside the tunica vaginalis so that on palpation it can be readily distinguished from and separated from the testis.

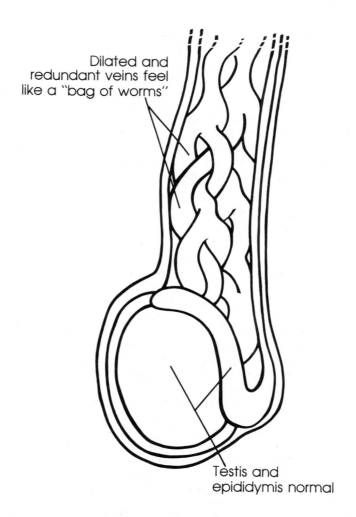

Dilated and redundant veins feel like a "bag of worms"

Testis and epididymis normal

Figure 11-10. Varicocele, a redundancy and dilatation of the veins within the scrotum.

proved fertility is the goal. Although varicocelectomy is often done in patients with infertility problems, it should be emphasized that there is no real scientific data to prove that such surgery is beneficial. Surgical repair consists of high ligation of the internal spermatic vein at or just inside the internal inguinal ring, which results in atrophy of the dilated and abnormal intrascrotal veins within several weeks of surgery.

HEMATOCELE

Hematocele results from trauma to the testis such as testis rupture and is a collection of blood between the layers of the tunica vaginalis (Fig. 11–11). The early stages consist of pain and tenderness associated with the trauma, and ecchymotic areas of the scrotum are often visible. During resolution, the mass is neither painful nor tender, but it usually presents as a very firm and nontransilluminating mass surrounding the testis. Palpatory findings of a hematocele are basically those of a hard mass within the scrotum completely surrounding the testis, therefore making the testis appear much larger than normal. It is impossible to palpate the testis with any degree of certainty because of the blood surrounding the testis. The epididymis is usually not distinctly palpable either. Carcinoma of the testis cannot be ruled out and surgical exploration is definitely indicated.

CARCINOMA OF THE TESTIS

In many ways, the purpose of the clinician becoming familiar with the various intrascrotal conditions to which men are prone is to be able to determine when a carcinoma of the testis is present. Inasmuch as carcinoma of the testis mandates surgery as promptly as possible, it is incumbent on the physician to know the palpatory findings of this condition (Fig. 11–12).

Although carcinoma of the testis may lead to a secondary hydrocele, epididymitis, or even a hematocele, rendering palpation of the testis difficult or impossible, in the vast majority of cases there are no obfuscating findings to detract from accurate preoperative diagnosis. The testis normally has a moderately firm but distinctly uniform feel throughout, and any areas of the testis suggesting greater firmness or greater hardness than other areas must be suspected of being carcinomatous. Additionally, any enlargement of a portion of the testis, such as one pole or the other, with or without corresponding hardness must also be suspect as carcinoma. In short, if palpation of the intrascrotal contents does not enable the examiner to feel an entirely normal testis throughout its surface the diagnosis of carcinoma must be considered. Moreover, if any firm or hard areas that are found within the scrotum cannot with certainty be determined to be distinct from and not part of the testis (as with an indurated and distinct epididymis), the diagnosis of carcinoma must again be considered. Whenever the diagnosis of testis cancer is considered, prompt inguinal exploration of the intrascrotal contents must be carried out.

There are many different palpatory sensations suggestive of carcinoma. A 1-cm area of firmness in the lower pole of the testis should make the clinician just as suspicious of carcinoma as a rock-hard feeling in the entire testis. Particularly important is that the clinician be able to differentiate the indurated epididymis of acute

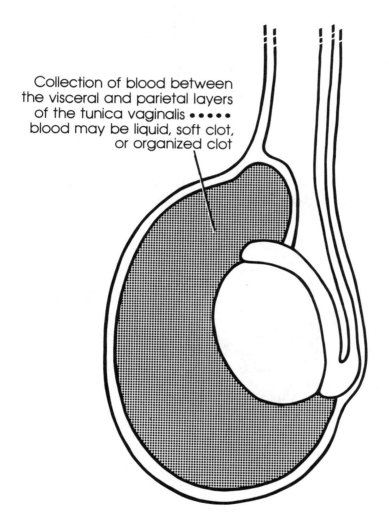

Collection of blood between
the visceral and parietal layers
of the tunica vaginalis ••••••
blood may be liquid, soft clot,
or organized clot

Figure 11-11. Hematocele, a collection of blood between the layers of the tunica vaginalis. It results from trauma and may be an accompaniment of testicular rupture.

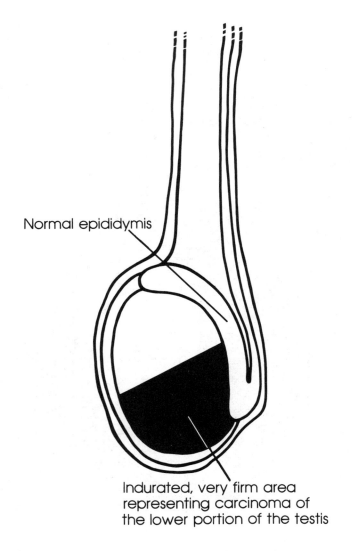

Normal epididymis

Indurated, very firm area
representing carcinoma of
the lower portion of the testis

Figure 11-12. Testis carcinoma, a condition in which there are few or no symptoms, but palpation of the testis usually suggests an induration, nodularity, abnormal firmness, or frank hardness. The epididymis is usually normal.

or chronic epididymitis from the testis itself, and if this is not possible, surgical exploration should be considered. The examining physician must further recall that cancer of the testis classically is painless, has few or no symptoms, and is most frequently diagnosed by the patient himself while feeling his own testes during a bath or shower. The frequency of early diagnosis and successful treatment of this extremely serious condition would be tremendously enhanced if examination of the testes were part of every physical examination and if clinicians maintained a high index of suspicion of this deadly condition.

When surgical exploration for a possible carcinoma of the testis is undertaken, the incision should be through the inguinal canal and not directly into the scrotal since the scrotal approach has a high risk for tumor spillage and local recurrence of the tumor in the scrotum. A more complete discussion of testicular cancer appears in Chapter 6.

REFERENCES

Donohue JP: Tumors of the testis. In Kendall AR, Karafin L (eds), Urology. Philadelphia, Harper and Row, 1980, vol 2, chap 8

Rous SN: Urology in Primary Care. St. Louis, Mosby, 1976

Rous SN: Treatment of testicular torsion. In Kaufman JJ (ed), Current Urologic Therapy, 1st ed. Philadelphia, Saunders, 1980, pp 362–365

12

Sexually Transmitted and Other Cutaneous Lesions of the External Genitalia in Males

EDUCATIONAL OBJECTIVES

1. Define phimosis and paraphimosis.
2. Define balanitis and balanoposthitis.
3. Recognize and identify balanitis and balanoposthitis.
4. Recognize and identify phimosis and paraphimosis.
5. Recognize and identify the following: primary chancre, chancroid, lymphogranuloma venereum, granuloma inguinale, and herpes progenitalis.
6. Discuss the differential diagnosis of genital ulcers in the male.
7. Differentiate between the cutaneous lesions of primary syphilis and herpes progenitalis.
8. List the symptoms of herpes progenitalis.
9. Recognize and identify verrucal warts (condyloma accuminatum) of the penis and of the distal urethra.
10. Recognize and identify sebaceous cysts of the skin of the genitalia.

Until about 30 years ago, the American Board of Dermatology was known as the American Board of Dermatology and Syphilology. This grandiose title reflected the thinking that cutaneous syphilitic lesions, and presumably all other cutaneous lesions of the external genitalia, came under the clinical purview of the dermatologist. Although the dermatologist still probably has the greatest expertise in the diagnosis of these various cutaneous lesions, more and more patients with these lesions are being referred to the urologist because of their anatomic location. There is no question, however, that it is the primary care physician who sees the vast majority of patients with cutaneous lesions of the external genitalia, at least initially, and it is incumbent upon this group of physicians to have at least a passing familiarity with the more common lesions.

HERPES PROGENITALIS (GENITAL HERPES)

This condition, caused by the genital herpes simplex virus, has been known and described in the medical literature for nearly 200 years. The enormous concern and anxiety that has been generated over the past few years because of this lesion, however, is a direct reflection of its ever-increasing incidence and prevalence and particularly because it is readily transmissible to sexual partners and there is no known cure.

The etiologic agent in genital herpes is the herpes simplex virus, which is related to several other herpesviruses that are pathogenic for man. There are two types of herpes simplex viruses: HSV-1, which is generally associated with infections about the face and mouth, such as the well-known "cold sore" or "fever blister"; and HSV-2, which is commonly associated with genital herpes lesions. However, a significant percentage of genital herpes may be caused by HSV-1 and HSV-2 may alternatively cause oral or pharyngeal infections. This "crossover" phenomenon can usually be attributed to oral–genital contact.

The symptoms of an initial infection are usually present within 2 to 21 days after a sexual contact with an infected person. Most patients experience a soreness and an itching in the region of the infection and about 75 percent of the patients develop enlarged or tender inguinal or femoral lymph nodes. About one third of infected patients experience some fever, malaise, and headache. Interestingly, about one quarter of men also have dysuria with a minimal urethral discharge as well as a urethritis, but most patients present with the classic skin ulcerations. In the initial infections, the skin ulcerations usually begin as vesicular, pustular lesions on the shaft of the penis. These pustular lesions last about 5 to 6 days and then usually turn into wet ulcers, and it is at this point that many patients seek medical assistance because the symptoms are most severe (Fig. 12–1). After about 12 days, lesions in men begin to crust over and total healing occurs in about 3 weeks. It is interesting to note that in about 20 percent of patients, herpetic lesions may simultaneously develop on the fingers, thighs, buttocks, or arms in addition to the penis. Although exact figures are not available because herpes progenitalis is not a reportable disease, some researchers in this field estimate that as many as 10 percent of the adult population of the United States have symptomatic genital herpes.

Diagnosis may be strongly suspected based on the clinical appearance of the lesions, particularly when they are in the wet ulcer stage. Definitive diagnosis is based upon isolation of the virus in tissue culture, a procedure that can be done in most virology laboratories. If cytologic methods are used, the scrapings from the base of the ulcer can be stained with Giemsa stain and the presence of multinucleated giant cells with large, eosinophilic intranuclear inclusions are usually diagnostic of a herpes simplex virus infection. Another diagnostic method is using an antigen detection technique and this incorporates the use of immunofluorescence. The sensitivity of the cytologic and antigen detection methods decreases as the infection becomes more long-standing and chronic.

When a herpex simplex infection is established in an otherwise healthy man, the immune system destroys most of the virus. What is not destroyed tends to migrate to nervous tissue, usually the sacral ganglia in the case of HSV-2. In immunocompromised patients, the viral infection may run rampant and become life threatening. In the newborn, herpes infections are usually contracted during passage of the infant through the infected birth canal, and the infection can readily disseminate widely, leading to neonatal death or permanent disability. For the majority of patients with normal immune systems, however, an initial HSV-2 infection will recur, generally at 2- to 4-month intervals. Most of these patients with recurrent disease have symptoms such as tingling or itching at the original infection site 1 or 2 days before the lesions actually reappear. These recurrent episodes tend to be less severe

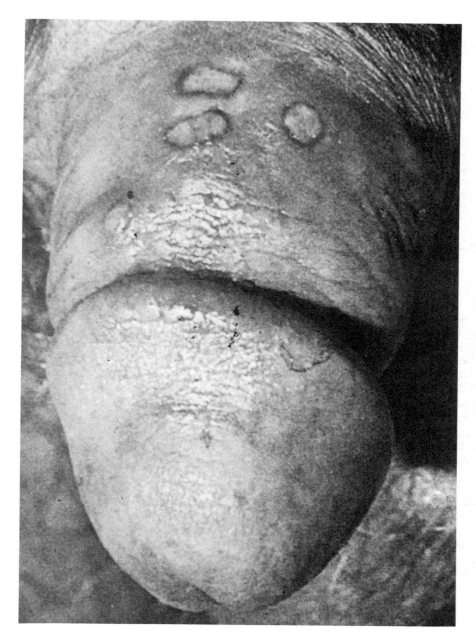

Figure 12-1. Herpes progenitalis, showing the typical herpetic lesions in the ulcerative stage when the symptoms are most severe. For a brief few days prior to becoming ulcerative the lesions of herpes progenitalis are usually vesicular.

than the initial episode, and somewhat shorter as well, generally lasting 10 to 12 days.

During the acute, or any recurrent episodes, patients should refrain from sexual intercourse, and this abstinence should continue until all visible lesions have completely healed. The antiviral agent, Acyclovir, has been shown to be clinically effective in both its topical and intravenous forms in primary initial genital herpes and in immunocompromised patients. It also is of benefit in recurrent cases of genital herpes, and in both the initial and the recurrent episodes Acyclovir shortens the duration of the cutaneous lesion by 2 to 3 days. It is definitely not a cure, however, and it certainly does not affect the incidence of recurrent lesions. Very recently, Acyclovir has been marketed in oral form, and this newest medication does indeed seem to greatly reduce recurrent episodes of herpes in some patients. Research towards developing a vaccine against herpes has been encouraging but is probably still some few years away from being a practical and clinical reality.

PRIMARY CHANCRE (SYPHILIS)

Even though syphilis is totally curable with our present methods of treatment, there is possibly no other cutaneous lesion of the external genitalia that causes more worry and anxiety to the sexually active male than the primary chancre of syphilis. This lesion is characteristically a painless, indurated ulceration that may vary in size from that of a small pin head to 1 cm or larger. It has a clean base and sharply demarcated borders and is usually associated with inguinal adenopathy (Fig. 12–2). The etiology is sexual intercourse with a person infected with the spirochete *Treponema pallidum*, and the incubation period between exposure and chancre averages 3 to 6 weeks. Diagnosis must be made by dark-field examination in which the organisms are scraped from the lesion and visualized microscopically. Serologic tests for syphilis may be negative at the time that the lesion first appears and diagnosis from observation of the lesion alone may be extremely difficult, particularly if there is a secondary coexisting infection. The principal differential diagnosis of the chancre is chancroid, a bacterial infection with which it may actually coexist.

Adequate treatment of the primary chancre consists of 4.8 million units of one of the long-acting forms of penicillin given intramuscularly. For individuals whose known sensitivity precludes the use of penicillin, oral administration of tetracycline, 500 mg by mouth four times per day for 15 days, or erythromycin in the exact same dosage schedule, provides the best alternate treatment. With proper treatment, the chancre usually disappears in 10 to 14 days. If no treatment is given, the chancre heals and disappears in 6 to 8 weeks and the generalized rash of secondary syphilis may appear anywhere from 1 to 3 months following the initial chancre.

CHANCROID

Caused by the gram-negative, pleomorphic bacillus (*Haemophilus ducreyi*), chancroid produces a severely inflamed ulcer that is usually multiple and a severe suppurative lymphadenitis. The ulcer itself is soft, painful, and purulent and the crater margins are irregular and not indurated (Fig. 12–3). Note the differences between chancroid and chancre. Diagnosis of this lesion is by microscopy of smears prepared

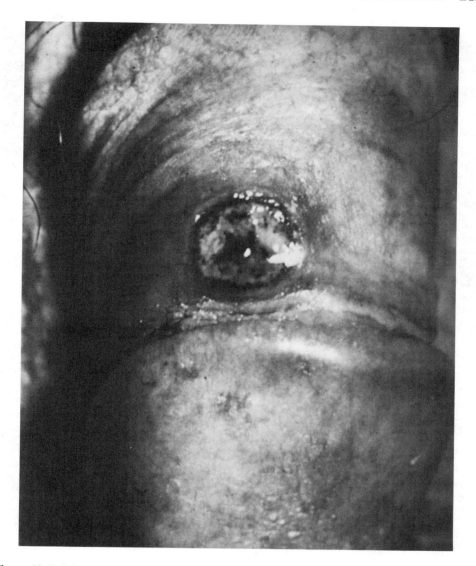

Figure 12-2. Primary chancre of syphilis, located just proximal to the glans penis in this patient. The lesion characteristically has a clean base, with sharply demarcated borders, and is usually painless and indurated.

from the undetermined ulcer edges in which the *H. ducreyi* organism may be seen. A dark-field examination should be performed at the same time to rule out the possible coexistence of syphilis. Appropriate treatment is tetracycline 500 mg four times a day for 2 weeks, and this, it should be noted, is effective against any incubating syphilis as well.

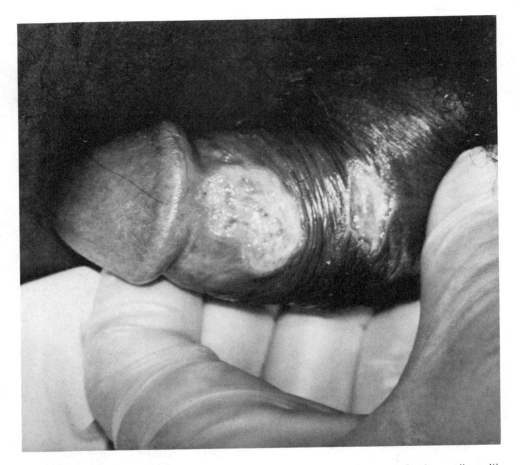

Figure 12–3. Chancroid characteristically produces a severely inflamed ulcer that is usually multiple and is soft, painful, and purulent. The crater margins are irregular and not indurated.

LYMPHOGRANULOMA VENEREUM

This is an uncommon sexually transmitted venereal disease that is much more frequent in blacks than in whites. The primary genital lesion is a few millimeters in diameter and painless. It is papular, erosive, or vesicular. The incubation is 2 days to 3 weeks and the very evanescent primary lesion disappears spontaneously within 3 to 4 days. The inguinal lymph nodes become enlarged, painful, and matted in appearance (Fig. 12–4) 10 to 30 days later, and this may lead to lymphatic obstruction and genital elephantiasis. Diagnosis is by the lymphogranuloma complement fixation test, which has a 97 percent accuracy level if determined within 4 weeks of the initial infection. Diagnosis may also be done by biopsy of the enlarged inguinal lymph nodes in which the organism may be found. It is a viruslike organism

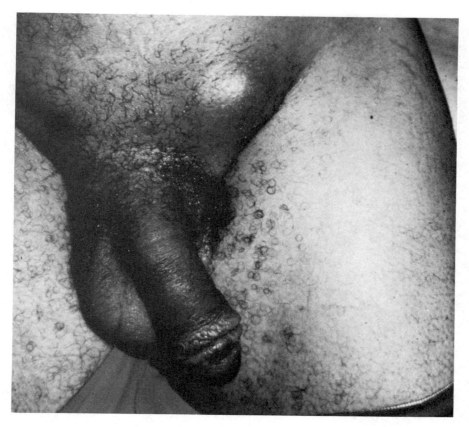

Figure 12-4. Lymphohogranuloma venereum is a very evanescent primary genital lesion that is just a few millimeters in diameter and is painless. It may be papular, erosive, or vesicular, but since the lesion is so evanescent the first lesion usually seen by the clinician is an enlarged group of inguinal lymph nodes that are painful and matted.

of the *Chlamydia* group. The treatment of choice is tetracycline, 500 mg four times a day for 3 to 6 weeks.

GRANULOMA INGUINALE

This lesion, caused by a gram-negative intracellular coccobacillus involves the skin and mucous membranes without producing any lymphatic obstruction, except very late in its course. It appears as a nodule on the penis or the groin that breaks down to become spreading, bright red, friable granulation tissue (Fig. 12–5). It remains superficial with contiguous spread and produces considerable itching. Diagnosis is by biopsy and by identification of the offending organisms, and the treatment of choice is tetracycline, 500 mg four times a day for 3 to 6 weeks.

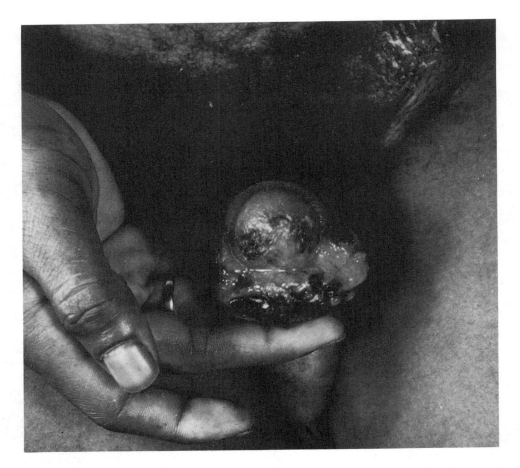

Figure 12-5. Granuloma inguinale starts as a nodule on the penis or the groin and breaks down to become spreading, bright red, friable granulation tissue.

DIFFERENTIAL DIAGNOSIS OF THE DISEASES PRODUCING GENITAL ULCERS

In sexually active men, herpes progenitalis, syphilis, chancroid, lymphogranuloma venereum, and granuloma inguinale are the diseases most likely to produce genital ulcers. The primary lesion of most acute genital ulcers is not an ulcer at all but rather is a vesicle, papule, or pustule. A papule is the first lesion of syphilis, granuloma inguinale, and sometimes chancroid and lymphogranuloma venereum. These latter two diseases may start also as pustules. Vesicles are the primary lesions of genital herpes, and when grouped on an erythematous base they present a picture that is quite diagnostic.

Genital lesions, whether papular, vesicular, or pustular, quickly erode to an ulcerative phase, but the different ulcer characteristics can be helpful in arriving at a diagnosis. A rolled, elevated border with a glistening pearly surface is characteristic of granuloma inguinale whereas the border of chancroid is ragged, undermined, and not indurated with a narrow zone of erythema surrounding it. The ulcer margins of syphilis and granuloma inguinale are firm and indurated whereas the ulcer margins of chancroid lesions are usually soft and maleable. A deep genital ulcer suggests chancroid whereas the ulcers of syphilis, herpes, and lymphogranuloma are more superficial. Purulent secretions suggest chancroid (or a secondary infection of almost any kind of ulcer) and a serous drainage is seen with herpes and syphilis. The most painful ulcers are those associated with chancroid and sometimes with herpes whereas the ulcers of syphilis and granuloma inguinalae are usually painless unless there is secondary infection present. The inguinal adenopathy produced by herpes is tender and that caused by syphilis is nontender and firm. The adenopathy associated with chancroid and lymphogranuloma venereum tends to be suppurative.

Recurrent genital ulcers that appear to be related to the ingestion of any particular medication is diagnostic of a fixed drug reaction, and it must always be borne in mind that traumatic ulcers should be included in the differential diagnosis, although these are almost invariably associated with some type of sexual activity.

SEBACEOUS CYSTS OF THE SKIN OF THE GENITALIA

Sebaceous cysts of the genital skin appear most commonly on the skin of the scrotum (Fig. 12–6) and are no different from sebaceous cysts anywhere else on the body. No specific therapy is needed for these cysts unless they cause the patient distress either because of their size or their appearance, in which case surgical removal of the cysts is indicated. If surgery is undertaken, it is necessary that the cysts be shelled out in their entirety and removed along with the cyst wall.

VERRUCAE (CONDYLOMA ACUMINATUM)

Verrucae (condyloma acuminatum) may occur anywhere on the penis or in the urethra as well as on the skin of the scrotum and surrounding perineum (Fig. 12–7). They may also appear just within the urethral meatus or anywhere within the urethra (Fig. 12–8). These lesions are caused by a papilloma virus and they are sometimes called venereal warts because they are spread through sexual intercourse. The incubation period may be anywhere from a few weeks to almost a year, making this condition particularly difficult to treat. Apparent recurrences of lesions already successfully treated may not be recurrences at all but may represent cutaneous manifestations of the virus that was still in a state of incubation during the initial and earlier therapeutic efforts. Continuing outbreak of new lesions may *also* represent an ongoing ping-pong effect of reinfection. Treatment with podophyllin 10 to 25 percent in tincture of benzoin has been a standard treatment for many years, and it is highly effective but very time consuming. The patient must be cautioned to wash the applied medication off within the prescribed time, usually 1 hour or less, lest it cause irritation and considerable discomfort to normal tissue underlying the warts. On occasion, one application of podophyllin is sufficient to cure the condition but much more commonly frequent applications over a period of several weeks are required because recurrence of the lesions from the delayed incubation periods are particularly troublesome. The duration of treatment is often directly related

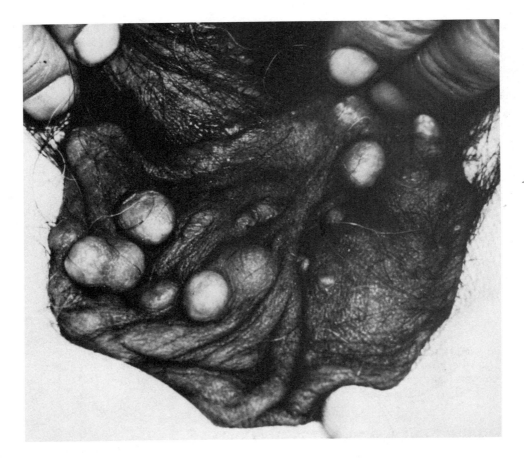

Figure 12-6. Sebaceous cysts of the skin of the scrotum are no different from sebaceous cysts anywhere else on the body. In this patient they were an incidental finding and did not require any particular therapy.

to the extent of the lesions because application of the podophyllin is tedious, time consuming, and requires meticulous care in order to avoid the use of large amounts of podophyllin at one time, as it is absorbed and it is toxic. Alternative therapies include cryotherapy, electrosurgery, surgical removal, and laser therapy. When the verrucae are located intraurethrally, podophyllin should not be used because of the risk of stricture and scar formation during the healing process. Intraurethral lesions may successfully be treated with 5-fluorouracil (5-FU) in ointment form instilled into the urethra, by sharp removal and fulguration, or by other forms of electrosurgery or laser therapy. Cystoscopy is indicated when intraurethral condyloma are found in order to detect the extent of the disease. Ideal therapy also warrants the use of condoms for several months after the last recurrence to preclude additional infection of the male organs or transmittal of this troublesome virus to its original female host or to another female contact.

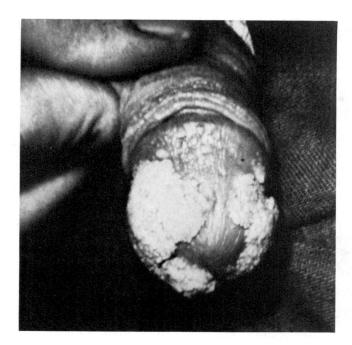

Figure 12-7. Condyloma acuminatum on the glans penis appears as a flat and cauliflowerlike growth that may involve any part of the external genitals in men and women. In this patient the lesion is confined to the glans penis.

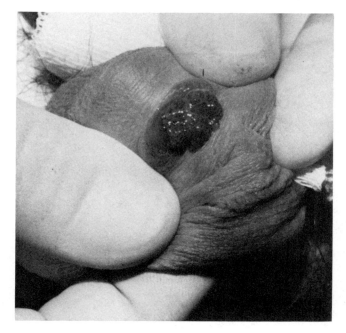

Figure 12-8. Condyloma acuminatum within the urethral meatus. This is a not uncommon location for this type of lesion. In the illustration, the urethral meatus is being forcibly everted so that the intraurethral condyloma is readily seen.

CANCER OF THE PENIS

Penile cancers are virtually all squamous cell carcinomas. Fortunately, they are relatively rare, probably accounting for less than 1 percent of all male cancers. This disease is found almost exclusively in uncircumcised males, and chronic irritation from phimosis or poor penile hygiene are considered to be predisposing factors. The lesions have many different appearances and no one type can be considered typical of penile cancer (Figs. 12–9, 12–10). However, the appearance of any undiagnosed and unexplained penile lesion mandates biopsy, as does any lesion that fails to heal within 2 to 4 weeks. It should be evident that physical examination of the male is totally inadequate unless the foreskin is fully retracted for the purposes of examining the glans. It is not unusual to have a carcinoma on the glans penis that is completely obscured from view by the foreskin (Fig. 12–11).

Metastases of penile cancer are primarily through the lymphatic system to the inguinal lymph nodes. Treatment consists of a subtotal or total penectomy, depending on the location of the lesion, and this may be combined with bilateral inguinal lymphadenectomy if there is tumor present in the nodes. The criteria for partial or total penectomy is that a 2-cm tumor-free margin be obtained; thus partial penectomy is satisfactory only if the carcinoma is on the distal portion of the penile shaft. Additionally, the use of Bleomycin as a chemotherapeutic adjuvant to surgical therapy has been beneficial in some cases.

It should be noted that there are some cutaneous lesions of the penis that, although very uncommon, are considered to be precancerous because they have a high frequency of malignant transformation. Conditions such as erythroplasia of Queyrat (Fig. 12–12) are considered premalignant and Bowen's disease may be

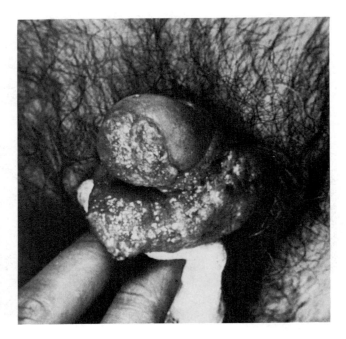

Figure 12-9. Cancer of the penis is seen virtually exclusively in uncircumcised men. It characteristically has several different appearances of which this is one.

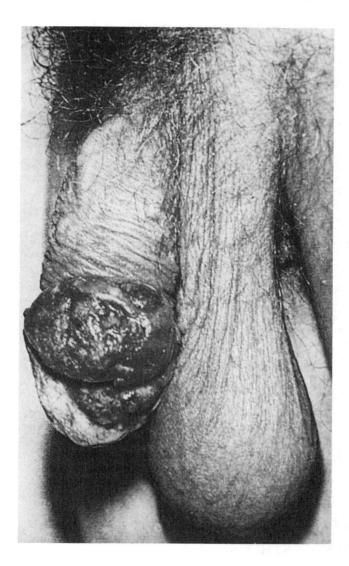

Figure 12-10. Cancer of the penis is another of its many presentations.

similarly considered (Fig. 12–13). Although these two conditions are histologically almost identical, the particular names applied to them are erythroplasia of Queyrat when the lesion is on the mucous membrane *anywhere* in the body (including the glans penis, which is not, strictly speaking, mucous membrane) and Bowen's disease when the lesion is on the skin *anywhere* in the body. These conditions, particularly Bowen's disease, are associated with a high incidence of internal malignancy not related to penile carcinoma. Management of these conditions involves their complete removal by one or another of various surgical techniques available, with additional long-term follow-up therapy, but penile amputation is usually not necessary.

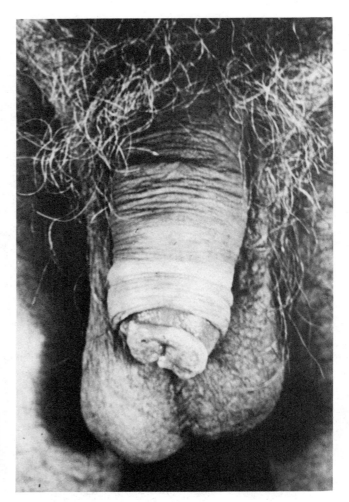

Figure 12-11. Cancer of the penis that was totally hidden under the foreskin and that would have never been found had the foreskin not been retracted during a physical examination.

BALANITIS AND BALANOPOSTHITIS

Balanitis is inflammation of the glans penis and is generally only seen in uncircumcised individuals. Its occurrence is usually caused by the intertrigo syndrome, a condition in which damp, moist areas are particularly predisposed to inflammatory changes (further examples of this syndrome would be inflammation and irritation in the groin or armpit areas). The glans penis is virtually always damp and moist when the foreskin is in its normal position covering the glans because there is almost always a drop or two of urine on the glans following voiding that serves as the source of wetness. Predisposition of the glans to such inflammation combined with poor or relatively poor personal hygiene such that the foreskin is rarely retracted for the purpose of thorough cleansing and drying of the glans, provides a situation particularly suitable to the development of balanitis. This situation, plus a secondary

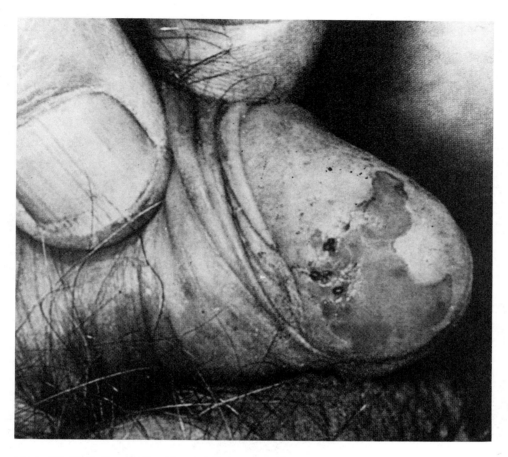

Figure 12–12. Erythroplasia of Queyrat is considered premalignant and may be present on the mucous membrane anywhere in the body or, as above, on the glans penis.

invasion with either *Candida* or *Mycobacterium smegmatis* (or both) provide an ideal setting for the resultant balanitis.

Balanoposthitis is the natural and common extension of balanitis, in which the inflammation of the glans penis also involves the undersurface of the overlying foreskin (Fig. 12–14). The causes of balanoposthitis are the same as those for balanitis.

Treatment of either of these conditions is essentially the same. Meticulous personal hygiene while keeping the glans penis absolutely clean and dry is mandatory. Ideally the glans penis should be exposed to the air, with the foreskin retracted, until the inflammatory process is resolved, but this is not always practical! Thorough cleaning of the glans with soap and water once or twice per day followed by careful drying and exposure to the air are the most beneficial. The use of a steroid ointment such as Mycolog (triamcinolone acetonide) is helpful because of its antiinflammatory effect, and the additional use of a topical antibacterial or antimycotic agent such as neomycin or mycostatin (Nystatin) is also helpful and should be applied a couple of times daily. The diabetic patient is particularly prone to balanoposthitis

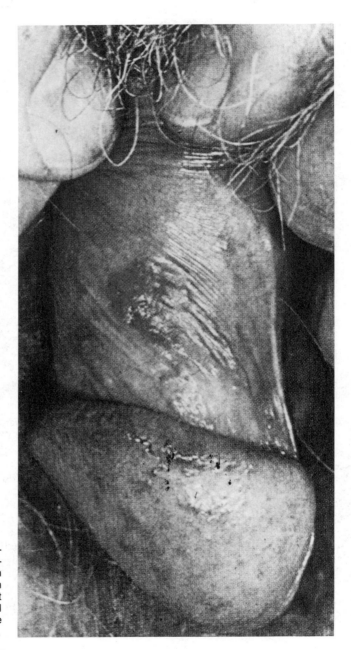

Figure 12-13. Bowen's disease is considered premalignant and may be found on the skin virtually anywhere in the body or, as here, just proximal to the coronal sulcus on the shaft of the penis.

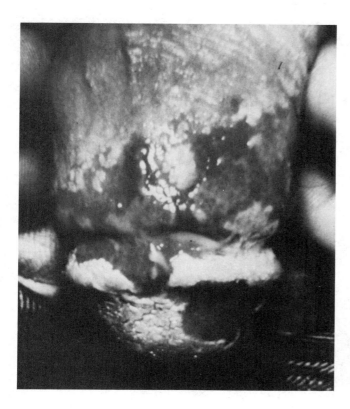

Figure 12-14. Balanoposthitis, showing severe inflammation of the glans penis as well as the overlying foreskin (retracted). When the lesion is confined to the glans penis it is known as balanitis.

and correction of glycosuria is essential to the improvement of this condition. In the author's experience, even though local and systemic therapy as just outlined brings about satisfactory results in most cases, balanitis and balanoposthitis are inevitably recurrent, and definitive therapy mandates circumcision in the vast majority of cases.

PHIMOSIS

Phimosis is a condition in which the penile foreskin cannot be retracted because of snugness or adhesions of the foreskin to the underlying glans. In some patients, it is not even possible to retract the foreskin enough to visualize the urethral meatus; in less severe cases adhesions of the undersurface of the foreskin to the coronal sulcus prevent complete retraction of the foreskin. If there is or has been coexisting inflammation of the glans and the undersurface of the foreskin (balanoposthitis), and if this inflammation is at all chronic in nature, the foreskin will be very much thickened and indurated. In these patients even visualization of the urethral meatus becomes extremely difficult or perhaps even impossible (Fig. 12–15).

In children, naturally occurring adhesions between the glans and the foreskin normally prevent retraction of the foreskin until the child is about 3 to 4 years of age. This is not unusual nor is it abnormal and there is no need for parental anxiety or for vigorous attempts to retract the foreskin, as this will only cause the child con-

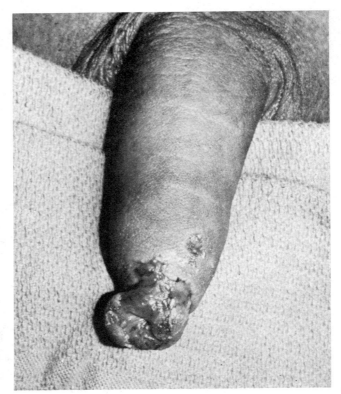

Figure 12–15. Phimosis, a relatively common condition, in which there is typically an inability to retract the foreskin. Some individuals may not be able to retract the foreskin sufficiently to expose the meatus whereas others can retract it almost to the coronal sulcus. In this patient, secondary infection of the redundant foreskin and trauma to the foreskin from repeated efforts to retract it required removal of the entire foreskin (circumcision).

siderable discomfort. However, once the adhesions between foreskin and glans have lysed, regular and daily hygiene should include complete retraction of the foreskin with careful cleansing of the glans and the coronal sulcus.

The treatment of phimosis consists of circumcision, which sometimes must be done as an urgent procedure when the patient is unable to void or when it is not possible to pass a urethral catheter in a patient whose medical condition requires it. Phimosis will never be present in an individual who has been circumcised.

PARAPHIMOSIS

In paraphimosis the retracted foreskin cannot be reduced (brought forward) to its normal position covering the glans. The foreskin becomes caught in its retracted position at the level of the coronal sulcus, resulting in edema of the glans penis, which makes reduction of the foreskin even more difficult (Fig. 12–16). If untreated, an ultimate vascular insufficiency of the glans may result. This condition is seen in uncircumcised individuals only and usually occurs when a relatively snug foreskin is vigorously or forceably retracted, as during sexual intercourse or in a bedridden patient with an indwelling urethral catheter, since the catheter itself tends to force the foreskin into a retracted position and the patient is often not aware of this and therefore unable to keep the foreskin properly reduced.

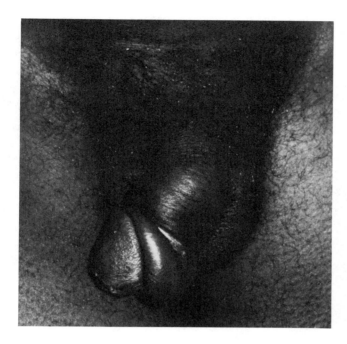

Figure 12-16. Paraphimosis, a condition in which a snug foreskin that has been retracted proximal to the coronal sulcus cannot be reduced to its normal state. Resulting profound edema of the foreskin makes reduction even more difficult and extremely painful. Treatment is usually a prompt dorsal slit followed by a circumcision when the edema has resolved.

Treatment of paraphimosis requires reduction of the foreskin to its normal position covering the glans penis. This reduction can be extremely difficult, particularly if there is significant edema of the glans and foreskin, which is common in the presence of a tight foreskin constricted around the coronal sulcus. Manual reduction of the foreskin is usually accomplished with the physician standing in front of the patient and forcing the glans in an inward position with the thumbs while attempting to pull the foreskin forward with the index and middle fingers of both hands. This often requires a most strenuous effort in order to reduce the glans and there is considerable patient discomfort, which usually requires sedation, ideally before the reduction of the foreskin is attempted. In some cases of advanced paraphimosis that have been unreduced for several hours or more, it may not be possible to reduce the glans manually and a dorsal slit may be required. In this operative maneuver, with the patient under penile block or general anesthetic, the dorsal surface of the entire foreskin is divided surgically to permit reduction of the foreskin. Circumcision is mandatory following this procedure, but it is best done several days later when the considerable edema of the foreskin has subsided. In patients in whom the foreskin can successfully be reduced manually, circumcision should be carried out electively as soon as possible.

REFERENCES

Korting GW: Practical Dermatology of the Genital Region. Philadelphia, Saunders, 1981

13
End-Stage Renal Disease, Hemodialysis, and Transplantation

EDUCATIONAL OBJECTIVES

1. List the most common kidney diseases that result in end-stage renal failure.
2. Discuss the approximate 1– and 2–year survival rates for patients on hemodialysis and postrenal transplantation.

END-STAGE RENAL DISEASE

By definition, end-stage renal disease refers to terminal or near-terminal situations in which renal function is not adequate to maintain life. There are many conditions that can lead to end-stage renal disease; however, since less than half of one kidney is adequate to maintain normal renal function, it is obvious that the pathologic process leading to end-stage renal disease must of necessity be bilateral. The exceptions to the rule of bilaterality might include a severe disease process such as renal cell carcinoma in a solitary kidney or severe renal calculus disease with progressive diminution of function in an individual whose contralateral kidney may already have been removed for the same condition. These examples notwithstanding, it is the chronic bilateral pathologic processes that ultimately lead to end-stage renal disease in the vast majority of patients, and glomerulonephritis is probably the greatest single cause of renal failure. Three other conditions that are responsible for significant numbers of patients having end-stage renal disease are pyelonephritis, polycystic kidneys, and nephrosclerosis. These severe chronic renal diseases ultimately lead to the anephric state in which life is not possible without hemodialysis or renal transplantation. When the creatinine clearance level is below 10 ml/min, and certainly when it is below 5 ml/min, end-stage renal failure has been reached and long-term hemodialysis or renal transplantation is required.

It is appropriate to mention that acute renal failure can lead, uncommonly, to end-stage renal disease. Such acute and irreversible failure can result from massive trauma, nephrotoxic drugs or poisons, acute infectious diseases, iatrogenic diseases, and fulminating glomerulonephritis. However, acute renal failure is usually reversible if the patient is given prompt and adequate treatment, which invariably in-

261

cludes the use of temporary hemodialysis. For this reason, the clinical condition induced by acute renal failure is not generally considered to be a forerunner of end-stage renal disease.

HEMODIALYSIS

The magnitude of chronic end-stage renal disease is underscored by an estimated 20,000 American deaths each year from this problem, most of which occur among patients on chronic hemodialysis or following renal transplantation.

Long-term intermittent hemodialysis as a lifesaving treatment for patients with end-stage kidney disease has been used since 1960. Although the artificial kidney had been developed and used in acute renal failure for 20 or more years prior to 1960, protracted (chronic) hemodialysis never achieved widespread usage because of the necessity of performing surgical cutdowns each time dialysis was carried out in order to establish a connection between the patient's circulation and the dialysis apparatus. In 1960, Dr. Belding Scribner developed the successful permanent indwelling plastic shunt (which bears his name) that made it possible to connect uremic patients repeatedly to artificial kidneys without the need to resort to specific surgical procedures on each occasion. Inasmuch as long-term dialysis is usually carried out three times per week, for months and years, the magnitude of the problem prior to the development of the permanent indwelling shunt is obvious.

The principle of hemodialysis, regardless of the type of equipment used, is the "washing" of a patient's blood to remove excess urea and uremic toxins. The patient is generally connected to the dialysis machine for 6 to 8 hours, during which time the blood is repeatedly and continuously circulated through the machine and returned to the system with some of the excess urea and uremic toxins removed with each circulation. At present there are about 70,000 patients with end-stage renal failure in the United States who are being kept alive with the aid of long-term hemodialysis. A small number of these patients undergo dialysis while awaiting transplantation, but the vast majority are not candidates for transplantation for one reason or another. The gross annual death rate for patients receiving protracted hemodialysis is approximately 16 to 20 percent and the most common causes of death are cardiac disorders, cerebral vascular disease, other vascular complications, and infections.

It must not be presumed that patients having long-term hemodialysis are able to lead an entirely normal life. Although they are frequently able to continue their normal occupations, the physical and emotional problems associated with dialysis are not minor. A measure of the severity of the emotional problems, for example, is the suicide rate of patients in protracted hemodialysis programs in the United States, which is 400 times higher than that of the general population.

More and more long-term hemodialysis is being done in the home setting (which generally requires that an able-bodied, intelligent individual be with the dialysis patient during each dialysis) and this is because of the significantly greater freedom of scheduling afforded to the patient on home dialysis. It is obvious that when the home situation is supportive, a patient is usually much happier than in the impersonal environment of a hemodialysis center. The cost of dialysis is approximately $25,000 per year in a dialysis center and about $20,000 per year in a home program. For the most part, federal funding supports the care of patients who are candidates for either protracted hemodialysis or renal transplantation.

RENAL TRANSPLANTATION

The patient with end-stage renal disease, whether child or adult, can be maintained only by hemodialysis or by renal transplantation. The fact that far more patients are maintained on dialysis than receive new kidneys is a reflection of the lack of availability of sufficient numbers of kidneys from living related donors and the difficulty in obtaining cadaver kidneys.

The first successful renal transplant was accomplished between identical twins in 1954 at Boston's Peter Bent Brigham Hospital. Since that time, over 50,000 transplant procedures have been carried out in the United States. At present, there are about 160 approved transplantation facilities in this country performing over 6000 renal transplants annually.

The standard technique for renal transplantation, except when the recipient is a very small child, is to place the donor's left kidney into the right iliac fossa of the recipient (or the right kidney into the left fossa). This is because when the kidney is "flipped over" in this manner the ureter is more anterior and is therefore less likely to kink when crossing the iliac artery. The renal artery is anastomosed end to end to the hypogastric artery and the renal vein is usually sutured end to side to the external iliac vein. The donor's ureter is implanted into the recipient's bladder by creation of a submucosal tunnel. In very small children the limited space available in the retroperitoneal iliac fossa usually mandates that an intraperitoneal location be used and end-to-side arterial and venous anastomoses are used, with either the aorta and inferior vena cava or the common iliac artery and vein, depending on where the kidney comfortably lies.

Immunosuppression

The graft recipient's natural mechanisms of defense that guard against a variety of invaders must be altered before a transplanted kidney, which contains tissue antigens foreign to the recipient, will be accepted. A regimen of suppression of the recipient's ability to mount a rejection reaction against the graft must be meticulously balanced against the obvious consequence of oversuppression and elimination of the recipient's defense against bacterial, viral, and fungal pathogens. The agents used to accomplish this clinical immunosuppressive therapy are azathioprine (Imuran), cyclosporine, heterologous antilymphocyte globulin (ALG), cyclophosphamide (Cytoxan), and corticosteroids in various combinations. Also well documented is the use of five to ten random blood transfusions given to the patient in the months prior to transplantation definitely lowers the likelihood of graft rejection. The ideal immunosuppressive agent, however, has not been developed yet, and all of the agents currently in use have the distinct disadvantage of being nonspecific, with resulting effects on biologic actions of the graft recipient other than those directed against the allograft itself. This nonspecificity enforces limitations of drug dosages and other biologic agents, thereby frequently preventing full efficiency of the immunosuppressive because of the side effects that might ensue.

Histocompatibility Typing

It was originally hoped that matching the prospective organ donor and the recipient through tissue typing might prevent or considerably reduce the high incidence of graft rejection. Unfortunately, many laboratories with extensive experience in the field have found correlations that are at times disappointing between the results of tissue typing and the clinical outcome of transplantation. The present status of tissue typing may be summarized as follows:

1. The ABO blood group must be compatible between the donor and the recipient.
2. The cytotoxic crossmatch which uses the serum of the recipient with the lymphocytes of the donor in the presence of complement must be negative. If it kills the recipient's cells, there is virtually a 100 percent likelihood of a hyperacute graft rejection, often before the surgery is even complete. If the cytotoxic crossmatch is negative, then HLA and B matching at the A and B locus is done. A four-antigen match (two at each locus) is ideal and the fewer antigens matched the greater the likelihood of graft rejection, particularly in living related donors.
3. A mixed lymphocyte culture (MLC) can only be done on living related donors, as it takes 7 to 10 days to perform.
4. Newer methods of measuring D-related antigens are being perfected using techniques such that the match can be done in cadavers. The significance of the D-related antigens is that it indicates mixed lymphocyte culture (MLC) compatibility.

In summary, it is obvious that the greater the number of matching antigens between donor and recipient, the greater the likelihood of a successful transplantation procedure being done. It must be emphasized that although a four-antigen HLA and B match is ideal, successful transplants have occurred with 0 and 1 antigen matches. The mixed lymphocyte culture, however, is a cellular test, and if this test suggests gross incompatibility at the D locus the odds of graft survival are not good. It should also be reiterated that the first two screening tests mentioned, the ABO group and the cytotoxic crossmatch, are just that; that is, if there is ABO group incompatibility between the donor and the recipient or if the cytotoxic crossmatch is positive (i.e., if it kills the cells) the graft procedure should not be carried out as it will be doomed to failure.

Results of Transplantation

The 1-year survival rate of patients with grafts still functioning (as opposed to surviving patients in whom the graft had to be removed and who are receiving hemodialysis) is about 85 percent with well-matched living, related donors, and 60 percent with cadaver donors. The 2-year survival rate for recipients of grafts from well-matched living, related donors is about 75 percent and it is about 45 percent from cadaver donors. In cases of death of the recipient, the most common cause is sepsis. If the recipient survives 2 years with a well-functioning graft, the chances of long-term survival are very good because the risk of graft rejection seems to decrease sharply after this time. It must be stressed that the failure of a graft does not necessarily result in the death of the patient, because protracted hemodialysis can be resumed pending another kidney graft.

The long-term survival statistics for patients with renal transplants is significantly better than for those on chronic hemodialysis and it is significant to note that the quality of life for the transplant patient is significantly better than it is for the dialysis patient, notwithstanding the fact that transplant patients must remain on long-term immunosuppressive therapy, with all of its attendant risks.

An interesting phenomenon observed in recent years has been the vastly greater risk of development of cancer in patients with transplants than in the population at large. This is presumably because the graft recipient's immune system has been altered by long-term immunosuppression and the immune mechanism is felt to be intimately involved with host resistance to cancer. The renal transplantation patient faces a 5 to 6 percent risk of cancer, an incidence approximately 100 times greater than in the general population of the same age range. It is interesting that the increase in tumor activity seems to be about 2 years after transplantation, with no further increase after that time. The malignancies are predominantly epithelial and lymphoproliferative in origin, with skin cancers (squamous or basal cell carcinomas) and lymphomas the predominant tumors.

REFERENCES

End-Stage Renal Disease Program Medical Information System. Faculty Survey Tables, 1982. Published by U. S. Department of Health and Human Services, Health Care Financing Administration, Bureau of Support Services, Washington, D.C.

Freier DT, Konnak JW, Niederhuber JE, Turcotte JG: Renal transplantation. In Kendall AR, Karafin L, (eds), Urology. Philadelphia, Harper and Row, 1981, vol 2, chap 27

Nelson RP, Rajagopolan PR, Fitts CT: Frustrations in renal donation. S Med J 71:1255, 1978

14
Sexual Problems, Incontinence, and Fertility Regulation

EDUCATIONAL OBJECTIVES

1. List the indications for vasectomy.
2. Discuss the comparative advantages of vasectomy and all other forms of birth control.
3. Define erectile dysfunction.
4. Discuss the evaluation and management of the patient with erectile dysfunction.
5. Examine and identify for viability the spermatozoa in a semen specimen.
6. Determine whether a patient understands nomenclature such as penis, urethra, testes, or labia or whether less clinical terms need to be used.
7. Instruct a man in the use of a condom.
8. Obtain a history of sexual activity from a man and a woman without being offensive or using language that cannot be understood.
9. Advise parents of 3-, 9-, and 15-year-old boys or girls about masturbation.
10. Define infertility.
11. Discuss the evaluation and management of the male patient with infertility.
12. Discuss the evaluation and management of the patient with erectile dysfunction.

SEXUAL PROBLEMS

Impotence

Impotence, or erectile dysfunction as it is more kindly called, is that condition in which a man is unable to have a sufficiently firm penile erection to accomplish penetration and/or ejaculation. The penis usually remains flaccid or semiflaccid in the truly impotent patient.

Functional Impotence. In at least half of the patients with erectile dysfunction, there is a functional basis for the problem. It may be related to physical or mental fatigue, to uncertainty, to fear or guilt feelings about the act of sexual intercourse for any variety of reasons, to aversion to the sex partner, or to virtually the entire spectrum of mental disease (particularly including problems of depression). Therefore, recognition of the functionally impotent patient very early in the diagnostic workup is most helpful and forestalls the necessity of expensive and time-consuming studies that might otherwise be undertaken in trying to find an organic cause of impotence.

A major step in the differentiation of functional from organic impotence can be taken with an accurate and careful history. Was the onset of the erectile dysfunction sudden, and can the patient specifically remember the particular time at which it first occurred? A sudden onset of erectile dysfunction suggests a functional etiology whereas a gradual onset over a period of many months or even years is more compatible with organic disease. Does the patient ever have a full and normal erection on wakening in the morning, during the night, or at *any* other time whether or not appropriate? The presence of erections of good quality occurring at *any* time strongly suggests a functional etiology for the impotence. Is the patient able to masturbate to orgasm and have a good erection while so doing? Obviously, if the patient can do this, the problem is not organic. Is the patient able to have successful intercourse with one woman (regardless of whether or not she is his wife), but not with another? Again, it should be obvious that successful intercourse with *any* woman precludes a diagnosis of organic dysfunction.

The treatment of functional impotence can be surprisingly simple or painfully difficult, depending on the underlying problem. In the author's experience, it is relatively common for a man to have an episode of erectile dysfunction with his wife (perhaps after he has been drinking too much), following by rebuke or ridicule, particularly when the marriage has been less than ideal. Perhaps this scenario occurs even more commonly with a woman who is not the patient's wife. In any case, the next time intercourse is attempted, the patient is fearful of failing again; this fear in turn promotes failure and a vicious cycle can be created. It is also not unusual for a middle-aged or even older man to have difficulty in obtaining an erection when he attempts to have intercourse with his wife but to have no problem at all with his girlfriend. Much of the battle is won if the patient can be made to realize that there is nothing organically wrong with him. Reassurance, compassion, and occasionally medication such as hormone replacement (if indicated) can help many men who are functionally impotent; however, when there are accompanying deep-seated psychiatric problems, long-term psychotherapy or even hypnotherapy may be required to restore potency, and even then success is not guaranteed. The author has been particularly impressed with the results of sensate-focus therapy in which couples are treated together.

Deep intramuscular injection of testosterone and the use of gonadotropins to stimulate the interstitial cells of Leydig to produce additional endogenous testosterone have both benefited considerable numbers of patients with functional impotence. These therapies probably have a placebo effect, because in the patient with a normal circulating testosterone level, additional testosterone, either exogenous or endogenous, does not make any difference in the physiology of erections. The placebo effect, however, is demonstrably powerful in many different situations and its advantages should not be summarily discounted if it seems to work. A strong note of warning is indicated for the physician whose patient is receiving exogenous testosterone or gonadotropin, with its resultant increase in testosterone production: cancer of the prostate gland is usually testosterone dependent and an unsuspected carcinoma in that gland may grow and spread rapidly as an effect of excess testosterone. Carcinoma of the prostate gland cannot always be ruled out by negative digital rectal exam, because small foci of carcinoma within the gland may be completely undetectable with this or any other means. Thus, irrevocable harm can be done to the patient with carcinoma, at least theoretically, by raising his circulating testosterone levels. The author personally shuns the use of this type of hormonal therapy in the man over 50 who has palpably normal testes and normal testosterone levels.

In addition to a careful history about the onset and the exact nature of the erectile dysfunction, the patient should be screened with serum testosterone, luteinizing hormone (LH), follicle stimulating hormone (FSH), and prolactin to rule out the possibility of an endocrine cause for the problem. In the author's experience, endocrine abnormalities are quite uncommon in this group of patients, but this must be determined and not surmised in each individual. Testing for vascular insufficiency to the penis is also part of the workup and auscultation of the penile blood flow is done using a Doppler stethoscope, and the penile blood pressure is determined at the same time. This pressure normally should be at least 80 percent of the brachial artery blood pressure. Again, in the author's experience vascular insufficiency is not a common problem, although it may actually be more common than we are able to determine with our present methods. Certainly, there may well be vascular problems related to abnormally rapid "emptying" of blood from the corpora cavernosa, or a "leak" in the tunica albuginea permitting premature detumescence. Both of these vascular problems would not be detected with the standard Doppler measurements. Corpora cavernosagrams may be helpful in diagnosing some of these abnormalities but they are not generally considered to be standard part of a workup for erectile dysfunction nor are they always diagnostic of underlying vascular problems. When it is not possible to readily differentiate organic from functional impotence by means of a careful history or any of the above noted studies, a nocturnal tumescence monitoring procedure is most helpful. This is based on the sound medical fact that men have frequent erections during the course of sleep and that if these are absent there is a strong likelihood of an organic basis for the erectile dysfunction. Although there are rather fancy (and rather expensive) machines available to monitor nocturnal erections, the author prefers the use of one of several varieties of "snap-off" devices that the patient can place around his penis at the time that he goes to sleep at night. These devices are not unlike miniature blood pressure cuffs (except that they do not measure blood pressure) and if the patient achieves a firm erection during the course of sleep, the device will snap off; when the patient finds that this has occurred during the night, he may safely assume that he has had a good erection. Obviously, a study like this is only indicated for the patient who claims that he literally *never* has any erections.

Organic Impotence. The percent of patients with erectile dysfunction having an organic etiology for this problem is perhaps directly related to the thoroughness, the diligence, and the excellence of the diagnostic workup, particularly in uncovering vascular problems that may or may not be readily discernible. As a general statement, however, probably somewhere between a quarter and a half of patients with erectile dysfunction have an organic basis for the problem. For example, the patient who says that he has never had an erection in his entire adult life, the patient who is unable to masturbate to orgasm, and the patient who does not have erections at *any* time should be prime suspects for true organic impotence. Diabetes is probably the most common organic cause of impotence, and every patient with symptoms suggestive of erectile dysfunction should have his urine checked for the presence of glucose. If indicated, this should be followed by a fasting blood glucose, 2-hour postprandial glucose, or glucose tolerance test. Diabetic neuropathy leading to erectile dysfunction can probably occur in as brief a time as 1 or 2 years after the clinical condition has been diagnosed, but the longer the time interval from when the diagnosis of diabetes was first made the greater the likelihood of erectile dysfunction due to diabetic neuropathy affecting the pelvic nerves S_2, S_3, and S_4 (the nervi erigentes). The prevailing clinical opinion is that the diabetic neuropathy is not based on the primary disease of the nerves as much as diabetic damage to the small blood vessels supplying the nerves with resulting secondary nerve involvement. Unfortunately, adequate clinical control of the diabetes does not usually restore potency to affected individuals.

There are other endocrinopathies associated with organic impotence, such as testosterone deficiency, which may be primary or secondary to gonadotropin deficiency. As a general rule, in these patients physical examination will reveal small (less than 3 cm in the greatest dimension), soft, or undescended testes that should make the clinician suspect testosterone deficiency. Erectile dysfunction may be irreversible if the testes have been destroyed by conditions such as mumps orchitis, torsion of the spermatic cord, or if they have been removed for reasons such as trauma, although replacement hormonal therapy may be considered and may be beneficial. General physical abnormalities such as dwarfism should alert the clinician to the possibility of pituitary gland failure. Chromosomal studies should be carried out in patients in whom organic endocrinopathy is suspected to rule out conditions such as Klinefelter's syndrome and a 24-hour urine for 17-ketosteroid levels along with serum levels of FSH, LH, testosterone, and prolactin should also be determined. These urine and serum studies will accurately reflect both pituitary and testicular functions; if these tests are normal, endocrine abnormalities are very unlikely. Low LH and FSH levels suggest pituitary failure for which human gonadotropic replacement therapy may produce beneficial results. In individuals with testicular failure, the FSH and LH levels may be normal or high but the testosterone levels are low, and replacement therapy with intramuscular injection of testosterone is often very beneficial. Prolactin producing tumors are not common but may be a definite cause of erectile dysfunction.

Lesions of the spinal cord, including the conus medullaris, are another cause for organic dysfunction. Such lesions include spinal cord tumors, tertiary lues and probably other rare and unusual lesions of the lower cord that affect the outflow tract of the pelvic nerves. Additionally, spinal cord injuries above the conus medullaris or involving the conus itself will produce varying degrees of erectile dysfunction depending on the severity and completeness of the lesion. With lesions of the upper spinal cord, impotence is often psychic; the patient's thought processes do not lead to an erection but direct penile stimulation does (reflexogenic erection). The majority of patients with complete lesions at the level of the conus or below usually are unable to have erections.

Other organic causes of impotence include previous priapism, severe penile trauma, the various vascular problems that can result in an inadequate inflow of blood into the corpora cavernosa, overly rapid emptying of the corpora following tumescence, and one or more small leaks in the tunica albuginea, which can produce a premature weakening of an otherwise firm erection. Another relatively common cause for erectile dysfunction is damage to the nerves controlling erections; this may occur during radical pelvic surgery that has been carried out in order to treat various forms of malignancy. Management of any of these numerous causes of organic impotence may theoretically be successful if it is possible to reverse or remove the underlying pathology but in practice this is not usually possible.

Surgical Management of Erectile Dysfunction.   Once it has been definitely established that the patient has an irreversible organic cause for his erectile dysfunction or even a functional etiology for his problem that is not amenable to conservative therapy, the surgical correction of the erectile dysfunction may be recommended with every confidence of a happy result.

Since the early 1970s the insertion of appropriately sized silicone prostheses into the paired corpora cavernosa has been done in many thousands of patients with almost uniformly excellent results in that the patient literally always has an erection that is firm enough for intercourse (Fig. 14–1). The prostheses are hinged so that when intercourse is not contemplated, the penis can be pressed into a "down" position where it lies along the patient's inner thigh and is not obtrusive or otherwise an embarrassment to the patient. It is then simply swung into the "up" position when intercourse is contemplated. An inflatable prosthesis has been available since the late 1970s for insertion into each of the corpora cavernosa. It looks like a long balloon and is inflated from a reservoir placed deep to the rectus abdominus muscle by the activation of a pump placed in the upper portion of the scrotum (Fig. 14–2). This type of prosthesis produces a very physiologic erection which increases the girth of the penis in addition to its length and rigidity. It may be fully deflated when intercourse is not contemplated and the casual observer would not suspect that the patient has had any surgical prosthesis inserted. The obvious advantages of the rigid prosthesis are that there are no valves or tubes to break down and require repair and the device itself is considerably less expensive than the inflatable model. On the other hand, the inflatable model more closely reproduces a physiologic erection, but about 10 percent of the patients need to have repeat surgery to repair various mechanical problems in the system.

There are many other models and varieties of penile prostheses that have come and are yet to come on the market, but all of them are simply variations of the two basic styles just mentioned and the degree of patient and spouse satisfaction following the insertion of either type is extremely high. Many patients want to know preoperatively if they will be able to have an orgasm and ejaculate postoperatively and the answer to this is "yes" if the patient is able to masturbate to orgasm and ejaculation preoperatively. If, however, the patient is not able to masturbate to orgasm and ejaculation prior to the implantation of the penile prosthesis, it is impossible to determine in advance whether or not he will be able to do so after surgery.

Premature Ejaculation

Premature ejaculation is a relative phenomenon. Its commonly accepted meaning is ejaculation either before vaginal insertion or from within a few seconds to a minute or two after insertion. It becomes a clinical problem when the timing of the man's orgasm, with resulting loss of erection, occurs before the woman's orgasm, leaving her physically or emotionally unsatisfied.

The treatment of premature ejaculation can be approached in two ways. First, efforts can be directed towards prolonging the time interval between erection and ejaculation. This can be a difficult process in some cases and the use of topical anesthetics applied to the glans penis may be helpful in selected and unusual situations. The technique that seems to achieve the most success is the "squeeze" technique in which the man goes through a training period with the assistance of his partner. In this technique, the man is brought to erection by the woman; just before he feels that he is going to ejaculate, she squeezes the glans penis for several seconds by applying her thumb to the ventral surface of the glans just distal to the coronal sulcus and her index and middle fingers to the dorsal aspect of the glans penis. Forceful squeezing in this area, primarily with the thumb over the distal urethra, will dissipate the desire to ejaculate. By repeated use of this method, the time interval between erection and ejaculation gradually can be lengthened sufficiently to allow for satisfactory sexual intercourse. As the time between erection and ejaculation becomes

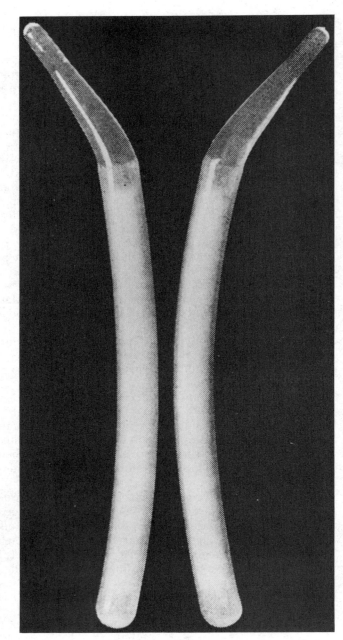

Figure 14-1. The Small–Carrion prosthesis. This pair of flexible, medical-grade silicone rods are inserted into the paired corpora cavernosa so that the penis is always rigid enough to permit intercourse. These rods are flexible so that the penis can be made to lie flat along the inner aspect of the thigh when intercourse is not desired.

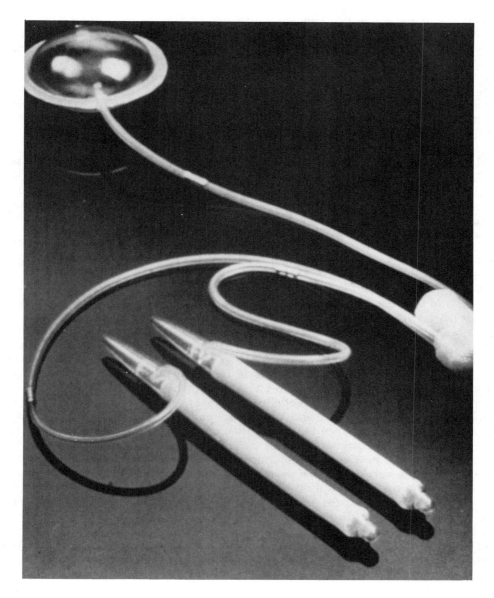

Figure 14-2. The inflatable penile prosthesis. The tubular cylinders are inserted into the corpora cavernosa and the fluid-filled reservoir (the round object at the top of the photograph) is placed deep to the rectus abdominus muscle. The pump (on the lower right side of the photograph) is placed in the superior portion of the scrotum and pressure on the pump drives the fluid from the reservoir into the tubular cylinders, thereby producing a physiologic erection.

lengthened, the man then begins to insert his penis into the vagina and withdraws it when ejaculation appears to be near while the woman applies the squeeze technique. This technique using increasing time periods of intromission before the "squeeze" is employed has brought gratifying results to many men in prolonging their ability to maintain an erection after insertion without premature ejaculation.

The alternative treatment of premature ejaculation can be directed toward ameliorating the woman's dissatisfaction. For example, any foreplay involving the penis can be eliminated; rather, efforts should be made to arouse the woman as much as possible using direct clitoral stimulation orally or digitally so that she is extremely close to orgasm or has actually achieved orgasm at the time of insertion, thereby minimizing the significance of any premature ejaculation that may occur.

Masturbation in Children

Masturbation in children of all age groups is a universal phenomenon that starts almost at the time that the child is old enough to be aware of his or her genitals. Parental concern and distress are almost equally universal, and the most important thing that the clinician can do is to reassure the parent of the completely normal and usual nature of the act, regardless of the age of the child.

Very uncommonly, masturbation may occur in other than normal situations. In the very young child of 3 to 4 years, the physician might elicit from the parents a history of any other behavior that the parents think unusual, such as whether the child is frequently or chronically irritable, whether he or she is difficult to get along with, and whether there is evidence of withdrawn behavior. In such situations, masturbation may actually be a symptom of an underlying emotional disorder and psychiatric guidance should be considered. Masturbation is equally normal in the slightly older child of 9 to 10 years provided, as just noted, his or her general behavior falls within the normal pattern.

To many parents, masturbation in the teenager is particularly alarming because of the persisting belief that the act can lead to insanity, organic disease, and future problems of sexual incompatibility. In actual fact, normal teenage boys probably masturbate at least once and more likely many times in each week, and, indeed, many teenagers masturbate more than once daily. It is quite possible that teenage girls masturbate frequently as well, but perhaps not to the same degree. After pointing out the normalcy of masturbation, the physician should inquire about the teenager's general emotional development and whether he or she appears excessively withdrawn or manifests signs of loneliness and isolation from his or her peers. In such circumstances it is very possible that masturbation is a reflection of an otherwise unhappy life situation rather than the cause of that unhappy life situation, as so many parents tend to perceive the problem. In summary, then, masturbation in all age groups is extraordinarily normal and as long as there do not appear to be any concurrent emotional problems the masturbation ought not to be criticized or condemned by parents.

PROSTHESES FOR INCONTINENCE

Incontinence has a multitude of etiologies that range, chronologically, from the physiological incontinence found in infants to the incontinence secondary to cerebral vascular accidents in older patients. Between these extremes are patients with urgency incontinence (most commonly due to infection or inflammation of the

trigone or bladder neck), overflow incontinence (usually secondary to bladder outlet obstruction), stress incontinence in women (usually due to a relaxation of the
normal vesicourethral angle), and also patients with a true damage to the
mechanisms of continence such as can occur following radical prostate surgery or
even transurethral prostate surgery and can also occur in patients with congenital
neurogenic deficits such as meningomyelocele.

For this latter group of patients with genuine damage to one or more of the
mechanisms of continence, there is now an excellent means of restoring continence
and that is using a surgically implanted artificial sphincter. Not too different in concept from the inflatable penile prosthesis, the artificial sphincter's most important
part is a very small cuff that is inflatable and is surgically placed either around the
vesical neck (in men or women) or the bulbous urethra (in men). There is a reservoir of fluid that is placed deep to the abdominal musculature and a pump
mechanism that is placed within the scrotum or the labia. When the cuff is inflated,
continence is maintained and when the cuff is deflated, urine can flow freely.
Although these inflatable sphincter devices are prone to various mechanical problems and failures, probably around 70 to 75 percent of the incontinent patients in
whom these devices are implanted can ultimately regain most or all of their continence even though one or more surgical revisions may be required to correct equipment failure. This is an enormous breakthrough in the treatment of these unfortunate
individuals and it is anticipated that as the years pass these devices will become
perfected to the point that the frequency of mechanical failure necessitating reopera-
tion will become significantly decreased.

FERTILITY REGULATION

Infertility

Infertility is said to exist when a couple has been trying to conceive for 2 or more
years without success. It affects about 15 percent of the couples of child-bearing
age and the male is responsible for the infertility in about half of the cases.

Semen Analysis. The first procedure in the workup of an infertile couple is to evaluate
the man's semen, inasmuch as this is far simpler than the determination of infertility in the woman. The author often obtains a semen analysis prior to even doing
a history or a physical exam because if the semen analysis is normal (as, not infrequently, it is) the patient is thereby spared the expense of a history and physical
examination. In men who have a normal semen analysis, it is the author's custom
to only do a cursory examination of the external genitalia to make certain that no
problems that might preclude successful delivery of semen well up into the vaginal
canal are present, for example, a severe hypospadias or any other sort of penile
deformity.

Following 3 days of sexual abstinence, a semen specimen should be deposited
(preferably by masturbation) into a clean, dry, wide-mouthed jar so that all the
ejaculated semen enters the jar and none is lost. The specimen should be maintained
at room or body temperature and sent to the laboratory within 1 hour of collection.
Condoms should never be used for semen collection because they frequently have
built-in spermicidal properties. The semen specimen should be evaluated
microscopically for motility, morphology, and sperm count as well as physical
characteristics such as color, liquefaction, volume, pH, and viscosity. A drop of well-

mixed semen is placed on a slide with an inoculating loop and is covered with a cover slip. Preparations are examined under both low and high powers of a microscope; five to ten fields are examined under each power and the average value for each field is obtained. Motility is rated from 0 (no motile cells) to 100 percent (all cells motile), rounded to the nearest 10 percent. Forward progression of motile sperm cells is rated from 0 (no forward progression) to 10 (all motile cells display a vigorous foward progression).

The sperm count, or sperm concentration, is determined by diluting the raw semen 1:20 with tap water in a white cell pipette and then placing the diluted semen in the four corner areas of a hemacytometer that is used for counting leukocytes. A sperm count of more than 20 million cells per milliliter is considered to be the lower limit of normal; a count of 80 to 100 million sperm cells per milliliter meets the "ideal" normal. When more than 50 percent of the cells examined are motile, the limits of normal have been met, and forward progression should be more than 5, on the scale of 0 to 10. The average volume is 1 to 5 ml and morphology should be normal in more than 60 percent of the cells examined. For determination of the sperm morphology semen smears are prepared, air dried, fixed in 10 percent formalin for 1 minute, rinsed in distilled water, stained in hematoxylin, and again rinsed in distilled water. Normal morphology is determined by counting 200 sperm cells and is recorded to the nearest percent. It should be recalled that the normal morphology of the sperm head is oval; therefore, only the oval-shaped cells are counted as normal. Additionally, the fructose level of the seminal plasma should be determined. Persistent agglutination of the semen (failure to liquefy) may indicate the presence of antisperm antibodies, which are, interestingly enough, found in 2 percent of fertile men.

Semen analysis is usually rather clear-cut, and a man's semen profile is either within the very broad limits of normal or it is distinctly abnormal. In abnormal profiles the most common finding is severe oligospermia (a count well below 20 million per milliliter) or azoospermia (no sperm visible). If oligospermia is found, the analysis should be repeated two or three times because there is a great deal of variability from day to day or week to week in the results of semen analyses. If oligospermia or azoospermia is found, then a detailed history and physical examination is indicated.

In obtaining a history for infertility, the patient must be carefully queried about any drug usage, particularly marijuana. The usage of even prescription medication should be carefully noted because some prescription drugs are known to have a deleterious effect on spermatozoa. Systemic illnesses, which also can have a harmful effect on spermatogenesis, should be noted, as should any exposure (past or present) to environmental or industrial toxins. A past history of possible epididymitis, orchitis, spermatic cord torsion, gonorrhea, mumps orchitis, Klinefelter's disease and any other entities known to have associations with decreased fertility should be obtained, as should a sexual history regarding the patient's potency, techniques of intercourse, and frequency of intercourse.

On physical examination any evidence of underandrogenization should be noted. This includes such things as scanty facial, pubic, or body hair, gynecomastia, or eunuchoid proportions. Examination of the genitals should include a check for hypospadias and palpation of the testes for size and consistency. Testes under 3 to 4 cm in greatest dimension may be considered to be smaller than average and may or may not represent hypogonadism. The descent or lack of descent of the testes should be noted, as should the presence of a varicocele, which must be checked for with the patient in the upright position.

Once it has been definitely established that the patient has oligospermia (or azoospermia) by means of at least two or three semen analyses, serum LH, FSH, and testosterone should be obtained, and, as these values fluctuate greatly during the course of a day, it is best to obtain three separate blood samples at least 20 minutes apart and then pool the blood, which is then sent to the laboratory. There are three broad classifications of male infertility and the values of these hormone levels is extremely helpful in making the differentiation.

1. *Pregerminal*, in which there is abnormal hormonal stimulation of the testes. This type of problem can sometimes be successfully treated.
2. *Germinal*, in which there is a lack of normal testis response (with spermatogenesis) to a normal hormonal stimulation. This type of clinical problem is by far the most common and is rarely, if ever, amenable to therapy.
3. *Postgerminal*, in which there is an inability to deliver normal, motile sperm into the urethra. This type of problem is most often seen in the postvasectomized patient but it is also found and potentially curable in patients with congenital or acquired obstruction anywhere along the transport mechanism between the testes and the urethra. It is this type of postgerminal obstruction that perhaps yields the highest number of therapeutic successes.

In the azoospermic patient there are four distinct hormonal patterns found:

1. Decreased testosterone, with elevated LH and FSH. This is a primary failure of the testes and the recommendation should be made to the patient and his wife for artificial insemination with a donor or for adoption.
2. A normal testosterone and LH, with an increased FSH pattern. This is primary germinal cell failure and the patient and his wife should be recommended for artificial insemination with a donor or for adoption.
3. Testosterone, LH, and FSH all decreased. This is hypogonadotropic hypogonadism and the patient should be tested for other hypopituitary conditions in order to help the clinician determine whether or not a panhypopituitarism exists. The patient should also be checked for a pituitary tumor by seeing if his prolactin levels are elevated and he should have a full neurologic and endocrine workup. Assuming the condition to be an isolated hypogonadotropic hypogonadism (and not a panhypopituitarism), treatment with human chorionic gonadotropin and human menopausal gonadotropin may yield beneficial results.
4. Normal testosterone, LH, and FSH. This is *either* retrograde ejaculation or *obstruction* of the ejaculatory system (postgerminal failure). Azoospermia without obstruction almost always shows an increased FSH. The seminal fructose should be checked, and if absent there is probably a congenital absence or obstruction of the seminal vesicles or vas deferens. On physical examination, care should be taken to try to palpate the vas deferens. However fructose is usually present and then the diagnosis is obstruction proximal to the ducts of the seminal vesicles. Exploration, vasograms, and testis biopsies are all indicated. This particular type of infertility, a postgerminal obstruction, offers by far the best chance for successful therapy of all the types of infertility.

There are four common hormonal patterns seen with *oligospermia*:

1. A decreased testosterone, with the LH and FSH increased. This is a primary gonadal insufficiency and recommendation to the patient and his wife is for artificial insemination with a donor or adoption. If the sperm count is around 20 million per milliliter, an attempt may be made to use the husband's semen for artificial insemination by using the split ejaculate technique and combining (pooling) several first portions of the ejaculate specimens and then using these for artificial insemination.

2. A normal testosterone and LH, with an increased FSH. This suggests germinal cell damage and the preferred recommendation again is artificial insemination with a donor or adoption.

3. A decreased testosterone, with the LH and FSH low to normal. This represents a *partial* gonadotropin deficiency and may be amenable to treatment with human chorionic gonadotropin and human menopausal gonadotropin.

4. A normal testosterone, LH, and FSH. This is by far the most common finding in oligospermic patients. If a varicocele is present, it should be repaired, and if it is not present, these patients are grouped under the heading of "idiopathic oligospermia." There are many forms of therapy, including the artificial insemination of the pooled first portion of split ejaculates, clomiphene citrate (Clomid), rebound therapy with testosterone, and human chorionic gonadotropin or human menopausal gonadatropin. No therapy is really beneficial with any degree of reproducibility and although there are reports of success in treating this problem, the really best come under the heading of "anecdotal."

Treatment of oligospermia is particularly successful when a varicocele is present and can be removed surgically. It should be noted that varicocelectomy for the treatment of infertility is neither scientifically valid nor reproducible to the degree usually required in scientific studies. Nevertheless, it is one form of treatment for infertility that has had enough support in the literature that it may indeed be recommended when it is found in infertile patients (see Chapter 11 for a further discussion of varicocele).

Contraception

Vasectomy. Vasectomy is usually performed in the physician's office under a local anesthetic. After the scrotum and surrounding areas have been carefully scrubbed and draped following a sterile technique, the vas deferens is palpated and immobilized between the physician's thumb, which is on the upper anterior surface of the scrotum, and the index and middle fingers, which are on the upper posterior portion of the scrotum. The portion of skin on the upper anterior scrotum where the vas has been localized under the thumb is then anesthetized by intradermal and subcutaneous infiltration of a local anesthetic such as 1 percent xylocaine. The vas is then immobilized by inserting a towel clip through the anesthetized skin of the scrotum underneath and around the vas, which is held securely in place by the fingers. A 1- to 2- cm-long incision is made within the curve of the towel clip and through the layers of the scrotum down to the vas, which is then grasped with an Allis clamp and dissected away from its surrounding tissues. The vas is then divided, and each end is securely ligated with absorbable suture material. The author prefers additionally to insert a fulgurating needle tip into the lumen of each cut end of the vas to destroy the lumen and thereby prevent spontaneous recanalization. Another method is to bend each cut end back on itself and ligate it in that position. Some physicians use a combination of these two steps. The scrotal skin and subcutaneous layers are then closed with absorbable suture material and the procedure is repeated on the other side of the scrotum. It is recommended that the patient wear an athletic supporter or tight underpants for several days. Most patients do not return to work on the day of surgery.

A desire on the part of a married couple not to have any more children is the primary indication for vasectomy. This decision may be based on medical, social, economic, or cultural considerations, or on any combination of these. When interviewing a patient who wants a vasectomy, the physician should insist on interviewing the patient's spouse also and should impress on the couple that for all intents and purposes the vasectomy must be considered irreversible. Although surgical recanalization of the cut ends of the vasa is not difficult and results in better than an 80 percent success rate, about half of the patients who have had a vasectomy for longer than 6 months seem to develop antibodies to their own sperm and this has a definitely deleterious effect upon conception even though sperm are able to reach the outside through the recanalized vasa. Most clinicians performing vasectomies have found that there will be more than an occasional unmarried man seeking vasectomy. Although each individual should be the master of his own body and should have the final say in determining what is and is not done to himself, it must be borne in mind that an unmarried individual may change his marital status and the sterile state brought about by vasectomy may be a source of much grief and unhappiness for both the man and his wife. For this reason, physicians should do all in their power to dissuade unmarried men from having vasectomies. Similarly, it is the rare married man who can see with great accuracy what the future holds, and a second marriage, either because of divorce or death of his spouse or the loss of his children, may quite commonly bring about a renewed desire to have children. For this reason, the author personally strongly discourages vasectomy and, in fact, refuses to perform the procedure except under most unusual circumstances. It is the author's opinion that an outpatient tubal ligation can be performed upon the wife with a level of safety and efficacy equal to that for a vasectomy and this makes infinitely more sense to a couple not desiring any more children since it is less likely that the wife's situation will change in the event of a divorce, that is, she is more likely to keep the children and thus less likely to be desirous of having more children.

The primary advantage of vasectomy as a means of birth control is that it need be performed only once for sterility to be pretty well assured. When vasectomies are properly done using the more recent techniques, the incidence of recanalization of the vas with resultant return of fertility is considerably less than 1 percent. The patient must be told, however, that he will not be sterile until he has had 10 to 20 ejaculations postvasectomy because it takes this long for spermatozoa already present in the vas, the ampulla, and the seminal vesicles to be cleared from the genital tract. The patient should have his semen checked for azoospermia before he assumes he is sterile.

Finally, it should be noted that no long-term deleterious effects have ever been reported, in other than an anecdotal sense, to substantiate the claims of some that vasectomies have long-term harmful effects in man. Although various researchers have reported untoward consequences of vasectomy in various other primates, the very considerable experience with vasectomized men in the United States has given no credence to the concerns of some that the cardiovascular system (or any other system) may be compromised as a result of vasectomy.

Oral Contraceptives. Pills taken by many women for control of fertility are virtually 100 percent successful if taken properly. This form of birth control has the great advantage of reversibility when the pills are no longer taken. Disadvantages include increased incidence of thrombophlebitis, as well as the remote but occasionally reported deleterious long-term side effects after a woman has been taking these pills for many years. Also, some individual women have immediate unpleasant side effects from the birth control pill, such as weight gain, edema, nausea, and headaches. There is no question that oral contraceptives are less than ideal for some women and may be contraindicated for other women.

Intrauterine Devices. Many intrauterine contraceptive devices are available. They are efficacious in preventing pregnancy in better than 90 percent of women who use them, although pregnancies have been known to occur even when such devices are properly in place. The principal disadvantage of the intrauterine devices is the grave risk to the woman's life should pregnancy occur while the device is in place. In the rare instances when pregnancy has occurred, septicemia and death have followed. The devices in general should not be shunned, but they should be used with caution and certainly not in any woman who would not be willing to undergo an abortion should she become pregnant. Additionally there is the risk of severe sepsis if a patient develops pelvic inflammatory disease while she is using an intrauterine device, and these devices are probably specifically contraindicated in the patient known to have such pelvic inflammatory disease.

Vaginal Foam, and Gels and Diaphragms. The main advantage of the various contraceptive foams and gels is their relative ease of use—neither a medical prescription nor even the assistance of a physician is required. Their disadvantages are the need to insert them within half an hour prior to intercourse and the fact that they are probably only 85 to 90 percent effective in preventing conception. When these gels and foams are used in combination with a diaphragm, they are successful in preventing conception about 95 percent of the time. The diaphragm can be left in place virtually indefinitely but should probably not be relied on as a sole means of birth control because of the possibility of it slipping from its proper location without the woman being aware of it. Insertion of a diaphragm is a simple matter that a woman can do herself after proper instruction from her physician.

Condoms. The condom in many ways represents a virtually ideal contraceptive device although it has not achieved nearly the widespread usage in the United States that it has in many European and Asian countries, where it is available in vending machines in virtually every public men's room in service stations, restaurants, and so on. Historically, condoms have been esthetically displeasing because they were made of a material so heavy in grade and texture as to markedly diminish pleasurable sensation for both the man and the woman; however, condoms made at the present time are exquisitely thin and commensurately strong and offer only minimally reduced sensation during intercourse. An additional and highly important advantage is that it offers the best possible protection against venereal diseases, the incidence of which has become rampant.

The younger generation of today has been brought up on oral contraception as the best and only method of birth control, so it is not too surprising to find that the condom is held in very low regard and rarely used by many young American men. As a matter of fact, many of these men are quite unfamiliar with condoms and their usage, and this is simply a reflection of the fact that the responsibility for birth control, which used to belong to the male, has now passed to the female almost exclusively. The physician counseling a young man on sexual matters might seriously consider determining if the patient has any concern, fears, or built-in antagonisms that might relate to misconceptions about condoms and their proper usage. There are many different kinds of condoms available on the commercial market, including lubricated and nonlubricated condoms, those with reservoir tips to collect the semen and those with built-in ridges to increase the pleasurable sensation for the woman. The physician who is able to discuss these various types of condoms with patients will better be able to communicte with them on all problems relating to sexual activity. It is very helpful if the physician is able to make the patient aware that only water-soluble lubricants, such as KY jelly or Lubafax, should be used with condoms; Vaseline and other petroleum products may make them ineffective because they have a harmful effect on the rubber. The patient should be taught that the condom is placed on the erect penis, leaving some space in the forward end in which the ejaculate can collect. If a reservoir-tipped condom is used, this end space is not necessary. The condom should be placed on the penis at the beginning of intercourse; it is not satisfactory to put it on just at the time of impending ejaculation because the pre-ejaculate fluid that usually seeps out of the urethra may very well contain spermatozoa. Following ejaculation, the condom should be held in place at the base of the penis with the man's fingers lest the condom fall off as the erection wanes and the penis is withdrawn from the vagina. Finally, it is helpful for the patient to realize that it is not necessary to test condoms by blowing them up or by filling them with water; this will only weaken them, and they are pretested anyway. There should be nothing embarrassing about purchasing condoms in a drugstore; a medical prescription is not necessary and they are universally available in pharmacies. There are several companies manufacturing condoms and almost all make a half dozen or more varieties to suit individual preference. It is helpful for the patient to familiarize himself with brand names (such as Ramses or Trojan) and to request them in the desired form (lubricated, nonlubricated, reservoir tip, no reservoir tip, and so forth).

REFERENCES

Amelar RD, Dubin L: Infertility in the male. In Kendall AR, Karafin L (eds), Urology. Philadelphia, Harper and Row, 1978, vol 2, chap 21

Cockett ATK, moderator: Symposium on infertility and male contraception. Contemp Surg 22:117, 1983

Cockett ATK, moderator: Symposium on the varicocele and its effect on fertility. Contemp Surg 24:111, 1984

Reed DM: Male sexual dysfunctions and counseling techniques. In Kendall AR, Karafin L (eds), Urology. Philadelphia, Harper and Row, 1982, vol 2, chap 30

Rous SN: Urology in Primary Care. St. Louis, Mosby, 1976

Spark RF, White RA, Connolly PB: Impotence is not always psychogenic. JAMA 243:750, 1980

Swerdloff RS, Boyers SP: Evaluation of the male partner of an infertile couple. JAMA 247:2418, 1982

Wasserman MD, Pollak CP, Spielman AJ, Weitzman ED: The differential diagnosis of impotence. JAMA 243:2038, 1980

15
Findings and Abnormalities in Urinary Composition and Output

EDUCATIONAL OBJECTIVES

1. List the causes of polyuria, oliguria, and anuria.
2. Identify and recognize squamous epithelial cells in the urine sediment.
3. List the causes for abnormal proteinuria.
4. List the causes for glucose in the urine.
5. List the cellular elements present in urine.
6. Identify and recognize the following elements in the urine sediment: white blood cells, red blood cells, white blood cell casts, red blood cell casts, hyaline casts, and granular casts.
7. Identify and recognize artifacts in urine sediment.
8. Obtain and examine clean-catch midstream urine specimens from men and women.
9. Discuss the relationship of the serum creatinine and BUN levels to renal function, urine flow rate, and nonrenal factors affecting plasma concentrations.
10. Discuss the methodology of obtaining a 24-hour urine specimen.
11. Calculate creatinine clearance.
12. Define specific gravity and relate it to a clinical situation.

Collection and examination of the urine is an essential part of diagnosing a suspected urologic problem or of screening an asymptomatic patient. The presence in urine of bacteria, pus, protein, glucose, blood, and other abnormal components is often a sign of disease. Abnormalities in the amount of urine produced and variations in the way it is produced and the amounts in which it is produced may also be reflective of a pathologic condition.

COLLECTION

The method of collection of urine, especially for the purpose of determining pyuria or bacteriuria (pus cells or bacteria, respectively, in the urine), is of utmost importance. Unless urine is properly collected and cultured, or refrigerated promptly while awaiting culture, diagnostic conclusions drawn from its study can be erroneous. Asymptomatic individuals in whom infection is erroneously diagnosed may be needlessly subjected to expensive, time-consuming, and often uncomfortable urologic investigations; or infection may be diagnosed and treated in symptomatic individuals when the real problem is simply inflammation, stone, or something more esoteric. Pus cells or bacteria in a random voided urine specimen, particularly in a woman, are of absolutely no consequence; however, absence of any bacteria or pus cells, regardless of the manner of urine collection, must be considered significant because false-negative specimens are most uncommon.

Female Patients

A large percentage of female patients, particularly girls, referred by the primary physician to the urologist because they are believed to have pus and infection in the urine in fact have neither. Because of the likelihood of vaginal, fecal, and external genital contamination, the random voided urine from the female of any age is absolutely useless for diagnosing urinary tract infection. The only satisfactory voided urine specimens from girls or women are clean-catch midstream collections obtained in the following manner: after thorough cleansing of the labia majora, labia minora, vestibule, and periurethral areas with hexachlorophene (pHisoHex), urine is voided and the midstream portion collected while the labia are retracted. If pyuria or bacteriuria persist after examination of more than one properly collected urine specimen from an asymptomatic female, a urine specimen obtained by catheter or by suprapubic needle aspiration should be cultured before a diagnosis of asymptomatic infection is made.

Male Patients

In men and in boys who are toilet trained, satisfactory urine collection involves thorough scrubbing of the glans penis with pHisoHex, after retraction of the foreskin (if present), followed by the accurate collection of the middle portion of the voided urinary stream. Catheterization or suprapubic needle aspiration are rarely necessary in the male who is old enough to void on command.

Very Young Children

In children who are not toilet trained, uncontaminated urine for culture is most satisfactorily collected by means of a suprapubic needle aspiration in boys and a suprapubic aspiration or catheterization in girls.

In the boy who is too young to void on command, a "spike," or collecting bag, may be placed over the penis to gather spontaneously voided urine. Culture of urine collected in this manner can be considered diagnostic only if it is negative. A positive culture may be caused by fecal contamination, and suprapubic aspiration is then indicated unless other signs and symptoms point to a urinary tract infection.

Three-Glass Urine Collections

The three-glass urine collection is a most important technique for diagnosing infection and for determining the source of hematuria in the male patient (see Chapter 16). In carrying out this procedure three sterile containers labeled "1," "2," and "3" are placed where the patient can conveniently reach them. The patient should be instructed to *initiate* his urine stream into container 1 (½ to 1 ounce of urine in this container is sufficient) and to *finish* the act of voiding in container 3, with the *middle* portion of the specimen voided into container 2.

Because at the very onset of voiding the urine traverses the penile portion of the urethra, infection or inflammation localized there will be washed out with the first portion of the urine and collected in container 1; bacteria or pus cells found in this container are presumed to have originated in the penile, or pendulous, urethra.

The urine in container 2 will have come from the middle portion of the voided stream, and anything present in this urine must therefore have been thoroughly mixed with the urine prior to voiding; the *source* of bacteriuria or pyuria in container 2 is located *above* the bladder neck and could include the bladder, ureter(s), or kidney(s). Pyuria or bacteriuria found in container 3 is generally considered to have come from the prostatic urethra or the bladder neck and is felt to have most likely arisen concurrent with the closing of the bladder neck at the end of voiding. After urine is collected in these three containers, the patient's prostate gland is massaged if the physician is attempting to determine whether or not a bacterial infection within the prostate gland exists. If no prostatic fluid for culture appears at the urethral meatus following the massage, the patient is asked to void again (only a small amount is necessary). This final voiding (container 4) will contain the secretions obtained from the prostatic massage and may therefore be presumed to be prostatic in origin. This technique, or the simpler one to differentiate between infections in the urethra and in the prostate described in Chapter 2, offers a helpful guide to the physician as to the source of bacteriuria, pyuria, or hematuria, but it is absolutely not a foolproof indicator of any of these. For example, it is possible for the purulent product of acute infection in the posterior urethra to run in retrograde fashion into the bladder and thoroughly admix with the urine. The midstream urine in container 2 would then be loaded with pus and bacteria, which would erroneously suggest that the origin and the infection was in the bladder, ureter, or kidney. Nevertheless, the three-glass urine collection is invaluable in directing the physician to *probable* sources of infection or hematuria.

The 24-Hour Urine Collection

Properly done, the 24-hour urine collection offers the clinician the most valid and reliable test for measuring creatinine clearance, which in turn is the best of the readily available methods of measuring glomerular infiltration. Moreover, a 24-hour urine collection offers the best means of determining total urinary protein excretion, which is important in determining the presence or absence of true proteinuria and certain related diseases of the kidney. The 24-hour urine determination is also crucial in measuring such things as calcium, oxalate, and uric acid in stone-forming patients. If the 24-hour urine collection is improperly done, grossly misleading findings may be obtained, with the resulting potential for serious mismanagement of the patient.

Ideally, a 24-hour urine collection is obtained on a day when the patient can be at home, thereby obviating the necessity of carrying around a large container for the urine. The patient is instructed to note the precise hour when he or she arises and then to void and discard the urine. All subsequent voidings are collected and saved right up to and including the time that the first urine was voided and discarded. For example, assume that the patient awakens and voids at 8:00 A.M. (and discards this urine). All urine that is voided thereafter (the next voiding might be about 10 or 11 A.M.), up to and including a voiding at precisely 8 A.M. the next morning (24 hours after the initial voiding and discarding of the urine), is saved and collected in a container large enough that all of the urine may be pooled (a 2-quart container will *usually* suffice). If the patient voids during the night this urine must be saved as well. Normal levels of creatinine clearance and total urinary protein excretion, as well as numerous other renal function determinations, are based on precisely 24 hours of urine production. If the patient miscalculates the time and saves less or more urine than is produced in 24 hours, the collection is not automatically invalid *provided* the precise time period of urine collection is noted so that calculation of the various parameters of renal function can be adjusted accordingly and correctly determined. A potential problem with this, however, is that the various parameters of renal function that are measured in the urine are not necessarily excreted at constant rate around a 24-hour clock and so one cannot always, with accuracy, adjust data to account for time periods greater or less than 24 hours and expect to find total accuracy.

REFRIGERATION AND CULTURING

Because bacteria in unrefrigerated urine doubles in number approximately every 20 minutes, the validity of any urine culture regardless of the mode of collection is extremely suspect unless the urine is cultured or refrigerated within 20 minutes following voiding. Furthermore, white blood cells in alkaline urine tend to disintegrate on standing, although refrigeration will retard and minimize this disintegration. Thus the absence of pyuria in unrefrigerated urine must be considered an unreliable finding.

Urine cultures require incubation for 24 to 48 hours. Any colony count of bacteria, however low, must be considered diagnostic of infection if the urine is obtained by urethral catheter or suprapubic needle aspiration. A colony count of under 10,000 organisms/ml in a clean-catch midstream urine specimen may be considered insignificant and a likely contaminant if the organism is a gram-negative organism and if the patient is asymptomatic. When the colony count is between 10,000 and 100,000 organisms/ml and is a gram-negative organism and the patient is symptomatic, the physician may suspect infection. Moreover, if gram positive, a colony count of even 1,000 to 10,000 organisms/ml may be indicative of clinical infection. A colony count of over 100,000 organisms/ml must be considered indicative of a true infection in the symptomatic patient.

EXAMINATION OF THE URINE SEDIMENT

A careful examination of the urine sediment in a freshly voided specimen is so important that it should be carried out by a trained laboratory technician or by the physician personally. To delegate the responsibility for examination of the urine sediment to any but the most known and trusted laboratory technician is to risk false-positive or false-negative interpretations, with resulting potential for patient mismanagement.

A portion of the collected urine is poured into a centrifuge tube and centrifuged for 5 minutes at high speed. The supernatant fluid is then decanted, leaving about 0.5 ml of fluid in which the urine sediment is thoroughly mixed by flicking the bottom of the tube with the finger. A drop of this sediment is then poured onto a slide and examined microscopically under low power ($\times 100$) and high power ($\times 400$), with or without the use of a cover slip. Staining the sediment with methylene blue or Gram stain is of inestimable value in searching for bacteria; the oil immersion lens is usually used for this examination. The cellular elements that may be found in urine sediment include white blood cells and red blood cells; casts (red blood cell, white blood cell, hyaline, waxy, and granular, both coarse and fine); squamous and transitional epithelial cells; and renal tubular epithelial cells as well as certain artifacts.

White Blood Cells

The presence of more than one to two white blood cells per high-power field is abnormal; however, the clinician must not make a diagnosis of urinary tract infection based solely on the presence of white blood cells in the urine sediment (Fig. 15–1). Both chronic and acute inflammation that affect the urethra, the bladder neck, or the trigone very commonly produce pyuria in absolutely sterile urine. Urinary tract infection should only be diagnosed following urine culture, but it may be diagnosed provisionally on visualization of bacteria when the urine sediment is stained with methylene blue or Gram technique and then examined under the oil immersion lens.

Red Blood Cells

In the urine sediment the presence of more than one to two red blood cells per high-power field is distinctly abnormal; if it is persistent a full urologic investigation is mandatory (see Chapter 16). For comparative purposes the clinician should realize that red blood cells are smaller than white blood cells when seen in the urine sediment and are extremely similar in appearance to yeast cells (Fig. 15–2).

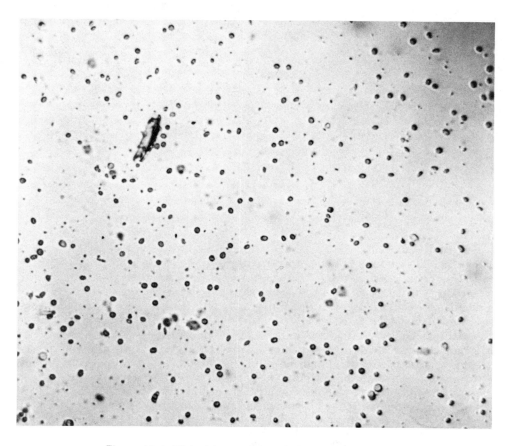

Figure 15-1. White blood cells. **A.** Low-power field (× 100).

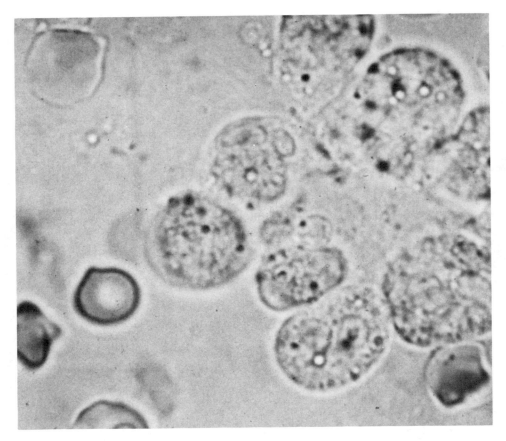

Figure 15-1 B. High-power field (× 450). The smaller cells seen are red cells.

Casts

The principal sites for cast formation are the distal convoluted renal tubules or the collecting ducts. Normal urine sediment does not have any casts, but the presence of certain types of casts, specifically an occasional hyaline cast, is not necessarily indicative of renal disease. It is rather common to find hyaline casts following exercise, when the urine is extremely concentrated, or when its pH is highly acid. Generally, however, casts tend to indicate intrinsic renal disease, and their presence is usually related to impaired function of nephrons. Proteinuria probably is also present when casts are found in urine sediment; therefore, abnormalities of protein filtration, reabsorption, or both may be suspected. With proteinuria, glomerular basement membrane damage is generally, but not always, present when casts are found. Factors that tend to predispose to cast formation are a decrease in urine flow rate, a high salt concentration, and abnormal protein amounts and constituents.

White Blood Cell Casts. White blood cell casts are always formed within the renal tubules and virtually always indicate intrinsic renal disease. Their presence demands

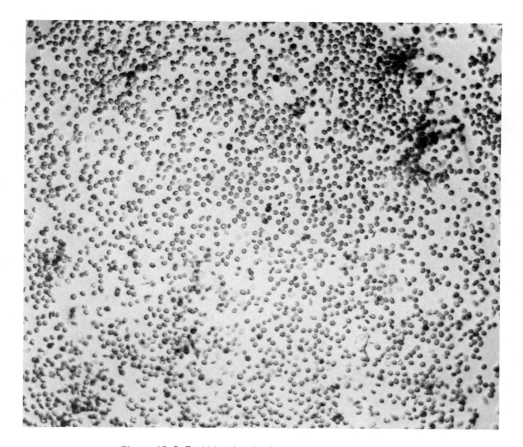

Figure 15-2. Red blood cells. **A.** Low-power field (× 100).

a urine culture and colony count as well as a full urologic investigation. In appearance, white blood cell casts may sometimes be confused with degenerating epithelial cell casts (Fig. 15–3).

Red Blood Cell Casts. The presence of red blood cell casts in urine sediment is distinctly abnormal and indicates bleeding into the nephron. The abnormality may be due to a glomerular or a vascular lesion or both, and it may at times be difficult for the clinician to identify these casts if the red cells are fused into a granular mass of cellular debris (Fig. 15–4).

Hyaline Casts. As already noted, small numbers of hyaline casts are not necessarily meaningful; large numbrs, however, usually indicate serious intrinsic renal disease. These casts are composed of protein with no inclusions and are a mixture of mucoid substance and a globulin that crosses the glomerular membrane (Fig. 15–5). Hyaline casts are only visible in acid urine and are not visible in alkaline urine; therefore, they are not seen in end-stage renal disease, even though present in large numbers,

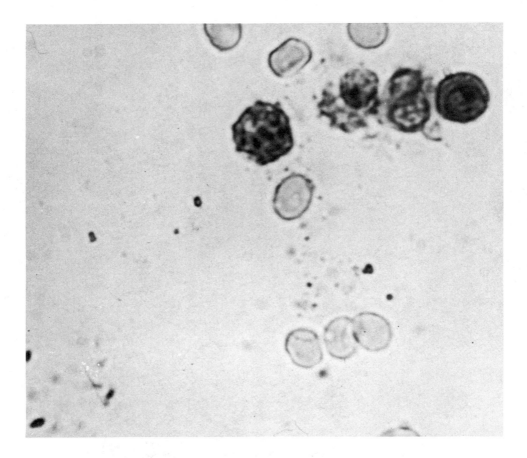

Figure 15–2 B. High-power field (× 400). The larger cells seen are white blood cells (which are stained).

because the kidney is no longer able to make the acid urine that is required for these casts to be seen.

Granular Casts. The composition of granular casts is varied and consists primarily of degenerated epithelial cells, white blood cells, red blood cells, albumin, fat, or any combination of these. The granular cast probably originates as an epithelial cell cast and rapidly disintegrates, becoming coarsely granular, then finely granular, and finally waxy in appearance as the deterioration continues. The presence of granular casts indicates intrinsic renal tubule disease, as does the presence of epithelial cell casts (Fig. 15–6).

Squamous and Transitional Cells. Both squamous and transitional cells are frequently seen in the normal urine sediment and are of no particular significance. Squamous cells come from the distal portion of the urethra; transitional cells arise from the normal urothelium of the bladder (Fig. 15–7). It is only when the specific histology of these cells becomes abnormal that disease should be suspected.

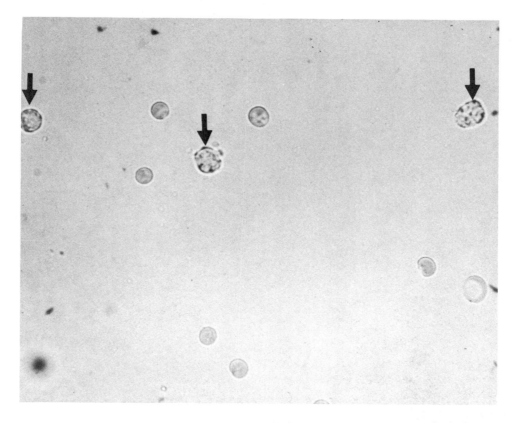

Figure 15-2 C. High-power field ($\times$ 400). The three larger cells (*arrows*) are white blood cells.

Artifacts

The only significance to be attached to artifacts is that they must be differentiated from true abnormalities of the urine sediment. Perhaps the most common artifact is simply dirt on the slide. Another extremely common one is starch granules from the powder that is sometimes found inside the surgical gloves used by the nurse or technician when obtaining a urine specimen (Fig. 15-8). Additional artifacts that may be found in urine sediment are ingested drugs such as aspirin, vitamin C, sulfa, antihistamines, and caffeine.

ABNORMALITIES OF URINE COMPOSITION

Proteinuria

Proteinuria is a condition in which abnormal amounts of protein are present in the urine. It is often thought that any amount of protein in the urine is abnormal, but this is not correct. Small amounts of plasma protein are able to pass through the glomerulus and do appear in normal urine. Between 50 and 150 mg of protein in the 24-hour urine collection is normal and in no manner a cause for concern. A

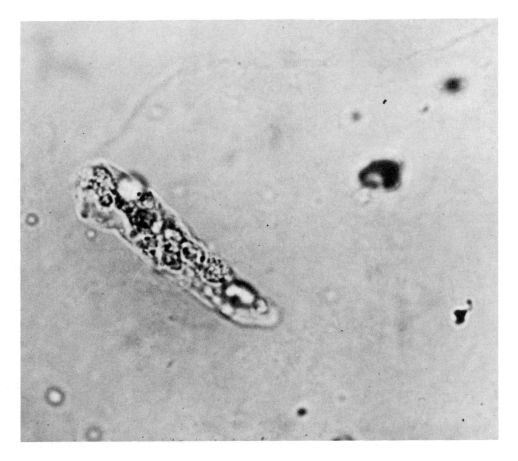

Figure 15-3. White blood cell casts seen in high-power field (× 400).

clinical problem that most frequently arises is diagnosis of false-positive protein-uria based on the use of a dipstick in a freshly voided urine specimen. It must be emphasized that dipstick findings represent an extremely gross determination of urine proteins and its use is therefore frequently responsible for needlessly alarming the clinician and the patient. The clinician should also bear in mind that if there is any microscopic or gross hematuria in the voided urine, proteinuria might be present and yet not necessarily related to any glomerular disease but merely to the presence of the blood itself. The safest rule to follow when the dipstick persistently reveals anything more than a trace of proteinuria is to have the patient collect a 24-hour urine for a quantitative determination of the actual amount of protein present in the urine. Another approach is to use the sulfosalicylic acid method of screening for urinary protein because it is less sensitive and has fewer false positives than the dipstick.

Small amounts of plasma protein are normally filtered at the glomerulus, but most of it is reabsorbed by the renal tubules, so the amounts of protein present in

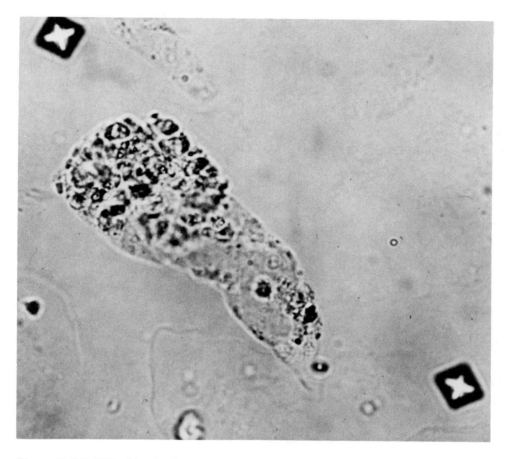

Figure 15-3 B. White blood cell cast in high-powered field (× 400). Note the calcium oxalate crystals in the upper left and lower right corners.

most individual's urine is in the vicinity of 50 to 150 mg per 24 hours. Under certain circumstances it is at least theoretically possible that the renal tubules may not be able to reabsorb the plasma proteins that are filtered by the normal glomerulus, and abnormal amounts of proteinuria may be present.

The most common cause for abnormal proteinuria (over 150 mg of protein for 24 hours) is renal glomerular disease such as may be seen in acute or chronic glomerulonephritis. In these conditions, as well as in other forms of glomerular disease, the glomeruli are unable to filter out the plasma proteins; thus they appear in the urine. When abnormal levels of proteinuria are found, it is invariably albuminuria that is being measured. There is a direct correlation between the degree of glomerular damage and the degree of proteinuria, and with severe glomerular disease, such as some cases of chronic glomerulonephritis, as much as 8 to 10 g or more of protein may be present in a 24-hour urine specimen.

A far less common cause of abnormal proteinuria is renal tubular disease in which the tubules abnormally secrete certain amino acids in unusually large amounts.

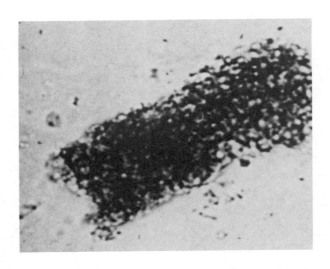

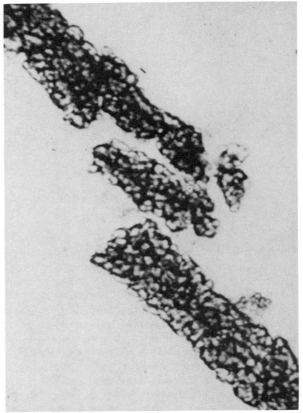

Figure 15-4. Two different types of red blood cell casts as seen in a high-power field (× 400).

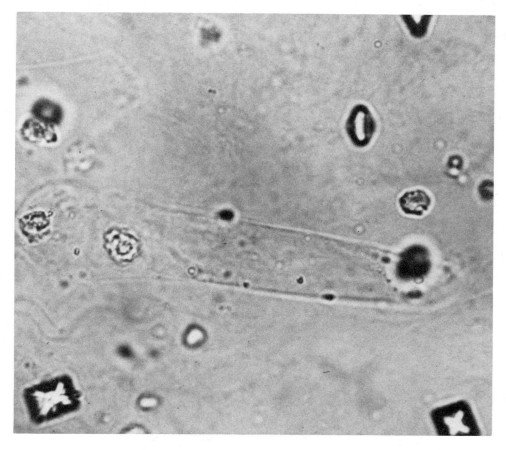

Figure 15–5. Hyaline cast seen in a high-power field (× 400). These casts are distinctive in that they are extremely difficult to see unless the illumination of the microscopic field is greatly diminished.

These are generally inborn errors of metabolism; that is, they are congenital renal tubular defects, and large amounts of amino acids such as cystine may be found in the urine. In these cases, the abnormal proteinuria is not albumin but it is nonetheless proteinuria.

When abnormal proteinuria has been diagnosed, it is almost always a symptom of an underlying renal disease, and diligent efforts must be made to search for the exact cause. Although such clinically exotic conditions as renal vein thrombosis are occasionally etiologic in the production of proteinuria, acute and chronic glomerulonephritis will be found in the vast majority of patients with abnormal quantities of protein in the urine. If a definitive diagnosis cannot be reached by clinical and laboratory means, renal biopsy may be indicated.

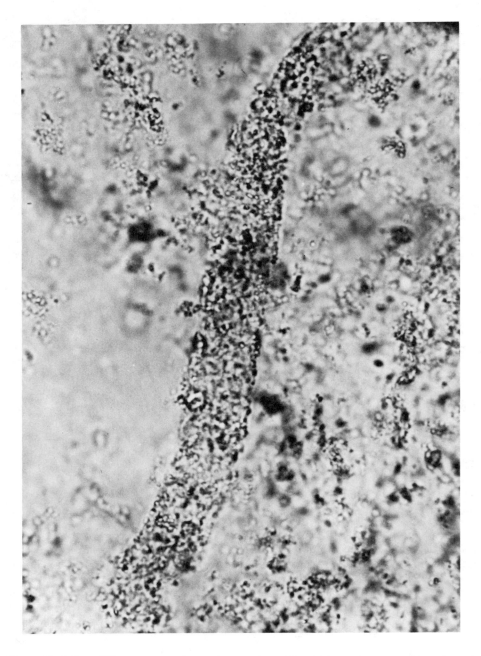

Figure 15-6. Two different types of granular cast (× 400), which can have considerable variation in size.

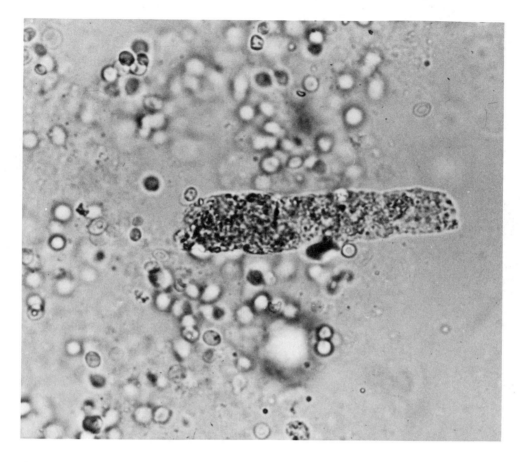

Figure 15-6 B. Note the presence of numerous red blood cells around the granular cast.

Glucosuria (or "Sugar in the Urine")

There are many kinds of sugar that may appear in the urine, but it is glucose that is referred to when one speaks of "sugar in the urine." Ordinarily there should not be any detectable glucose in the urine. Its presence, as determined by the use of a dipstick or one of the other qualitative tests performed on voided urine, generally indicates the presence of diabetes mellitus. In order for circulating blood glucose to spill into the urine, given normal renal tubular function, it must reach a blood level of 180 mg/dl or higher. When this occurs, diabetes mellitus may be said to exist.

In a minority of cases of glucosuria, renal tubular disease may be the cause. The ability of the tubule to reabsorb glucose filtered at the glomerulus is impaired, and glucose may appear in the urine despite the fact that the blood glucose level is under 180 mg/dl. In these cases diabetes mellitus may or may not exist.

Glucose is normally filtered at the glomerulus, but as long as the blood glucose level is under 180 mg/dl, reabsorption of glucose by the normal renal tubules is assured and it will not be present in urine. Therefore, when glucosuria exists, the

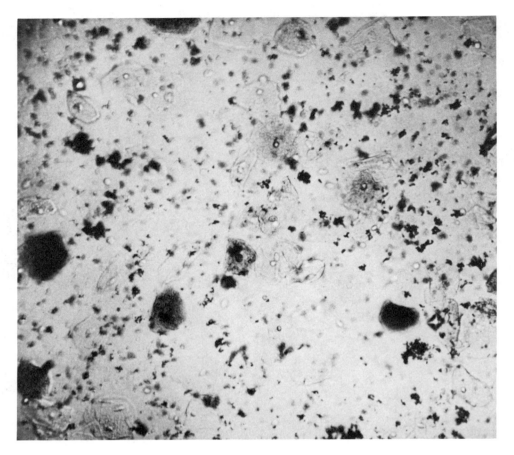

Figure 15–7. Squamous cells, frequently seen in the normal urine sediment. Transitional cells may also be seen in normal urine sediment. **A.** low-power field (× 100).

likelihood of diabetes mellitus is great. Fasting and 2-hour postprandial blood glucose tests and possibly a glucose tolerance test are indicated in these circumstances; if these studies appear normal, various glucose loading tests to determine the reabsorptive capacities of the renal tubules are indicated.

Variations of Urine Specific Gravity

The specific gravity of urine is based on the relative molecular weights of the solutes present in the urine. The more solutes present, the higher the specific gravity. Osmolality of urine is based on the number of particles present in the urine. Specific gravity and osmolality are usually closely related, but in certain circumstances may not be. For example, following an excretory urogram the injected contrast medium present in the urine will elevate the specific gravity markedly, but the osmolality of the urine will not be correspondingly elevated.

Clinically, the specific gravity of urine is related to the tubular function of the

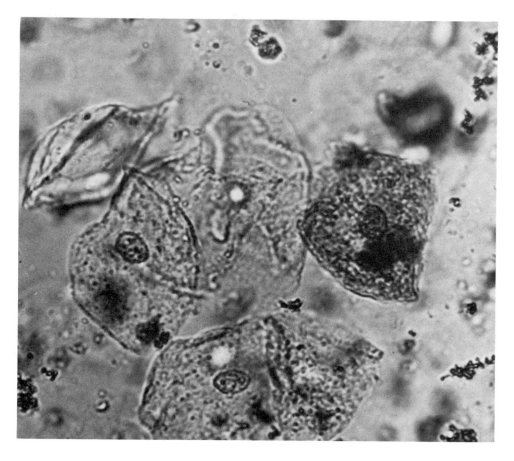

Figure 15-7 B. Squamous cells in high-power field (× 400).

kidneys. One of the principal functions of the renal tubules is to reabsorb water and return it to the general circulation. Only about 1 to 1½ liters per day of urine are normally produced, representing about 1 percent of the total glomerular filtrate. Thus the difference between the amount of fluid filtered at the glomerulus and the amount actually produced as urine represents the fluid that is reabsorbed by the renal tubules, or about 99 percent of the entire glomerular filtrate. If the renal tubules are not functioning properly in reabsorption, then a greater amount of less concentrated urine will result and will have a relatively low specific gravity. When severe chronic renal disease exists, for example, the specific gravity may be fixed at 1.010, which is the specific gravity of the plasma filtrate. In this situation, the tubular function is very definitely diminished, specifically as regards the diminished reabsorption capacity of the tubules. A normal individual can concentrate urine to 1.030 or 1.040, depending on the state of hydration. The inability to concentrate urine is sometimes one of the earlier renal tubular functions that is lost in chronic renal disease.

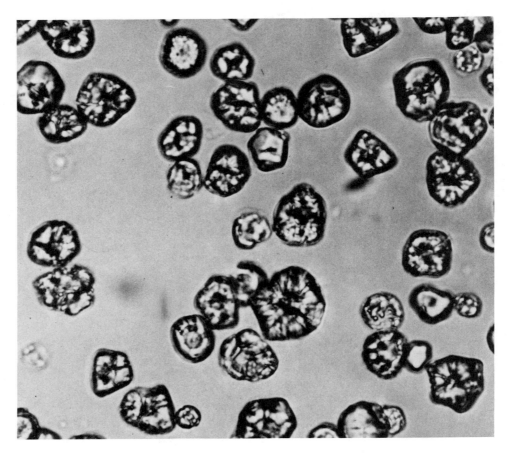

Figure 15–8. Artifacts (× 400). The artifacts seen here are starch granules from powder inside a surgical glove. Numerous other artifacts may be present in urine at any time.

MEASUREMENT OF GLOMERULAR FUNCTION

Serum Creatinine and Blood Urea Nitrogen (BUN) Levels

Serum creatinine and blood urea nitrogen (BUN) levels are two of the more common chemical determinations used to measure glomerular filtration. The creatinine level is much more reliable as a parameter of glomerular filtration because the creatinine is only minimally secreted by the renal tubules and for all intents and purposes may be considered as though it were neither secreted nor reabsorbed by the renal tubules. Thus, its determination can provide an accurate measurement of glomerular filtration.

In the dog, the creatinine level offers a virtually perfect measurement of glomerular filtration because it is neither secreted nor reabsorbed by the tubules. In humans, however, the only agent that is neither secreted nor reabsorbed at all by the renal tubules is inulin; this, therefore, is the most accurate substance to use for the precise measurement of glomerular filtration. Inasmuch as inulin is an exogenous substance, however, its use entails much more difficulty than the measurement of the endogenous creatinine level, which is accurate for all practical purposes, particularly if it is measured as a 24-hour creatinine clearance.

Urea, on the other hand, is significantly reabsorbed by the renal tubules, and the rate of reabsorption is directly related to the rate of urine flow through the renal tubules; therefore, the slower the flow rate, the more urea is absorbed by the tubules and returned to the general circulation, and the higher the resulting blood urea nitrogen level becomes. For example, if the urine flow rate were slowed, as it would be if a significant back pressure from the bladder were transmitted to the ureters and into the renal collecting system, the measurement of the blood urea nitrogen level would be considerably elevated because more of it would be reabsorbed into the general circulation. Although this is of clinical importance to the physician, it does not necessarily represent any intrinsic renal disease, and for this reason the measurement of the creatinine level is much more valid. Because it is not reabsorbed and really only minimally secreted by the renal tubules, creatinine determinations offer the clinician a far better measurement of the actual glomerular function in terms of whether any significant glomerular disease exists. If the back pressure on the kidneys just noted were of sufficient magnitude that the glomerular filtration were actually decreased, the serum creatinine and blood urea nitrogen levels would rise. The creatinine level, however, rises more slowly and only when there is an actual *decrease* in the glomerular filtration, whereas the urea, which is absorbed by the renal tubules, rises more readily and rapidly when there is simply a slowing of blood flow through the kidneys, thereby allowing more urea to be reabsorbed and sent back into the general circulation where its increase can be measured. This does not mean that blood urea nitrogen level is not a valid determination but only that its abnormal elevation does not necessarily indicate the presence of intrinsic renal disease.

There are, moreover, numerous nonrenal factors that can affect the plasma concentration of blood urea nitrogen but leave the level of serum creatinine relatively unaffected. First, bleeding into the gastrointestinal tract will lead to an increased breakdown in red blood cells, with increased absorption of protein producing the same net effect as though the individual patient were on a high-protein diet. This high-protein diet would cause an increase in the blood urea nitrogen level, whereas a low-protein diet would cause a decrease in the blood urea nitrogen level. Second, dehydration of the patient would bring about a hypovolemia and a very slow flow rate through the kidneys, thereby leading to an increased reabsorption of urea from the renal tubules and an increased concentration of blood urea nitrogen by means of the mechanism already discussed. Although severe dehydration can also result in a rise in the serum creatinine without any intrinsic renal disease being present, the fact remains that creatinine levels are not nearly as sensitive to the vagaries of hydration and dehydration as are the blood urea nitrogen levels. Also, severe liver failure will bring about a *decrease* in the blood urea nitrogen levels because the liver is unable to produce even normal amounts of urea.

Creatinine, although not subject to as many extrarenal vagaries as is blood urea nitrogen, is definitely a function of and proportional to the muscle mass of the individual. The normal serum creatinine level for a large, muscular man would be expected to be higher than that for a small, unmuscular woman. The large, muscular man would also be expected to have a higher serum creatinine level than the average man; if he is found instead to have a normal or a low normal serum creatinine level, muscle wasting or a general debilitating condition should be suspected and investigated.

Renal function does not remain a constant throughout the full spectrum of life, and with advancing age glomerular filtration tends to decrease, leading to elevation in the normal serum creatinine levels for different age groups. Above age 70 years, for example, the normal creatinine level can be around 1.8 mg/dl without representing a disease process.

It should also be understood that the laboratory determination of serum creatinine levels is a colorimetric determination, and other chromogens may be present in the serum that could adversely affect this determination and give falsely elevated values. This possibility must always be kept in mind, and when a seemingly healthy individual has an unexpectedly high creatinine level, a repeat determination and probably even a 24-hour creatinine clearance test should be done.

The foregoing discussion has been primarily intended to alert the clinician to the various factors, renal and nonrenal, that could potentially affect the serum concentration levels of creatinine and blood urea nitrogen. It is in no way intended to deprecate the value or validity of these studies, which remain as reliable and as commonly used as any current measurements of renal function.

Calculation of Creatinine Clearance

An important measurement of glomerular filtration is creatinine clearance. This refers to the number of milliliters of creatinine that can be cleared by the kidney(s) in 1 minute. Although it is usually sufficient for the clinician to be aware of the normal values for creatinine clearance based on a 24-hour urine collection (approximately 120 ml/min for both kidneys in the normal adult, corrected to 1.73 m^2 of surface area), it is also of extreme importance that the derivation of creatinine clearance be understood so that the clinician can interpret the raw data received from the hospital laboratory. Errors of calculation based on accurate measurement of raw data and inaccurate mathematical interpretation of these data (often by the lab) may frequently result in grossly erroneous creatinine clearance determinations that in turn lead to the patient's having additional needless, expensive, and often unpleasant diagnostic studies.

Creatinine clearance (an estimate of glomerular filtration rate) is best determined on a 24-hour urine collection in order to minimize errors in measuring urine flow rate. The formula for creatinine clearance is

$$C = \frac{UV}{P}$$

where C is the creatinine clearance in milliliters per minute, U is the concentration of creatinine in the urine, expressed as milligrams per either milliliter or deciliter (mg/ml or mg/100ml), P is the concentration of creatinine in the plasma in milligrams per either milliliter or deciliter, and V is the urine flow rate in milliliters per minute (24-hour volume divided by 1440 min/day). To calculate creatinine clearance properly, the values for P and U must be in the same units so that they cancel each other:

$$C \text{ ml/min} = \frac{(U \text{ mg/dl}) (V \text{ ml/min})}{P \text{ mg/dl}}$$

In addition to U, V and P, some laboratories report the 24-hour creatinine excretion as

Excretion (mg per 24 hours) $= (U \text{ mg/ml})(V \text{ ml per 24 hours})$

Creatinine clearance in milliliters per minute can be calculated from the value by dividing by P (mg/ml) and 1440 min per 24 hours.

Creatinine clearance should also be corrected to 1.73 m² of surface area (the ideal in a person weighing 70 kg). This is necessary inasmuch as creatinine clearance is traditionally expressed in milliliters per minute and the figure obtained is then corrected to 1.73 m², on which the normal value range of creatinine clearance is based. There are tables in virtually all textbooks of renal physiology in which the height and weight of a given person are tabulated to give his or her dimensions in square meters. This figure can then be compared with the 1.73-m² standard. In a practical sense, this last calculation is necessary only for children and inordinately small adults, so that a false impression of their renal function is not given.

ABNORMALITIES IN URINE OUTPUT

Polyuria

Polyuria is said to exist when the total 24-hour urine output significantly exceeds 1200 to 1500 ml, which is considered average for an adult. Normal output for children, and therefore also polyuria, varies with the child's size and age. True polyuria cannot be determined without accurate measurement of 24-hour urine volume. Most patients tend to equate frequent voiding with an abnormally high urine output, which is not necessarily or even usually the case. An output of over 2000 ml per 24 hours may be indicative of polyuria but not necessarily of disease.

The most common cause of polyuria by far is a *very high fluid intake,* and this must be determined by the clinician when a patient has documented polyuria. It is not only the total amount of fluid ingested that predisposes individuals to polyuria but the type of fluid as well. For example, coffee is a known diuretic; the ingestion of 3 liters of coffee per day would produce polyuria to a greater degree than the ingestion of 3 liters of water per day. In treating someone with a provisional diagnosis of polyuria, the clinician should have the patient accurately monitor both daily intake (including the type of fluid) and urine output as well as the precise times of voiding over an exact 24-hour period (see above). When these measurements are carefully determined and totaled, it will be evident that in the vast majority of cases either true polyuria does not exist or it simply reflects a high fluid intake with no pathologic condition present.

In a clinical setting the complaint of *frequency* is an extremely common one and most patients mean that they are voiding more often than formerly. Strictly speaking, frequent voidings of large amounts of urine so that the 24-hour total represents a true polyuria is not really a true frequency at all. When the clinician is confronted with a patient complaining of "frequency," an excellent and rapid screen for possible polyuria is the specific gravity of the random voided urine sample produced in the office. The lower the specific gravity value is (below 1.010) the greater the likelihood that a true polyuria exists, and this must be confirmed or ruled out by having the patient prepare one or two very accurate 24-hour intake and output sheets as noted above. Without question the "frequency" caused by a true polyuria should be well up on any list of differential diagnoses in patients who simply complain of frequency. It is worth noting, parenthetically, that when a patient has the symptoms of frequency *only* during the daytime and has no nocturia at all, the odds are excellent that the frequency is being produced by anxiety and there is no organic problem at all.

Diabetes mellitus is one of the most common pathologic causes of polyuria and the related frequency. The elevated blood glucose level seen with this condition exceeds the renal tubular reabsorptive capacity; thus, sugar enters the renal tubules and then the urine. It is this sugar within the renal tubules that acts as an osmotic diuretic, pulling along water with it and therefore increasing the total urinary output (polyuria). There is an accompanying and compensating water intake. Diagnosis is based on the presence of sugar in the urine, followed by the finding of abnormal elevations of the blood glucose level.

Certain forms of *chronic renal disease* can also lead to polyuria. This is based in part on severe renal tubular damage so that the tubular reabsorptive capabilities are impaired. In these cases, a so-called high-output renal failure results, with ensuing polyuria. It is very rare for polyuria to be the initial finding of this type of chronic renal disease, however, and it usually occurs in an individual previously known to have chronic renal disease and occurs late in the course of the disease. Definitive diagnosis is based on history of known renal disease and elevated blood creatinine and urea nitrogen levels.

Diabetes insipidus is another cause of polyuria. This condition may be divided into three distinct classifications: pituitary, nephrogenic, and psychogenic diabetes insipidus.

The posterior pituitary gland secretes antidiuretic hormone (ADH) that acts on the collecting ducts of the kidney to promote water reabsorption at that point, thereby serving to concentrate the urine and to decrease the actual urine output. Failure of the pituitary gland to secrete ADH in sufficient amounts therefore results in increased urine production. *Pituitary diabetes insipidus* can be ruled out if the second voided morning urine specimen (which represents a fasting or dehydrated urine) has a specific gravity higher than 1.020. The normal morning voiding will have a moderately high specific gravity if the posterior pituitary hormone secretion is present in normal quantities. If this second voiding of the day has a specific gravity less than 1.020, it is strong presumptive evidence that there is insufficient ADH present. A therapeutic trial of parenteral administration of pituitary ADH will confirm the diagnosis by causing a cessation of polyuria and a resulting increase in the specific gravity of the morning voiding.

Nephrogenic diabetes insipidus is caused by a failure of the end organ to respond to ADH; that is, the pituitary gland secretes ADH normally, but the receptor cells of the collecting ducts of the kidney are unable to respond to the stimulus of the hormone by increasing water reabsorption, so that polyuria results. This end-organ unresponsiveness to ADH is frequently a hereditary condition for which no specific therapy is readily available. Nephrogenic diabetes insipidus may be diagnosed in the individual with polyuria by a clinical failure of response when ADH is administered parenterally to the patient whose early morning voided specimens show persistently low specific gravity (below 1.020).

Psychogenic diabetes insipidus is induced by abnormal ingestion of very large amounts of fluid, resulting in polyuria. In this condition, ADH is secreted normally and acts normally on the collecting ducts of the kidney, but the fluid load presented to the kidney by massive fluid ingestion is so great that polyuria ensues. Diagnosis is based on the results of placing the patient in a controlled environment, such as a hospital, where water restriction is possible. When fluid intake is restricted, polyuria ceases and specific gravity of the urine rises. Care must be exercised, however, not to employ diagnostic fluid deprivation in a patient with true pituitary diabetes insipidus.

Finally, as already noted near the beginning of this section, by far the most common cause of polyuria is simply a large fluid intake, voluntary in nature, and with no pathologic condition present. The patient often is not aware that he or she is ingesting unusually large volumes of fluids until this is graphically demonstrated as a result of the 24-hour intake and output flow sheets. Once the patient realizes the reason for his or her problem (frequency), the patient can then decide whether he or she wants to continue with the frequency or cut down on the fluid intake.

Oliguria

Oliguria is said to exist when the 24-hour urine output is less than 500 ml. This abnormal condition may be due to a low renal blood flow, certain types of chronic renal disease, partial ureteral obstruction, or a combination of these. Low renal blood flow results when the blood pressure is too low to permit adequate renal perfusion, such as in clinical shock. It is felt that if the systolic blood pressure is under 80, renal perfusion will be minimal and oliguria will result. Shock may result from acute blood loss or from one of many other etiologies, but it inevitably leads to a transient oliguric state.

Chronic renal disease with poor glomerular function, such as that seen in chronic glomerulonephritis can also produce an oliguric state. When oliguria is secondary to chronic renal disease and poor glomerular function, supplementary hydration does not relieve the oliguria; rather, the patient becomes overhydrated and heart failure and pulmonary edema may result.

Another cause of oliguria is acute renal failure from glomerular, tubular, or vascular damage. Tubular damage is probably the most common finding with acute renal failure and may be produced by heavy metal poisoning, incompatible blood transfusion, drug reactions, and the like.

Partial ureteral obstruction can produce oliguria that may be iatrogenic in etiology, as from inadvertent partial ligation of one or both ureters during pelvic surgery. It can also result from ureteral obstruction from extrinsic sources such as metastatic carcinoma or retroperitoneal fibrosis. Unilateral ureteral obstruction in the presence of a normal contralateral kidney will not produce oliguria; the ureteral obstruction must be bilateral in the presence of two otherwise normal kidneys. A combination of factors can also lead to oliguria. For example, unilateral partial ureteral obstruction combined with chronic renal disease on the contralateral side could exist, although chronic unilateral disease is not nearly as common as chronic bilateral disease.

Anuria

Anuria is the complete or virtually complete absence of urine over a 24-hour period. It is extremely uncommon and never occurs as a result of chronic renal disease, because even the most severe renal disease will allow for the production of some urine. The clinician must realize that a significant number of patients with severe chronic renal diseases have a very *high* urine output, referred to as high-output renal failure.

Basically, there are only two or three conditions, or combinations of them, that can lead to true anuria and they should be diligently searched for and treated in the patient with clinical anuria. A bilateral renal arterial embolism or renal vein thrombosis can produce total or virtually total anuria, as can the same pathology if it is unilateral on the side of a solitary functioning kidney. Ureteral obstruction, either bilateral or unilateral on the side of a solitary functioning kidney, that is complete enough to result in anuria may be due to (1) an obstructing ureteral calculus or a bilateral ureteral calculus; (2) iatrogenic occlusion of one or both ureters from a misplaced suture ligature; (3) severe retroperitoneal fibrosis that is including one or both of the ureters; (4) metastatic carcinoma to retroperitoneal lymph nodes that occludes the ureters, such as might occur from carcinoma of the cervix; (5) direct extension of carcinoma that occludes the ureters, such as might occur with carcinoma of the prostate gland; and (6) severe fibrosis and scarring of the periureteral tissues secondary to radiation therapy (an extremely unusual and rare finding).

REFERENCES

Carroll HJ, Oh MS: Water, electrolyte and acid-base balance. In Kendall AR, Karafin L (eds), Urology. Philadelphia, Harper and Row, 1980, vol 1, chap 19

Rous SN: Urology in Primary Care. St. Louis, Mosby, 1976

Rous SN: Understanding Urology. Basel, Karger, 1973

16
Hematuria

EDUCATIONAL OBJECTIVES

1. List the causes of gross and microscopic hematuria.
2. Describe the workup and management of a patient with gross or microscopic hematuria.
3. List the most likely etiologies for hematuria in males and females under age 40 and over age 40.
4. List the most likely etiologies for hematuria in the neonate, in infants, and in children.
5. List the specific diagnostic studies that can be used to determine the etiology of microscopic or gross hematuria.

Hematuria is the presence of blood in the urine; it can be either gross or microscopic. It cannot be stressed strongly enough that the clinical difference between these two types of hematuria is quantitative, not qualitative, and that it is only a matter of degree of pathology rather than type of pathology that differentiates them. *Any* lesion that can cause gross hematuria can cause microscopic hematuria and the clinician must *never* be lulled into a state of diagnostic inactivity on the grounds that "only microscopic hematuria" exists.

ESTABLISHING THE PRESENCE OF HEMATURIA

It is axiomatic that not all red-colored urine is bloody urine, and the patient who says that he or she has hematuria is not necessarily correct. Other possible causes of red-colored urine include myoglobinuria associated with strenuous exercise and resulting muscle pain and tenderness, hemoglobinuria that may be secondary to intravascular hemolysis, porphyria, ingestion of laxatives containing phenolphthalein, use of phenothiazines or rifampin, and dietary intake of beets or rhubarb. Vaginal bleeding also may be confused with bloody urine and the clinician must be certain that an uncontaminated urine specimen is being examined. The presence of red blood cells in the urine sediment, as seen under low- or high-power microscopy, definitely establishes a diagnosis of hematuria.

SITES OF ORIGIN OF HEMATURIA

Although in the vast majority of cases, microscopic or gross hematuria originates within the genitourinary tract, there are two principal sources of hematuria outside of the genitourinary tract that must be borne in mind. First, a "systemic," or "medical," disease such as a blood dyscrasia or coagulopathy may exist. Vitamin C or vitamin K deficiencies are examples that can produce blood in the urine. Cardiac disease with embolization and infarction of the kidneys and drug reactions from anticoagulants and nephrotoxic drugs are other examples of medical or systemic disease. Sometimes included in this group and of particular concern to the clinician, is the presence of one of the nephritides, of which acute post streptococcal glomerulonephritis is the most common. This condition in particular must always be considered as a very likely cause of hematuria, particularly in the patient under 20 years of age.

The other principal site of origin of hematuria is any structure adjacent to the urinary tract that has a lesion and is in direct contact with part of the urinary tract, usually the bladder or a ureter. Examples of this would include diverticulitis, salpingitis, and colonic carcinoma. Such lesions, because of their proximity and direct contact with the bladder or ureter, can be responsible for hematuria.

The vast majority of patients with hematuria, however, have a urologic lesion within the genitourinary tract itself, and this includes the kidney, (glomerulonephritidies may logically be included in this group), ureter, bladder, prostate gland, and urethra. Lesions in other portions of the genitourinary tract, such as the seminal vesicle and the testes are virtually never a source of hematuria.

HISTORY AND INTERPRETATION

It is of great importance to ascertain if hematuria is initial, total, or terminal. When taking a history this differentiation is significant only for gross hematuria; however, the serendipitous finding of microscopic hematuria on routine examination can be analyzed in the same context by means of a three-glass urine collection (see Chapter 15). With initial, gross hematuria the blood is present either immediately before or during the initial stages of voiding, after which the urinary stream appears to clear and to return to its normal color. Such initial hematuria arises from a lesion within the penile or bulbous portions of the urethra and the flow of urine probably serves as the stimulus to start the bleeding. As the flow of urine continues, it tends to "wash clear." Lesions in those portions of the urethra that could cause initial hematuria include foreign bodies, severe inflammation, and carcinoma.

In total hematuria, blood is present in the urine throughout the entire act of voiding. The source of bleeding must be higher than the bladder neck in order for the blood to mix thoroughly with the urine prior to the onset of voiding. Examples of such lesions would be carcinoma of the bladder, ureter, or kidney, stones in the kidney or ureter, severe infection in the kidney, ureter, or bladder, and tuberculosis of the kidney.

In terminal hematuria, the urinary stream is visibly clear until the end of voiding when the last part of the urine is visibly bloody or some blood is passed from the meatus after the patient thinks that urination has ceased. The origin of the bleeding is considered to be the prostatic urethra and the bladder neck and it is probable that the contraction and "snapping shut" of the posterior urethra or bladder neck at the conclusion of voiding serves to bring about the onset of bleeding. Lesions in this region that could produce terminal hematuria include acute inflammation of the posterior urethra, carcinoma of the bladder on a long stalk that projects into the posterior urethra, and benign prostatic hyperplasia, among other conditions.

It must be stressed that the interpretation of initial, total, and terminal hematuria should serve only as a point of departure for the clinician in guiding the diagnostic thinking pattern because the rules of thumb just noted are not hard and fast. Total hematuria, for example, can occur if bleeding from a site in the posterior urethra runs back into the bladder and mixes with the urine prior to voiding. In short, it is very useful to determine the type of bleeding that has occurred, but interpretation must be done in a very guarded manner. Additionally, it is often not possible for a female patient to determine whether her bleeding has been initial, total, or terminal, and the interpretation of such history of bleeding, if offered, must therefore also proceed in a guarded manner.

In continuing with the patient's history, the presence or absence of pain accompanying gross or microscopic hematuria should be determined. Pain may be present during the act of voiding or it may be seemingly unrelated, but it must always be noted. Pain over the costovertebral angle may be associated with a renal calculus, tumor, or infection. Pain along the course of the ureter, posteriorly or anteriorly, is most often associated with passage of a ureteral stone. Pain occurring during the act of voiding is the most common finding with acute bladder infection. The presence or absence of other urinary tract symptoms should be determined. The existence of bladder outlet obstruction, for example, would lead the clinician towards a diagnosis of benign prostatic hyperplasia as the source of the bleeding. The absence of all symptoms except hematuria should lead the clinician to suspect the presence of a possible bladder carcinoma.

The presence of associated symptoms such as fever, chills, malaise, nausea, or vomiting should alert the physician to the possibility of an infectious process such as acute pyelonephritis.

PHYSICAL EXAMINATION

Physical examination of the patient with gross or microscopic hematuria is usually remarkable because of the absence of abnormal physical findings. Nevertheless, certain procedures are indicated because, if positive, they may provide an insight into the cause of the bleeding. Abdominal and flank palpation should be carried out to determine if the kidneys are palpable. Normally, it is not possible to palpate either kidney unless the patient is extraordinarily thin or the kidney is extremely mobile. Palpation of the lower pole of the kidney should usually suggest the possibility of an abnormally large kidney, possibly with renal tumor or hydronephrosis. Percussion of the costovertebral angle should be performed to ascertain if there is an inordinate or unusual tenderness in this area that might suggest edema of the renal parenchyma or dilatation of the renal collecting system against a fairly rigid renal capsule. This is a reasonably constant finding with acute pyelonephritis or with an obstructed kidney secondary, for example, to an obstructing stone in the ureter. The suprapubic region should be palpated superficially and deeply for any evidence of a suprapubic mass or tenderness. An unexpected finding of bladder distension may suggest a diagnosis of benign prostatic hyperplasia as the direct cause of bladder distention and hematuria. Suprapubic tenderness to deep palpation may be found in cases of acute bladder infection. Rectal examination should always be carried out. An enlarged prostate gland might suggest benign prostatic hyperplasia as a likely source of hematuria and the classic finding of a rock-hard prostate gland from carcinoma is also a condition to which one could conceivably ascribe hematuria. The corpus spongiosum and the urethra should be palpated carefully for any evidence of a urethral mass that could suggest a diagnosis of urethral carcinoma or urethral diverticulum with calculus or infection. In females, the urethra should be palpated vaginally to search for these conditions also.

GENERALITIES ABOUT THE CAUSES OF HEMATURIA

Although it is always risky to indulge in broad generalities, certain statements regarding hematuria may be helpful to the clinician in choosing the most appropriate initial diagnostic steps after formulating a very provisional differential diagnosis.

Based on signs and symptoms alone, an adult with gross hematuria and no other genitourinary tract symptoms *probably* has a bladder tumor; an adult with gross hematuria and a vague sense of flank discomfort or a vague feeling of flank mass *probably* has a kidney tumor; an adult with very scanty bleeding, or microscopic hematuria, and severe pain in the flank or anterior or lower abdomen is *probably* passing a stone.

Broad generalities regarding hematuria that are based on the age of the patient serve as another information base that may aid the clinician. In neonates (see Chapter 5), bleeding tendencies, congenital problems leading to sepsis such as ureteral pelvic juncture obstructions, and renal vein thrombosis or renal artery embolization are the most identifiable common causes of gross hematuria, and it must be remembered that gross hematuria is idiopathic about one third of the time and overall it is very uncommon in neonates. Gross hematuria is rarely seen in children but when it or microscopic hematuria does occur, the most common cause is acute poststreptococcal glomerulonephritis and the principal differential diagnosis must include porphyria, bleeding tendencies, and infection in the urinary tract. Appropriate diagnostic studies for glomerulonephritis should be undertaken before any urologic procedures such as cystoscopy or excretory urography are contemplated. A urologic lesion (as opposed to an intrinsic renal lesion such as glomerulonephritis) is a relatively rare source of hematuria in children, and when it is found it is usually due to infection secondary to obstruction, which more often than not is congenital in etiology. For example, ureteropelvic junction can obstruct the outflow tract of the kidney, leading to stasis, infection, and ultimately to hematuria. Pyelonephritis and cystitis must also be considered very uncommon causes of hematuria in children. Tumors are even more uncommon as the cause of hematuria, and even Wilms tumor, the most common of childhood tumors, is only very rarely responsible for hematuria. Meatitis, a relatively common finding in circumcised infants and young boys, may often cause a small amount of blood to be seen on diapers or underwear and it may be diagnosed visually.

In patients up to age 40 gross hematuria is most often due to infection in some part of the genitourinary tract, and there will usually be accompanying symptoms. After age 40, in men and women, bladder tumors are the most common cause of hematuria, followed by calculi and inflammation. After age 60, prostatic lesions (BPH) and bladder tumors in men and inflammation and bladder tumors in women are the most common causes of hematuria.

The diagnostic workup of patients with gross hematuria should begin as soon as possible after the first episode in men or boys and probably in women and girls (see Chapter 5 regarding girls with infection) as well except in those cases (in adult females) where bacterial cystitis has been documented and it is presumed that a bacterial hemorrhagic cystitis has been causative of the hematuria. Even with such documentation, the author feels that the second bout of hemorrhagic cystitis in adult females warrants a full investigation to be certain, for example, that a necrotic tumor that has become infected is not the underlying source for both the hematuria and the infection. Diagnostic methodology for boys with hematuria includes inspection for meatitis, appropriate medical workup for glomerulonephritis and porphyria, and a blood profile to determine predisposition to bleeding. If all studies are negative, then a complete urologic workup, including excretory urograms and cystoscopy, should be undertaken.

Diagnostic workup for any individual with hematuria should consist of several urinalyses to check for red blood cells in the sediment and to be certain about the existence of hematuria. A careful search (of the urine sediment) should again be carried out more than once for red blood cell casts, which may indicate that the patient has glomerulonephritis. A high-dose or drip infusion urogram with voiding films should be done to visualize the kidneys, ureters, bladder, and urethra so that the clinician can check for inflammation, neoplasm, foreign body, tuberculosis, congenital lesions, or trauma. Cystoscopy of the bladder and the entire urethra should be carried out following the infusion urogram to complete the examination of the genitourinary tract because lesions in the bladder or urethra cannot always be detected by urograms alone. Additional diagnostic modalities that are helpful and may be indicated in workup of the patient with hematuria (see Chapter 1) are urinary cytology, nephrotomography, retrograde ureteropyelography, ureteroscopy and ureterorenoscopy, selective renal angiography, ultrasonography, CT scanning, and sometimes even surgical exploration, biopsy, or both.

As a rough guideline to the clinician regarding the likely sources of gross hematuria, in one series of 6000 cases of gross hematuria the kidney was the source in 42.7 percent of the cases, the bladder in 29.6 percent, the prostate in 14.1 percent, the ureter in 8.7 percent, and the urethra in 4.6 percent. Inflammation, neoplasia, and foreign bodies in that order are the three most common disease processes causing gross hematuria and together account for over 80 percent of all cases.

In the author's university, when 110 consecutive patients admitted to the hospital with a chief complaint of gross hematuria were thoroughly examined, fully one fourth were found to have a malignancy in the genitourinary tract. Infection (inflammation), however, was the most common etiologic category for the hematuria.

ASYMPTOMATIC MICROSCOPIC HEMATURIA

As noted at the beginning of this chapter, microscopic hematuria differs from gross hematuria only in a quantitative sense, and it may be the harbinger of disease that is every bit as serious as that heralded by gross hematuria. The individual with completely asymptomatic microscopic hematuria, detected perhaps on routine physical examination, frequently poses a dilemma for the clinician because the patient is extremely reluctant to undergo any tests to determine a condition that is neither visible nor causing any discomfort. In an effort to determine the significance of asymptomatic microscopic hematuria, two large series were reviewed. One reported on 200 consecutive patients with asymptomatic microscopic hematuria and the second had 100 similar patients, and the conclusions reached from both studies was that 20 percent of the patients with asymptomatic microscopic hematuria had highly "significant" lesions and 65 percent of those with "highly significant" lesions actually had cancer of the genitourinary tract. Presented in another way, 13 percent of the 200 patients with totally asymptomatic microscopic hematuria were found to have cancer in the genitourinary tract. Another 64 patients (32 percent of the total number of patients) were found to have a "moderately significant lesion," such as a stone obstructing a ureter or a stone in the renal pelvis. "Insignificant lesions" (such as trigonitis or urethritis) were found in about half of the patients studied. It is significant to note that renal biopsies were not done in this study although it is recognized that, undoubtedly, subclinical and chronic glomerulonephritis would have been found to be the etiology for the hematuria in at least some of the patients. Another very important finding was that there is no relationship whatsoever between the grade (degree) of the microscopic hematuria and the severity of the lesion found.

Given the above, it is obvious that asymptomatic microscopic hematuria must absolutely never be ignored and it must be diligently pursued until a diagnosis is made.

CHECKLIST OF CAUSES OF MICROSCOPIC AND GROSS HEMATURIA

It is fundamental to the making of a diagnosis in clinical medicine that an entity cannot be diagnosed if it is not first considered. For this reason, a list of some of the more and some of the less common causes of hematuria is included here, grouped by the source of the hematuria, so that the clinician may be aware of the very large number of conditions that can and do produce hematuria.

1. Kidney: transitional cell carcinoma of the collecting system, renal cell carcinoma, Wilms' tumor, sarcoma, acute and chronic glomerulonephritis or one of the other nephritides, acute or chronic pyelonephritis, tuberculosis, sickle cell disease (almost always limited to blacks), calculus disease, arteriovenous malformations or other vascular anomalies, renal vein thrombosis, renal arterial thrombosis, or embolism.
2. Ureter: transitional cell carcinoma, ureteritis, tuberculosis, and calculus disease.
3. Bladder: transitional cell carcinoma, squamous cell carcinoma, adenocarcinoma, calculus disease, acute and chronic cystitis, interstitial cystitis, schistosomiasis, alkaline encrusted cystitis, trigonitis, tuberculosis, foreign bodies, and diverticulum with carcinoma or stone.
4. Prostate: benign prostatic hyperplasia and carcinoma.
5. Urethra: urethritis in females, posterior urethritis in males, foreign bodies, diverticulum and inflammation, carcinoma or stone, tuberculosis, transitional cell carcinoma, and squamous cell carcinoma.

It is to be emphasized strongly that the above list is not intended to be all inclusive but to merely serve as a guide for the clinician.

REFERENCES

Carson CC III, Segura JW, Green LF: Clinical importance of microhematuria. JAMA 241:149, 1979

Carter WC III, Rous SN: Etiology of gross hematuria in 110 consecutive adult urology hospital admissions. Urology 18:342, 1981

Rous SN: Urology in Primary Care. St. Louis, Mosby, 1976

17
Educational Objectives for Undergraduate Urology: Self-Assessment and Evaluation

No matter how well an author knows and presents his material, a textbook must be considered a failure if the reader has not increased his or her fund of knowledge as a direct result of having read it.

Listed below, and at the beginning of each chapter as well, are the educational objectives for urology mentioned in some detail in the introduction of this book as being "necessary" for every graduating medical student. Following this listing of the educational objectives, self-assessment exercises are offered so that the reader may evaluate his or her grasp of the material covered in this text. If the reader is able to accomplish all of the responses sought in the exercises, and in all instances these responses and the accompanying thought processes should be compared with those outlined in the appropriate chapters of the book, he or she may feel with some certainty that sufficient knowledge has been acquired to understand the various urologic disease entities, the diagnosis of these entities, and their therapy. The prudent physician, however, will always seek expert urologic consultation to assist in the management of certain clinical situations in which he or she is not absolutely certain of his or her own ability to manage specific problems in the best possible manner for the patient.

EDUCATIONAL OBJECTIVES

In order for the graduating medical student to have a firm understanding of those urologic conditions deemed "necessary" (see Introduction), he or she must be able to accomplish the following:

1. List the various symptoms that a patient might have in connection with the following kidney diseases: infection or inflammation, stones, kidney cancer.
2. Explain specifically why each of the symptoms just listed occurs.
3. List the symptoms that a patient might have in connection with infection or inflammation of the bladder.

313

4. Explain why each of the symptoms just listed occurs.
5. Examine a penis and scrotum (and contents) for normalcy.
6. List the symptoms that a patient might have in connection with the following diseases of the prostate: benign enlargement, acute infection, chronic infection.
7. Explain why each of the symptoms just listed occurs.
8. Discuss the procedure to be used in attempting to palpate the kidney.
9. Explain the procedure to be followed in doing a digital rectal examination of the prostate.
10. List the specific things to be looked for in doing a digital rectal examination of the prostate.
11. Explain the significance of the bulbocavernosus reflex.
12. List the indications for an excretory urogram.
13. Recognize and identify a normal excretory urogram.
14. Explain the significance of a unilateral delay in visualization on the nephrogram phase of the excretory urogram.
15. List the indications for cystoscopy.
16. List the indications for bladder catheterization.
17. Pass a catheter into the bladder atraumatically.
18. List the indications for radioisotope studies of the kidneys (renal scanning).
19. List the indications for CT scanning of the kidneys.
20. List the indications for ultrasonography in urology.
21. List the indications for renal angiography.
22. Describe the two basic functions of the detrusor (bladder).
23. List, in broad terms, the innervation of the detrusor.
24. Discuss the location and the specific type of muscle found in each of the two urinary sphincters.
25. List the available tests that are used to quantitate voiding (urodynamics).
26. Explain and give an example to illustrate the statement that voiding dysfunction may be a result of disease processes originating outside of the urinary tract.
27. Estimate the level of anxiety of a patient over procedures involving manipulation of the genitalia.
28. Discuss the significance and the management of asymptomatic bacteriuria.
29. Discuss the management of acute pyelonephritis in a man and in a woman.
30. Discuss the management and therapy of chronic or recurrent pyelonephritis in a man and in a woman.
31. List the symptoms and the physical (including any urine test) findings of acute pylonephritis.
32. List the symptoms and physical (including urine test) findings of chronic pyelonephritis.
33. List the diagnostic tests needed to make a diagnosis of renal tuberculosis.
34. List the symptoms of renal tuberculosis.
35. List the symptoms of acute cystitis.
36. Discuss the management of postcoital cystitis in a young woman.
37. Discuss the pathogenesis of acute cystitis in males and females.

38. Describe the management of acute cystitis in males and females.
39. Describe what is meant by "bacterial adherence" in terms of lower urinary tract infections in women and girls.
40. Discuss the rationale of collecting urine from a man sequentially in three glasses to localize the source of infection.
41. List the antimicrobials effective against the most common organisms that cause cystitis.
42. List the symptoms of acute prostatitis.
43. Discuss the management of acute prostatitis.
44. Discuss the use of prostatic massage in the management of chronic bacterial prostatitis and prostatostasis.
45. Discuss the causes of acute prostatitis.
46. List the symptoms of chronic bacterial prostatitis and prostatostasis.
47. List the symptoms of posterior urethritis.
48. Explain, on an anatomic basis, why the symptoms of prostatitis and posterior urethritis may be so similar.
49. Describe how to "strip" a prostate gland to obtain prostatic secretions for microscopic and bacteriologic studies.
50. Describe the differential diagnosis between chronic bacterial prostatitis, chronic nonbacterial prostatitis (prostatostasis), and prostatodynia.
51. List the methods used in the treatment of acute epididymitis.
52. List and discuss the theories of etiology of pyelonephritis.
53. List the symptoms and the causes of epididymitis.
54. Explain how the infecting organism in epididymitis varies with the age of the patient.
55. List the methods used in the treatment of orchitis.
56. Describe the palpatory findings used to differentiate epididymitis from orchitis.
57. Obtain and examine a smear from a urethral discharge to find pus and bacteria.
58. List the symptoms and findings and common urologic causes of gram-negative sepsis and gram-negative shock.
59. Describe the management of patients in gram-negative shock.
60. List the criteria for making the diagnosis of gram-negative sepsis (shock).
61. List the common and preferred antmicrobials against *Escherichia coli.*
62. List the common and preferred antimicrobials against coagulase-negative staphylococci.
63. List the common and preferred antimicrobials against *Proteus.*
64. List the common and preferred antimicrobials against *Pseudomonas.*
65. List the common and preferred antimicrobials against *Enterococcus.*
66. Describe the "big bang" theory and explain the impact of this theory on the treatment of vesicoureteral reflux.
67. List the causes of enuresis.
68. Discuss the role of urodynamic studies in evaluating the enuretic child.
69. Discuss the management of functional enuresis.
70. Discuss the management of acute pyelonephritis in a girl and in a boy.
71. Discuss the management and therapy of chronic or recurrent pyelonephritis in a girl and in a boy.
72. Discuss the etiology of acute glomerulonephritis.

73. List the clinical symptoms occurring with acute glomerulonephritis.
74. List the physical and laboratory (urine and blood) findings of acute glomerulonephritis.
75. List the methods used in making a diagnosis of acute glomerulonephritis.
76. Discuss the short- and long-term management of acute glomerulonephritis.
77. Discuss the common causes of cystitis in little girls.
78. Describe the management of cystitis in little girls.
79. List the clinical symptoms associated with Wilms tumor.
80. List the most common causes of hematuria in children for the following age groups: neonates (first month of life); infants (1 month to 1 year of age); children (1 to 16 years of age).
81. Discuss the pros and cons of neonatal circumcision.
82. List the most common causes of abdominal masses in infants and children.
83. Describe what is meant by "a dysfunctional voider."
84. List the clinical symptoms associated with hypernephroma.
85. List the symptoms of bladder cancer.
86. List a differential diagnosis for hard areas of the prostate gland as noted on rectal palpation.
87. List the symptoms of early carcinoma of the prostate gland.
88. List the causes of scrotal mass.
89. Discuss the management and prognosis of hypernephroma.
90. Discuss the relationship of estrogen and testosterone in carcinoma of the prostate gland.
91. List the late symptoms of carcinoma of the prostate gland.
92. Discuss the hormonal treatment of carcinoma of the prostate gland.
93. Palpate a significantly enlarged lower pole of a kidney.
94. Palpate a prostate gland that has hard nodular areas suggestive of carcinoma and identify it as such.
95. Palpate a prostate gland that is diffusely hard, as in carcinoma, and identify it as such.
96. Describe the diagnosis and management of carcinoma of the bladder.
97. List the symptoms of carcinoma of the testis.
98. Describe the diagnosis and management of carcinoma of the testis.
99. Discuss with a patient and his family the implications of surgery for carcinoma of the prostate gland necessitating orchiectomy and treatment with Stilbestrol.
100. List the symptoms associated with benign prostatic hyperplasia.
101. Discuss the reasons why hesitancy, frequency, nocturia, intermittency, hematuria, urgency, and foul-smelling urine may occur in benign prostatic hyperplasia.
101a Discuss the anatomic relationship and the pathophysiology of BPH.
101b List the indications for the surgical treatment of BPH.
102. Discuss the causes of stones in the bladder.
103. Discuss with a patient and his family the implications of surgery for prostatic hyperplasia and subsequent complications.
104. Determine if a patient is delirious postoperatively.
105. Discuss the management of a patient who is delirious postoperatively.
106. List the most common metabolic causes of renal stone formation.
107. Discuss the relationship of obstruction and infection to stone formation.
108. List the common types of urinary tract stones.

109. Discuss the medical management of recurrent stone formation for calcium oxalate stones, calcium phosphate stones, and uric acid stones.
110. Discuss the management of the patient with a 5-mm stone in the ureter.
111. Discuss the management of the patient with a 1.5-cm stone in the ureter.
112. List the indications for surgical intervention when there is a stone (1) in the kidney; and (2) in the ureter.
113. List the symptoms of stones in the bladder.
114. List the steps to be taken in determining the etiology of stone formation in the patient with recurrent urolithiasis.
115. Discuss the mechanism by which a narrowed renal artery may produce hypertension.
116. Discuss the actions of cortisol.
117. Discuss the steps taken to determine if hypertension is of adrenal origin.
118. Describe the mechanism of action of aldosterone.
119. List the symptoms associated with failure of the adrenal cortex.
120. Discuss the relationship of the adrenal glands to hypertension.
121. List the symptoms of pheochromocytoma.
122. State the anatomic and pathologic differences between intraperitoneal and extraperitoneal bladder rupture.
123. Discuss the diagnosis and the management of blunt and of penetrating trauma to the kidney.
124. List the indications for excretory urography and for renal angiography in blunt and in penetrating renal trauma.
125. Discuss the symptoms, the diagnosis, and the management of trauma to the urethra and to the bladder.
126. Discuss the diagnosis and the treatment of torsion of the spermatic cord.
127. Discuss the differential diagnosis of torsion of the spermatic cord and acute epididymitis and epididymoorchitis.
128. List the symptoms of torsion of the spermatic cord.
129. Discuss the causes and the treatment of hydrocele.
130. Describe the findings and management of torsion of the appendix testis and the appendix epididymis.
131. Palpate a scrotal mass and correctly identify: a hematocele, a hydrocele, a spermatocele, epididymitis, epididymoorchitis, torsion of the spermatic cord, testis carcinoma, and inguinoscrotal hernia.
131a List the early symptoms, physical findings, and differential diagnosis of testis cancer.
132. Define phimosis and paraphimosis.
133. Define balanitis and balanoposthitis.
134. Recognize and identify balanitis and balanoposthitis.
135. Recognize and identify phimosis and paraphimosis.
136. Recognize and identify the following: primary chancre, chancroid, lymphogranuloma venereum, granuloma inguinale, and herpes progenitalis.
137. Discuss the differential diagnosis of genital ulcers in the male.
138. Differentiate between the cutaneous lesions of primary syphilis and herpes progenitalis.
139. List the symptoms of herpes progenitalis.
140. Recognize and identify verrucal warts (condyloma accuminatum) of the penis and of the distal urethra.
141. Recognize and identify sebaceous cysts of the skin of the genitalia.

142. List the most common kidney diseases that result in end-stage renal failure.
143. Discuss the approximate 1- and 2-year survival rates for patients on hemodialysis and postrenal transplantation.
144. List the indications for vasectomy.
145. Discuss the comparative advantages of vasectomy and all other forms of birth control.
146. Define erectile dysfunction.
147. Discuss the evaluation and management of the patient with erectile dysfunction.
148. Examine and identify for viability the spermatozoa in a semen specimen.
149. Determine whether a patient understands nomenclature such as penis, urethra, testes, or labia or whether less clinical terms need to be used.
150. Instruct a man in the use of a condom.
151. Obtain a history of sexual activity from a man and a woman without being offensive or using language that cannot be understood.
152. Advise parents of 3- , 9- , and 15-year-old boys or girls about masturbation.
153. Define infertility.
154. Discuss the evaluation and management of the male patient with infertility.
155. List the causes of polyuria, oliguria, and anuria.
156. Identify and recognize squamous epithelial cells in the urine sediment.
157. List the causes for abnormal proteinuria.
158. List the causes for glucose in the urine.
159. List the cellular elements present in urine.
160. Identify and recognize the following elements in the urine sediment: white blood cells, red blood cells, white blood cell casts, red blood cell casts, hyaline casts, and granular casts.
161. Identify and recognize artifacts in urine sediment.
162. Obtain and examine clean-catch midstream urine specimens from men and women.
163. Discuss the relationship of the serum creatinine and BUN levels to renal function, urine flow rate, and nonrenal factors affecting plasma concentrations.
164. Discuss the methodology of obtaining a 24-hour urine specimen.
165. Calculate creatinine clearance.
166. Define specific gravity and relate it to a clinical situation.
167. List the causes of gross and microscopic hematuria.
168. Describe the workup and management of a patient with gross or microscopic hematuria.
169. List the most likely etiologies for hematuria in males and females under age 40 and over age 40.
170. List the most likely etiologies for hematuria in the neonate, in infants, and in children.
171. List the specific diagnostic studies that can be used to determine the etiology of microscopic or gross hematuria.

EXERCISE NO. 1

You are an internist in a large urban medical center. On Tuesday morning, June 27, your nurse gives you the following information sheet about your next scheduled patient.

Patient status:	First visit
Name:	Sarah Heiman (Mrs.)
Age:	23
Address:	16271 Fairfield Street
Phone:	671-2254
Occupation:	Chemist
Place of employment:	Petromac Chemical Corp. *Phone:* 421-6178
Spouse:	Israel Heiman
Occupation:	Seminary student *Phone:* 671-4590
Insurance:	Blue Shield
Present complaint:	Dysuria, urgency, and frequency of urination

- *What are five possible diagnoses that could account for the symptoms Mrs. Heiman has?*
- *For each possible diagnosis, what are two or three questions you would ask while taking the history? What diagnostic laboratory procedures would you use to rule out or confirm each possibility?*

Mrs. Heiman tells you that she has experienced increasing frequency and urgency of urination, which began about 4 days ago. Usually, she only goes to the bathroom once or twice during the day, but lately it seems she is always in the bathroom. About 2 days ago urination began to be painful, and she noticed that, even though she felt the need to urinate, very little volume was produced. Last night the pain became more severe, and this morning she noticed some blood in the toilet bowl and some on the toilet paper when she wiped herself.

When she first experienced discomfort, she says, it was like the pressure of a full bladder. In the last 2 days, this pressure has become an almost constant throb that increases in intensity when she finishes urinating. There is also some burning around the urethra during urination.

Mrs. Heiman also tells you that she was married 6 weeks ago and that she sometimes notices vaginal soreness after intercourse. She had had no previous sexual experience and thought perhaps the soreness derived because intercourse is somewhat new to her. She has not used any douches or medications for vaginal discomfort. She does not remember if she usually voids after intercourse. She customarily wipes herself from front to back after bowel movements.

Mrs. Heiman's family history is noncontributory. She states there is no family history of diabetes, tuberculosis, or known drug allergies.

The results of the physical examination are unremarkable. All vital signs are normal, as is the examination of the head and neck, ears, lungs, breasts, and abdomen. There is a very definite suprapubic tenderness to deep palpation but no evidence of any bladder distention on percussion in the suprapubic area.

Laboratory test results were as follows:

CBC

HGB: 12 g/100 ml
PCV: 40 vol%
RBC: 5.1 million/mm³
WBC: 9000/mm³
Diff: Stabs 3%, segs 59%, lymphs 33%, monos 5%

Urinalysis (Clean-catch midstream sample)

Color: Dark yellow
pH: 6
Spec. grav.: 1.029
RBC: 60-80 per high-power field
WBC: 40-50 per high-power field
Casts: None

Remainder of urine specimen before centrifugation was sent to the laboratory for culture and sensitivity studies.

- *What is the differential diagnosis for Mrs. Heiman? What plan of management would you develop?*

In view of Mrs. Heiman's past and present history, you have decided the most likely diagnosis is acute (probagly postcoital) cystitis and give her sulfisoxazole (Gantrisin), 2 g stat. and 1 g q.i.d.

When you speak to Mrs. Heiman 48 hours later, she states that virtually all her symptoms are gone. The urine culture report is back and shows a growth greater than 100,000 colonies/ml of *Escherichia coli,* and the organism is sensitive to sulfa. Two weeks later, a follow-up urine culture is sterile, and she is entirely asymptomatic. She has been taking the sulfa therapy for 10 days.

- *What would you tell Mrs. Heiman at the time of the follow-up visit about the cause and management of postcoital cystitis? Try to anticipate the questions she would ask, and give your answers in vocabulary that would clearly communicate your ideas to Mrs. Heiman.*
- *Cystitis occasionally presents other clinical problems than those of Mrs. Heiman. What would your management have included had the following clinical situations occurred?*
  1. *The urine culture was negative.*
  2. *Symptoms persisted after 2 to 3 days of sulfa (Gantrisin) therapy.*
  3. *The organism cultured was not sensitive to sulfa.*
  4. *All symptoms returned in a few weeks.*

Author's comment. A proper understanding of this case is greatly facilitated if the clinician understands the relationship between sexual intercourse and lower urinary tract infection in women. The cause of the infection must be considered, as well as the rationale of voiding before and after intercourse. The rationale of frequent voiding (every 2 hours) should also be understood as a means of preventing recurrent lower urinary tract infections. Finally, it is incumbent on the clinician when confronted with a patient with a history of lower urinary tract infection to be absolutely certain that the cause is not a focus of infection within the upper urinary tract that is periodically seeding the bacteria into the bladder. See Chapter 2 for answers to this exercise.

EXERCISE NO. 2

It is Tuesday, March 3, and you are relaxing at home after a moderately busy day. You are a family physician in a small town of about 5000 in central Minnesota. There is a 100-bed hospital in the town, with an emergency facility. At about 10:30 PM you get a call from Susan Jenson. Susan is 27, married, and has two children. She and her family have been your patients for 3 years. Susan is calling you because she has acute pain in her belly. You quickly rummage through your brain for relevant information. To your knowledge neither Susan nor her family have any prior history of abdominal or stomach problems, and she made no mention of pregnancy on her last visit 2½ months ago when she had a sore throat.

- *What questions would you ask Susan at this time (no more than 10)?*

Susan tells you over the phone that the pain is really terrible—like labor pains without any relief. The pain began about ½ hour ago without any prior symptoms and is located in the lower right part of her abdomen. She has had no fever, nausea, or vomiting. You ask her to meet you in the emergency room at the hospital. While driving to the hospital you think about the information you have.

- *What are the three most likely diagnoses that would explain Susan's problems?*

When you see Susan at the hospital, she is obviously in acute distress and is not able to lie still because the pain is so severe. She denies any prior history of similar pain. She specifically points to the right lower quadrant of her abdomen as the focus of most of her discomfort, but adds that there is some mild discomfort in the region of her labia majora, and she thinks there is some discomfort in her back in the region of the right costovertebral angle, although this is minimal. She repeats that the pain came on suddenly. Susan tells you that she took two aspirins shortly after the pain began, but has had no relief. She has tried to find a body position that relieves the distress, but nothing seems to help. Neither the quality nor the location of the pain have changed significantly since it began. You ask Susan about frequency of urination since the pain started. She responds that she frequently feels as if she has to urinate, but almost nothing comes out. She adds that she noticed a tiny bit of dark urine several hours ago before the pain started.

- *In the light of this new information, what other possible diagnoses are there? What cues suggest them? Why are diagnoses you have ruled out, if any, no longer appropriate?*
- *What physical examination procedures and laboratory tests will you do in order to evaluate possible diagnoses? Remember that you are in the emergency room and be careful to focus on the patient's immediate problems.*

Physical examination reveals the following findings:

Weight:	127 lb	*Respiration:*	20 breaths/min
Height:	5′ 4½″	*Temperature:*	99 F
Blood pressure:	120/80 mmHg		

On physical examination of the abdomen, there is definite and severe tenderness over the right lower quadrant. The abdomen shows no guarding or rigidity. There is no rebound tenderness. There is minimal tenderness to percussion over the right costovertebral angle (CVA).

Auscultation of the heart and lungs reveals no abnormality. There is no joint or back pain except over the right CVA. Breast examination reveals no abnormalities. Pelvic examination is not remarkable except that tenderness is noted again on the right side of the abdomen.

- *Before proceeding, answer the following questions relevant to data learned from history and physical examination:*
  1. *What would be a reasonable differential diagnosis of this patient's abdominal right lower quadrant pain?*
  2. *Why do you think this patient experienced frequency and urgency of urination?*

By the time you complete the physical examination the following data are available:

CBC

HGB: 14.2 g/100 ml
PCV: 45 vol%
RBC: 5.0 × 10⁶/mm³
Diff: Stabs 3%, segs 60%, lymphs 30%, monos 7%

Urinalysis

Color: Dark brownish yellow
pH: 6
Spec. grav.: 1.020
RBC: 20-30 per high-power field
WBC: 5-10 per high-power field

- *What are the likeliest reasons for the red blood cells in the urine? What other condition(s) in the differential diagnosis could produce the microscopic hematuria?*
- *A differential diagnosis of abdominal right lower quadrant pain could include apprendicitis or tubal pregnancy. Why are these unlikely in this patient?*
- *Would you order an excretory urogram at this time? If your answer is no, why not? If your answer is yes, why and what would you expect to learn from it?*

Your orders for Susan include the following:

General

Bedrest with bathroom privileges (BRP)
Forced-fluid diet

Dx. Excretory urogram

Rx. Meperidine (Demerol) 50 to 100 mg q4h p.r.n.

Wednesday afternoon you get the abdominal x-ray film and the results of the excretory urogram, which shows a normal left kidney and ureter and a 5-mm stone in the lower third of the right ureter, which is producing a minimal delay in function of the kidney and a minimal dilation above the stone.

- *What is your diagnosis now? How would you manage the 5-mm stone revealed by the excretory urogram?*
- *Give three alternative plans of management that might be appropriate. What are the assets, drawbacks, and probable results of each alternative listed?*

You continue to hydrate Susan with the forcing of fluids orally. In 2 days the stone is spontaneously passed.

- *What measures would you recommend to Susan to reduce the likelihood of recurrence of this problem?*

- *On Friday, March 6, Susan is discharged from the hospital. Write a discharge summary for Susan.*

Author's comment. The key to this case is the clinician's including ureteral calculus disease in the differential diagnosis of right lower quadrant pain, particularly when this pain is accompanied by some frequency and urgency. The clinician should also be able to state why diagnoses such as appendicitis and tubal pregnancy are not as likely as stones (because a true surgical abdomen was not present). Of particular importance in any case where the diagnosis is in question is the obtaining of urologic x-ray films, and the clinician must be fully aware that a KUB (flat plate) is absolutely not sufficient to confirm or rule out a ureteral calculus; excretory urography must be done. See Chapter 8 for answers to this exercise.

EXERCISE NO. 3

You are a physician in a private practice of internal medicine.

Today you are seeing Joe Mallory for his annual physical examination. He has neither seen nor consulted you since his last physical examination 14 months ago. Mr. Mallory is 63 years old. He owns an auto repair shop and lives in a middle-class suburban community with his wife; his two daughters are married. The most significant event he can think of in the last year is the birth of a grandson.

Mr. Mallory says that he is in excellent health. Review of systems is unremarkable. However, Mr. Mallory tells you that for the past 7 years he has been awakened once or twice a night with a desire to urinate. You quickly note that no mention was made of this during his last physical examination.

- *What diagnostic possibilities (no more than 5) might you consider at this point. Be sure to include those conditions that are not strictly urologic?*
- *What questions (no more than 10) would you ask to further clarify Mr. Mallory's complaint?*

On further questioning, Mr. Mallory tells you that for about the past year he has noticed that it takes him a little bit longer to start his urine stream. Additionally, he says that his stream will sometimes stop in the middle and then start again. He tells you that sometimes he feels he empties his bladder, but at other times he is not so sure about this, although in general he thinks he empties his bladder well. About 6 months ago, he had to urinate about every 30 minutes for a day and a half and, when he had the urge, he had to go right then or else he feared he might wet himself. He also noticed at that particular time that his urine had a foul smell. He said that all of these acute symptoms cleared up in a couple of days after he got some pills from his druggist. He does not remember the name of the pills. Mr. Mallory tells you that for the most part he is not too unhappy with his voiding, but as long as you have been asking him these questions he is answering them as best he can.

- *With this new data, revise your possible diagnoses. Explain why those possibilities you add or carry over seem likely, using the new information from the history. For those possibilities you have now dropped, explain why they no longer seem likely.*
- *What would be the focus of your physical examination, and what would you expect to find?*

Physical examination discloses a questionable suprapubic mass; the penis and testes appear to be within normal limits. On rectal examination the bulbocavernosus reflex is positive, and the rectal mucosa feels normal. The prostate gland appears only very slightly enlarged, if at all, and you would probably grade it as − 1. One small area in the right lobe of the prostate gland, towards the apex, is somewhat harder and almost nodular, and you estimate it to be about ½ cm in diameter. All other physical findings are within normal limits.

- *What laboratory tests would you order at this time?*

You explain to Mr. Mallory that his prostate gland appears to be enlarged and that you would like to see him again in a couple of days when the results are back from the lab. An appointment is set up for 2 days later.

- *For the following symptoms and signs, what is the pathophysiology of nos. 1 and 2 and the pathology and pathologic anatomy suggested in nos. 3 and 4?*
    1. *Hesitancy, intermittency, nocturia*
    2. *Frequency, urgency, foul-smelling urine*
    3. *Near-normal size of prostate gland as determined by palpation rectally*
    4. *Palpation of suprapubic mass*

When Mr. Mallory returns to your office, you have the following test results available.

CBC

HBG: 16.2 g/100 ml
PCV: 47 vol%
RBC: 5.9 million/mm³
WBC: 7000/mm³
Diff: Stabs 4%, segs 57%, lymphs 30%, monos 7%, eos 2%

Urinalysis

Color: Deep yellow
pH: 5.6
Spec. grav.: 1.017
WBC: 0-2 per high-power field
RBC: 2-4 per high-power field
BUN: 22 mg/100 ml (N = 6 − 23 mg/100 ml)
Creatinine: 1.3 mg/100 ml (N = 1 − 2 mg/100 ml)

You explain to Mr. Mallory that your findings and his history are consistent with benign prostatic hyperplasia. He asks you what that means. How would you explain in words he can understand?

- *How would you explain this in layman's language?*
- *What would you do now?*

It is appropriate at this point to schedule Mr. Mallory for an excretory urogram and refer him to a urologist for further evaluation (particularly cystoscopic) and management.

The excretory urogram shows a normal upper urinary tract and an elevation of the base of the bladder suggestive of an enlarged prostate gland.

- *With this new information, record a differential diagnosis, assessment, and plan.*

The urologist sends you reports on cystoscopic examination and biopsy.

Cystoscopic evaluation immediately after voiding discloses residual urine of 95 ml, a grade 2 bladder trabeculation, and a middle lobe enlargement of grade 2. The lateral lobes of the prostate gland do not appear significantly enlarged.

Transrectal needle biopsy of the nodular area of the prostate gland discloses a small adenoma.

- *Given these results, surgical management is indicated. Of the surgical procedures listed below, which is most appropriate in this case and what is the reason(s) for your choice?*
  Retropubic prostatectomy
  Transurethral resection
  Perineal prostatectomy
  Suprapubic prostatecomy

Mr. Mallory expresses concern about hospitalization and asks you to explain to him what the procedure involves. He also wants to know what kind of differences he will notice afterwards; if urination will be different or feel different; if it will be painful for awhile and, if so, for how long.

- *How would you answer these questions?*

After you have finished explaining the surgical procedure and results to Mr. Mallory, he says, somewhat embarrassed, "Doctor, ah, you know my wife and I still have sex sometimes. Will this operation affect that?"

- *How will you respond to his concerns?*

A transurethral prostate gland resection was successfully performed on Mr. Mallory 2 weeks later.

- *What is your prognosis for this patient?*
- *Briefly outline your plan for long-term follow-up.*

Author's comment. The key to a proper understanding of this patient management problem rests in a comprehension of the pathophysiology of benign prostate hyperplasia and therefore a comprehension of the meaning of each of the symptoms expressed by the patient. It is also important to recognize that prostatic enlargement as palpated rectally may or may not be significant, because an enlarged middle lobe of the prostate gland, which can produce severe obstructive symptoms, cannot be palpated rectally. Another key point for the clinician to observe is that the one episode of severe frequency and urgency accompanied by foul-smelling urine reported by the patient in this case almost certainly indicates a bladder infection. When this occurs in a man, it should warrant a full urologic investigation, regardless of whether any other symptoms are present. See Chapter 7 for answers to this exercise.

EXERCISE NO. 4

You are an emergency medicine resident working in the emergency room of a 200-bed general hospital. It is 4:30 PM and quiet on Tuesday, August 19. You are chatting with a fellow resident when a two-car accident is called in. The ambulance attendant on the scene states that two people were injured and will be brought in. One appears to have only cuts and bruises, the other is "pretty banged up." He is conscious and his blood pressure and pulse are good; but there is damage to the upper abdomen and left flank, with a large ecchymotic area visible in the suprapubic region. The patient cannot walk and is experiencing pain in the abdominal and pelvic regions.

- *While awaiting the arrival of the ambulance, what plans would you make to ascertain the extent of injuries to the person just described to you?*

The ambulance arrives, and your patient, David Seeley, is placed in an examination room. You observe that he is conscious and oriented as to time, person, and place. He is having no respiratory difficulty. His vital signs are as follows:

Radial, temporal, femoral, and pedal pulses: 90/min and stable
Respiration: 20 breaths/min
Blood pressure: 130/80 mmHg
Temperature: 98 F

David tells you that he is having pain in his left side and abdomen as well as in the pelvic area. Inspection confirms the presence of numerous contusions across David's upper abdomen and left flank as well as the previously reported large ecchymotic area in the suprapubic region. Palpation reveals marked suprapubic tenderness. Diffuse tenderness to palpation is noted over the entire abdomen. When asked to void, the entire urine stream is noted to be grossly bloody.

- *What are some possible causes for bloody urine that would be compatible with other findings in this patient?*
- *What diagnostic studies would you perform in order to rule out or confirm the problems listed above?*

Before you obtain a brief history from David and complete the physical examination, you order the following studies: Pelvic x-ray films, urinalysis, CBC, and blood type.

You retake David's blood pressure and find that it has remained stable. Because his pain is quite severe, you prescribe meperidine (Demerol) 100 mg by hypodermic injection.

You obtain the following information from David before sending him to the x-ray department:

Name: David Seeley
Age: 22
Address: 1452 Pine Street
Occupation: Telephone installer
Marital status: Married (wife, Judy; no children)
Height: 6'1"
Weight: 175 lb
Insurance: Blue Cross

David has no drug allergies, is currently taking no medications, and has not recently been ill or hospitalized.

As the nurse comes in to take David to the x-ray department, he asks you if anyone has called his wife; you ask the nurse at the reception desk to do so.

Results of the urinalysis confirms the earlier impression of gross hematuria. CBC is normal; blood type is O + .

Pelvic x-ray films show two fractures of the rami of the pubic bones.

- *Using this new information, what are some other possible causes for bloody urine in this patient and what further tests would you order?*

Completion of the physical examination reveals the following:

General appearance: Well-developed white male in acute distress
Head and neck: Some stiffness noted in neck; no external injuries to head or neck
Eyes: Conjunctivae normal, pupils equal and react equally to light and accommodation; funduscopy shows no abnormality
ENT: External ears unremarkable, tympanic membranes and canals normal; teeth in good repair, no injury to mouth or jaw

Chest and lungs: No respiratory difficulty; no evidence of damage to thoracic cage

Heart: Left border of cardiac dullness is 8 cm left of midsternal line in fifth intercostal space; heart sounds normal, rhythm regular, no murmurs heard

Abdomen: As noted previously

External genitalia: No external injuries, circumsized penis, testes normal in size and consistency, no sign of trauma

Rectal: No abnormalities noted

Musculoskeletal: No abnormalities except as noted earlier

Neurological: DTR's brisk and symmetrical; abdominal reflexes intact; sensation intact over abdominal, inguinal, femoral, and pudendal regions

You admit David to the hospital's urologic service and tell his wife that David may have to have surgery if further studies document damage to his genitourinary tract. You reassure her that, although David is pretty banged up, he is not in critical condition and will probably be OK. She agrees to check back with you sometime the next afternoon.

- *You should have ordered either an excretory urogram or a drip infusion urogram. In this case, what is the advantage of drip infusion urography over excretory urography?*
- *Can significant renal trauma be ruled out in this patient if the results of the urography are normal?*
- *Regardless of the results of the excretory urograms, what further diagnostic studies, if any, should be done to determine the presence of possible renal trauma? What additional information will be provided by this testing?*

The results of the infusion urogram, renal angiograms, and excretory cystogram are available shortly after admission:

Infusion urogram: Right kidney normal; left kidney shows slight delay in visualization, with no gross abnormalities seen.

Excretory cystogram: Extensive extravasation of contrast medium into the abdomen suggests intraperitoneal bladder rupture.

Renal angiogram: Severe laceration and fracture of lower pole of left kidney.

A repeat CBC done at 9:30, approximately 6 hours after David was brought in, shows a drop in hemoglobin of 3 g.

- *Given this information, write a differential diagnosis for David, with assessment and plan. If you cannot, what further information is necessary and how will you obtain it?*

A retrograde cystogram is indicated to confirm the provisional diagnoses based on the excretory cystogram. A catheter is passed into the bladder, and injection of contrast medium confirms intraperitoneal extravasation.

In this patient the bladder rupture was most likely secondary to the fractures of the pubic bone, with probable perforation of the bladder by a bony fragment.

- *What are the anatomic delineations that make a bladder rupture either intraperitoneal or extraperitoneal? What is the significance and treatment of each of these two types of bladder rupture?*
- *Briefly describe the x-ray appearance of:*
  1. *Intraperitoneal rupture*
  2. *Extraperitoneal rupture*

After consulting with you, the urologist schedules David for emergency surgery.

- *Describe briefly surgery done for:*
  1. *Repair of bladder*

2. Partial nephrectomy of lower pole of left kidney
The surgery is successfully performed, with no postoperative complications. What kind of postoperative management is appropriate for David, and what measure of full recovery would you predict? What problems might he encounter, and what can he do to avoid them?

Author's comment. The clinician must suspect renal injury anytime there is blunt or penetrating trauma involving an area anywhere near the kidney. An infusion urogram is an absolute requirement, and it is particularly important to realize that a perfectly normal urogram does not rule out renal trauma. If clinical signs or physical findings point to the possibility of renal trauma, a renal angiogram is indicated even in the presence of a normal excretory urogram. Additionally a bladder rupture will very frequently occur when there is a traumatic break of the bony pelvis. Diagnosis as to the presence or the kind of bladder rupture is dependent on a retrograde cystogram. See Chapter 10 for answers to this exercise.

EXERCISE NO. 5

You are a physician with a family practice in a suburban clinic. On February 20, George Coleman, a new patient, comes for his 3 PM appointment. The nurse has begun a chart for Mr. Coleman with the following information:

Name: George F. Coleman
Birth date: 9-4-20
Address: 14587 Farmington Road
Phone: 476-2581
Race: Negro
Occupation: Sales Executive
Education: B.A. in business
Insurance: Blue Cross/Blue Shield
Marital status: Married 1946
Wife's name: Opel J. Coleman
Birth date: 1936
Race: Negro
Occupation: Housewife
Education: 2 years of college
Children: James, age 17; Darla, age 14

A checklist of Mr. Coleman's prior medical history indicates the following:

____Kidney disease	____Nervous and mental
____Heart disease	____Diabetes
____Hypertension	____Thyroid dysfunction
____Rheumatic fever	____Phlebitis, varicosities
____TB	____Epilepsy
____VD	____Drug sensitivity
____Gyn disorder	__X__Allergies: hay fever
__X__German measles: age 6	____Blood dyscrasia
____Rh, ABO sensitivity	____Blood transfusions
__X__Mumps	__X__Operations, accidents: T&A, age 8;
__X__Chicken pox	broken leg, age 15
____Measles	

You and Mr. Coleman engage in the following dialogue.

You: Good afternoon, Mr. Coleman. Please have a seat. (Mr. Coleman sits in the chair in front of your desk.) Can you tell me what brings you here?

Mr. C: Well, my wife I guess. I feel fine but she's been after me for awhile to come and see you. (Hesitates) About 6 weeks ago while we were getting ready for bed both of us were in the bathroom, and she noticed that there was blood in the toilet when I urinated. The next morning it was clear and I felt fine, but she's been worried about it. (Hesitates again) I noticed blood in my urine once before that, maybe 3 months ago. It was the same sort of thing: you know, clear the next day. I didn't tell my wife about it that time.

- *What are five possible diagnoses, in reasonable order of probability, based on the information Mr. Coleman has given you?*
- *What further questions will you want to ask Mr. Coleman to better characterize his symptoms?*

You: Was the entire stream bloody, do you remember?

Mr. C: Yes, I think so, on both occasions.

You: When during urination did you notice blood in the stream?

Mr. C: Oh, right away. I noticed it right away, and it stayed bloody until I finished.

You: Have you experienced any pain or burning or other discomfort at any time while urinating?

Mr. C: None whatsoever!

You: Have you noticed any interruption of your stream whenever you void or any change in the force of the stream?

Mr. C: No.

You: Has frequency of urination changed at all?

Mr. C: No, not that I've noticed.

You: After you've finished voiding and closed up your trousers, do you ever notice that you've wet yourself a little bit?

Mr. C: No.

You: Do you ever get up at night to urinate?

Mr. C: Once in awhile, if I've had a few beers or a lot of coffee. No more now than in the past several years, though.

You: How many times will you have to get up in a night?

Mr. C: Oh, just once.

You: Have you had any back pain?

Mr. C: No.

You: Any kidney trouble of any sort? Or has anyone in your family had kidney trouble?

Mr. C: No.

You: Have you experienced any injuries to your back or side or abdomen in the last 3 months? Any trauma at all?

Mr. C: No.

You: Is there anything that you can think of that happened that might be related to the blood on either occasion?

Mr. C: Can't think of anything.

You: Do you have sickle cell disease?

Mr. C: Not that I know about.

- *Mr. Coleman's family and social history and review of systems are non-contributory. What possible diagnoses are you considering, and why are you considering them, based on information obtained thus far?*
- *What would you look for on physical examination to help confirm or rule out your possible diagnoses?*

Physical examination findings are within normal limits: external genitalia normal; rectal, bulbocavernosus reflex normal; prostate gland enlarged to grade I but benign.

Office laboratory data tests show no abnormalities in CBC or differential data.

Urinalysis shows 5 to 10 RBC per high-power field and 1 to 2 WBC per high-power field. Other values normal.

- *Based on the information you now have, give a differential diagnosis and present a diagnostic methodology. Are there any further diagnostic tests you would use to evaluate Mr. Coleman's condition? For each test you list, give a justification and describe the procedure; state what you hope to learn from each test ordered.*

You explain to Mr. Coleman that the results of the excretory urogram and excretory cystogram suggest that he probably has a bladder tumor. You would like to refer him to a urologist, who will probably admit him to a hospital for an excisional biopsy for the purpose of confirming the diagnosis and determining the stage of the tumor. Cure depends on the grade and stage of the tumor. Mr. Coleman asks what you mean by grading and "staging" and why curing him depends on this.

- *How would you explain these terms and implications for prognosis in language understandable to an educated layperson?*

Mr. Coleman also states that he does not know what an excisional biopsy is and asks for a straightforward assessment of the seriousness of his condition.

- *How would you answer these questions?*

Mr. Coleman concedes you are probably justified in wanting to refer him to a urologist who will probably hospitalize him for testing. He is scheduled to be admitted the following Monday, February 24.

Late Monday afternoon you visit Mr. Coleman in the hospital. He is doing well and is anxious to know the results of his tests.

By 5:00 PM the following test results are available.

Sickledex: negative
Repeat urinalysis: Unchanged since done in office; sample reserved for culture (including TB), sensitivity, and cytology
Residual urine: 30 ml
Urinary cytology: Strongly suggestive of malignant cells
Excretory urogram: Upper urinary tracts normal
Excretory cystogram: Filling defect seen in right side of bladder, without any evidence of ureteral obstruction.

On Tuesday morning, you receive urine culture and sensitivity reports showing normal results.

- *Revise your differential diagnosis. Give an explanation for dropping any possible diagnoses considered earlier or for adding any new possibilities.*
- *Are any further diagnostic tests needed to confirm a diagnosis? If so state what they are and explain what results you expect.*

You schedule Mr. Coleman for cystoscopic examination on Wednesday, February 26, at 7:30 AM. At that time an area of the bladder is removed, biopsied, and identified as grade 1, stage A transitional cell epithelioma.

- *What prognosis would you expect for Mr. Coleman; what sort of follow-up is indicated?*

Later, when Mr. Coleman is out from under the anesthetic, he is very concerned. You listen while the urologist tells him the results of the cystoscopic examination and surgery and assure him that the survival rate for this type of bladder cancer is very high (the 5-year survival rate for the type he had is 90 percent). Mr. Coleman is visibly relieved and admits that "he was pretty scared."

- *What is your final diagnosis(es)? Be sure to include plans for discharge and long-term follow-up.*

Author's comment. The key to the correct diagnosis in this patient management problem is in recognizing that gross, total, painless hematuria in a 54-year-old man, in the absence of any other genitourinary tract symptoms, is most likely caused by bladder cancer. A second choice for the etiology of the bleeding should be benign prostatic hyperplasia. Although other strong possibilities also exist to explain the hematuria, the likelihood of bladder cancer being the existing condition absolutely mandates that an excretory urogram and cystoscopy be carried out. The excretory cystogram phase of the excretory urogram is frequently adequate to make the diagnosis of bladder tumor, but such a patient should always be referred to a urologist for cystoscopic evaluation. See Chapter 6 for answers to this exercise.

EXERCISE NO. 6

You are a young physician working in a clinic for migrant workers. One of the many patients who have come to the clinic today is a young Mexican-American, Julio Sanchez. He states his age as 18, although you suspect he is close to 3 years younger. He voices his complaint: "Hey, Doc, it hurts when I pee!"

- *What are five possible diagnoses that could account for Julio's problem? For each possibility, list pertinent questions you will ask Julio in taking a history and the kinds of diagnostic procedures you would use to rule out or confirm it.*
- *How will you determine when taking a history whether Julio understands the usual medical nomenclature or requires less technical language?*

Julio understands the terms penis and testicles, although he uses different words for both. He is not familiar with other technical terms like urethra, prostate gland, and glans, but it is easy to communicate with him as long as you keep your language very simple.

Julio gives you the following information. He, his father, mother, and five siblings have been in the area about 2½ years. They live in a four-room cottage in the same area as the other farm workers. Julio is the fourth of eight children, two of whom have left home. Julio is supposed to be in school, but he only goes sporadically. Sometimes he works with his parents, and sometimes he just "hangs around." He drinks alcohol and smokes "pot" sometimes, but does not use any other drugs. He remembers having pneumonia when he was little (about 6 or 7 years old) and was hospitalized. Otherwise, he has been healthy and has not seen a doctor for anything. About 3 days ago he first noticed a slight burning sensation on urination. For the last 2 days the burning has gotten worse, and he has noticed a purulent yellowish discharge from the urethral meatus.

Julio has said nothing to his parents about this, though he is not sure why. He responds positively when you ask him if he feels embarrassed about discussing these kinds of things, but says: "I can't talk to my father, but it's OK to tell you."

In response to questions about his sexual behavior, Julio tells you that the first he ever "did it" was about 6 months ago when he was apparently seduced by an older woman he met in the park one day. He never saw her again. More recently he has been "making it" with a girl he met about 2 weeks ago. He has used no contraception and does not know if the girl did.

Julio has no known allergies and is on no current medications. Review of systems reveals no abnormalities other than the present complaint. Other items of the history were noncontributory.

Before you physically examine Julio, your nurse takes urine and blood samples for urinalysis and CBC, and you take a smear of the discharge material from the urethral meatus for staining and microscopic examination.

Physical examination reveals no physical abormalities, with the exception of numerous dental caries, a possible need for corrective glasses, and the urethral inflammation and discharge noted previously.

Results from the laboratory were as follows:

CBC

HGB: 16 g/100 ml
PCV: 49 vol%
RBC: 5.9 million/mm³
WBC: 8000/mm³
Diff.: Stabs 2%, segs 61%, lymphs 30%, monos 4%, eos 3%

Urinalysis

Color: Deep yellow
pH: 6
Spec. grav.: 1.021
WBC: 4–5 per high-power field
RBC: 0–2 per high-power field

Microscopic report of urethral discharge smear showed numerous pus cells with intra- and extracellular gram-negative diplococci.

- *Write a differential diagnosis with assessment and plan.*

You have diagnosed acute gonorrhea and, after double-checking to discern that he has no known penicillin allergy, prescribe 4.8 million units of aqueous penicillin given intramuscularly with 1 g of probenecid given orally. You ask Julio to come back for a checkup in a week. You tell him to refrain from intercourse during this time, explaining to him simply your diagnosis and reasoning. Because the girl mentioned previously is probably infected, you ask him to please have her come in for treatment as soon as possible. He has already indicated to you that he knows very little about contraception. He now says: "You know, Doc, I heard of rubbers, but I don't know where to get them or anything." After you discuss generally the various methods of contraception available, Julio asks you if he can get a condom from you and how it works.

- *How would you instruct Julio in the use of a condom?*

The day following Julio's visit, the girl he mentioned comes to the clinic to be treated. She has no idea where she picked up the disease, but gives you the names of three other youths with whom she has had contact. She tells you she is taking birth control pills that her older sister got for her. She subsequently becomes your patient. Julio comes back for his scheduled checkup and is found to be infection free.

EXERCISE NO. 7

You are a pediatrician in private practice in a small southern town. You are talking with Mr. and Mrs. Johnson in your office regarding two of their three sons, whom you have just examined. The boys are in the waiting room examining various playthings. You tell the Johnsons that Greg, age 3, and Steven, age 9, are both in excellent physical condition and developing normally. (The oldest boy Michael is now 13, and you have not been his physician for about 3 years.)

The Johnsons are pleased to hear that their sons are healthy. Mr. Johnson rises to leave, but Mrs. Johnson hesitates as though she would like to say something. You encourage her to express her concern.

"Well, Doctor," she frets, "its' Steven. I've caught him playing with himself several times in the last 2 or 3 months." She pauses; you notice that Mr. Johnson looks surprised and embarrassed and quickly finds something to attract his attention on the street below the window. Mrs. Johnson continues: "We never had this kind of trouble with Michael, and I just don't know how to stop him." She looks at you uncomfortably, clearly wanting a response.

- *What kinds of things will you want to know before responding to Mr. and Mrs. Johnson? Include questions about the history of Steven's behavior as well as that of the other two boys and questions relating to the nature of the Johnsons' concerns and beliefs about masturbation.*

During the subsequent conversation Mrs. Johnson does most of the talking, occasionally asking Mr. Johnson if he agrees with something she has said. Mr. Johnson seems very unwilling to participate in the conversation.

Mrs. Johnson tells you that Steven is harder to understand than Michael. He is quieter and keeps to himself more. He doesn't like sports; Michael does. He does well enough in school, in fact has about an A average and reads a lot, but doesn't have as many friends. He seems to be kind of a stranger to them. Michael is very different. He, too, is a good student, but he is always doing something and isn't moody like Steven. He's just easy to get along with and always on the go. Mrs. Johnson says she has never had this kind of trouble with Michael. Twice she found Steven playing with himself in the bathtub and once lying in the grass in the back yard. She has told him that it is not good for him—she doesn't believe that it will make him crazy like some people used to think, but it certainly isn't nice or normal. Greg is still pretty much a baby, so there is no problem with him. He is pretty easy going, not as moody as Steven was when he was Greg's age. Greg is in nursery school 2 days a week and gets along fine with other kids. Mrs. Johnson is afraid that Greg will learn bad habits from Steven.

Mrs. Johnson tells you that there is a girl in the neighborhood whom Michael sometimes goes around with, but he doesn't have a girlfriend. She seems surprised and offended when you ask her if, to her knowledge, Michael is sexually active. Mr. Johnson continues to be quiet and uncomfortable throughout this conversation.

- *What detailed response would you give to Mr. and Mrs. Johnson? Consider the following in your response:*
    1. *The development of sexuality in childhood, adolescence, and early adulthood*
    2. *Changing views about masturbation*
- *Would the information you sought or your discussion of sexuality and masturbation have been different had the Johnsons had three girls? If so how?*

Author's comment. See Chapter 14 for answers to this exercise.

EXERCISE NO. 8

Hematuria, both microscopic and gross, can be divided into three diagnostically significant categories: initial, total, or terminal. The significance of each of these three categories of hematuria also depends on the age and sex of the patient.

On the chart on pp. 336 please list at least one likely etiology for each category of hematuria as it occurs in males and females of different ages. If you consider a certain type of hematuria to be totally inappropriate (for example, initial hematuria in a neonate), state this. Further, explain the significance of the findings in terms of the pathology, pathophysiology, or both, and possible treatment.

Please list the diagnostic tests you would perform, in order of importance, to determine the exact etiology of the hematuria in a given patient. Do this according to age and sex and the three categories of hematuria as listed. It is not necessary to do this for both microscopic and gross hematuria. Do it for gross hematuria (because this is the more likely symptom) but recognize that *any* condition causing gross hematuria can cause microscopic hematuria.

NOTE: In females the classification of initial, total, and terminal hematuria does not apply because it is very difficult to determine. This classification likewise does not apply to microscopic hematuria in males.

See Chapter 16 for answers to this exercise.

EXERCISE NO. 9

You are a pediatrician in a small northern city. On Wednesday, October 11, 1975, Mrs. Sloan brings her son Joey to see you. Joey is almost 8 years old and has been your patient for 3 years. Mrs. Sloan tells you that he has begun to wet the bed frequently, something he has not done since he was 4 years old.

- *What are five possible causes for enuresis in a child Joey's age? For each possibility, briefly indicate the procedure you will follow, including laboratory testing, to confirm or rule out that possibility.*

Your records contain the following information about Joey:

> *Patient:* Joseph Jeramie Sloan
> *Date of birth:* 12/7/67
> *Parents:* Susan R. and Donald B. Sloan
> *Siblings:* Brother (Jeffrey, born 1970; see separate file)
> *Address:* 2417 Pine Street
> *Phone:* 889–3725
> *Pregnancy/labor/birth:* Normal, no difficulties
> *Neonatal development:* Normal

Review of Joey's most recent visit tells you the following:

> *Date of visit:* 7/21/75
> *Chief complaint:* Routine physical
> *Nutrition:* Diet and appetite good, no deficiencies
> *Development:* Normal for size and age
> *Growth:* Height 4' 2½"; weight 67 lbs.
> *Habit disorders:* None
> *Review of systems:* No abnormalities
> *Physical examination:* Normal physical findings for size and age

As you talk with Mrs. Sloan about Joey's current problem, she tells you that she has noticed no particular change in appetite and no weight loss or excessive thirst. Joey is eating well, is active, and does not tire easily. He has not complained of any burning or discomfort on urination. This is confirmed by Joey. Neither of them has noted that Joey is troubled by frequency or urgency during the day.

Mrs. Sloan tells you that Joey tends to wet in the early part of the night. "He usually goes to bed before 9:30, and if he doesn't wet the bed before midnight he is likely to stay dry." He urinates before going to bed, and lately she has not been letting him have any milk or water after about 8:00 PM. Mrs. Sloan says that Joey wets three or four nights a week and that this began just before school started. She tells you also that she and her husband have been separated since the early part of August, and she thinks Joey is upset about it. She has filed for divorce. Joey is more affected then Jeffery because he is close to his dad. She thinks maybe Joey is being more aggressive with is brother and playmates than he used to be, but isn't sure if that is because he is getting older.

A review of systems reveals no changes or abnormalities other than bedwetting.

- *Given this additional information, are there any changes in your possible diagnoses and method of workup? For any possibilities you have ruled out, indicate why. For any new possibilities, list those cues that support them.*

You proceed with the physical examination and find no abnormalities. The following growth changes are noted.

Height: 4' 3"
Weight: 69½ lbs

You ask Mrs. Sloan to stop at the central laboratory in the medical arts building and have a blood count and urinalysis tests done on Joey, telling her that the nurse at the desk will give her the appropriate slips. You also ask her to set up an appointment for Friday afternoon, at which time you will run some tests to determine if there are any urinary abnormalities present.

On Friday when Mrs. Sloan and Joey return you have received the following results of the laboratory tests:

CBC

HBG: 13 g/100 ml
HCT: 39 vol%
RBC: 4.79 × 10⁶/mm³
WBC: 5000/mm³
Diff: Stabs 4%, segs 59%, monos 5%, lymphs 29%, eos 3%

At this time you perform an excretory urogram with a voiding cystourethrogram.

You tell Mrs. Sloan that happily you have found no physical abnormalities and that Joey is in excellent physical condition. Mrs. Sloan says in a stricken voice: "Does that mean that Joey needs a psychiatrist?"

- *How will you respond to Mrs. Sloan's concern?*
- *Write a differential diagnosis with assessment and plan.*

You tell Mrs. Sloan that it is entirely normal for many boys Joey's age to wet the bed occasionally, and most especially if they are under some kind of emotional stress. He will probably outgrow the bedwetting soon enough, and, although it is annoying, there is no cause for alarm. You tell Mrs. Sloan that you are going to

	Hematuria	Likely etiologies	Significance
Children (boys and girls)	Initial		
	Total		
	Terminal		
Women to age 40*	Initial		
	Total		
	Terminal		
Men to age 40	Initial		
	Total		
	Terminal		
Women 40 to 70 years of age*	Initial		
	Total		
	Terminal		
Men 40 to 70 years of age	Initial		
	Total		
	Terminal		

Continued.

	Hematuria	Likely etiologies	Significance
Women 70 years and older*	Initial		
	Total		
	Terminal		
Men 70 years and older	Initial		
	Total		
	Terminal		

*Although women theoretically can identify initial, total, and terminal hematuria, in practice this is extremely difficult.

prescribe a drug called Ditropan, (5 mg to be taken 1 hour before bedtime). Mrs. Sloan asks you what the drug does.

- *How would you answer Mrs. Sloan's question?*

Mrs. Sloan checks back with you a week later to report that the drug you prescribed seems to be having some positive effect. She asks how long Joey will need to continue taking the medicine and how long the bedwetting is likely to continue.

- *How will you respond to Mrs. Sloan's long-range concerns?*

Author's comment. See Chapter 5 for answers to this exercise.

EXERCISE NO. 10

On pages 338–339 is a six-column chart relative to intrascrotal problems. The first column, Conditions, list all problems that can cause intrascrotal palpatory findings. In the second column describe the palpatory findings for each condition you have listed. In column 3 list one or two principal aspects of the differential diagnosis for each condition listed. In column 4 give the significant laboratory findings (urine and blood) for each condition listed; if there are none, indicate so. In column 5 give the significant x-ray findings; if there are none, indicate so. In column 6 briefly state what treatment is indicated and under what circumstance(s); if there is none, indicate so.

See Chapter 11 for answers to this exercise.

Conditions	Description of palpatory findings	Differential diagnosis

EXERCISE NO. 11

You are a general practitioner in a suburban village. Your practice includes a variety of medical problems and a lot of physical examinations and "patch jobs" for the local high school athletic team. You have lived in this village for 10 years and know just about everybody. On August 25, 1975, Norma Haglund comes in for her annual physical examination. Norma, aged 31, and her two children, aged 6 and 3, have been your patients since they moved here 5 years ago. Norma teaches second grade in the local elementary school; she has been divorced since 1972.

Norma's medical history is as follows:

Significant lab findings (urine and blood)	Significant x-ray findings	Indicated treatment (list circumstances)

Name: Norma Haglund

Address: 1324 Dogwood Drive, Ada, Michigan

Phone: 676–5023

Date of birth: April 12, 1944

Children: Susan, Eric (see separate files)

Marital status: Divorced 1972

Occupation: Teacher, second grade, Ada Elementary School

Office visits: Sept. 2, 1970 (first visit)

Physical examination; all results within normal limits; pelvic and Pap smear normal. ℞: Ortho-Novum 1 mg, 12 mo.

Jan. 19, 1971
Sore throat; cultures positive for β-hemolytic streptococcal infection. R: Penicillin orally, 10 days.

Aug. 28, 1971
Physical examination: findings normal; pelvic and Pap
smear normal. R: Ortho-Novum 1 mg, 12 mo.

Nov. 20, 1971
Anxiety; marital problems. R: Valium 5 mg, 100 tablets,
refill once. Referral to counselor.

Mar. 3, 1972
Broken arm (simple fracture of radius). Simple
reduction.

Sept. 5, 1972
Physical examination: normal findings; pelvic and Pap
smear normal. R: Ortho-Novum 1 mg, 12 mo.

Aug. 26, 1973
Physical examination: all findings normal; pelvic and
Pap smear normal. R: Demulen 1 mg, 12 mo.

Dec. 10, 1973
Flu. R: Bed rest and fluids.

Aug. 30, 1974
Physical examination: all findings normal; pelvic and
Pap smear normal. R: Demulen, 12 mo.

You talk with Norma for a few minutes in your office. She tells you that she is feeling fine, is happy, and has no complaints. A quick review of systems reveals no changes or reported abnormalities.

Norma then goes into the examining room with your nurse, who takes Norma's vital signs and prepares her for examination. As you enter the examining room, you read Norma's vital signs as recorded by the nurse:

Weight: 122 lbs
Height: 5' 5"
Temperature: 98.5 F
Blood pressure: 180/110
Pulse: 80/min
Respiration: 18 breaths per min

You immediately again check Norma's blood pressure in both arms, getting the same value of 180/110. You know that Norma has been normotensive up to and including last year's physical examination.

- *What are five possible causes of Norma's hypertension?*
- *For each diagnostic possibility, what would you look for in the physical examination, and what diagnostic tests would you order to confirm or rule out that possibility?*

The results of the physical examination are as follows:

General appearance: No change since last visit
Head and neck: No masses in neck, no lymphadenopathy, no neck stiffness
Eyes: Pupils equal, round, react equally to light and accommodation; EOM
normal bilaterally; slight thickening of arterioles on fundoscopy

ENT: External ear skin clear, tympanic membranes normal, buccal and nasal mucosa normal; pharynx shows no abnormalities; tonsils present, not inflamed or enlarged; teeth in good repair

Chest and lungs: Normal to inspection, percussion, and auscultation; no masses or tenderness in breasts

Heart: Heart sounds normal, rhythm regular, no murmurs; PMI in fifth left intercostal space, 8 cm from midsternal line, inside midclavicular line

Abdomen: Soft, no masses or tenderness; liver and spleen not palpable; no rebound or CVA tenderness; normal bowel sounds; faint bruit heard over left side of abdomen anteriorly

Inguinal area and genitalia: No inguinal lymphadenopathy; external genitalia normal to inspection

Pelvic: Cervix and uterus normal in size and shape; no masses or tenderness; ovaries normal in size and shape

Musculoskeletal: Upper and lower limbs symmetrical and well nourished. Peripheral pulses present and symmetrical in the posterior popliteal, tibial, and dorsalis pedis arteries; no edema

Laboratory tests show the following:

CBC

HGB: 14.8 g/100 ml
PCV: 40 vol%
RBC: $5.2 \times 10^6/mm^3$
WBC: $7200/mm^3$
Diff.: Segs 61%, lymphs 32%, monos 5%, eos 2%

URINALYSIS

Color: Yellow
Spec. grav.: 1.020
pH: 5.8
RBC: 0–2 per high-power field
WBC: 0–2 per high-power field
Protein: Trace
Epithelial cells, casts, bacteria, crystals, or bile: None

- *With this new information, how would you revise your diagnostic possibilities? List them in order of likelihood. For any possibilities you discard, state why they are no longer appropriate. For any new ones you add, what information in the physical examination or laboratory data suggests them?*

The faint bruit heard over the left side of the abdomen suggests to you the possibility of a renal arterial lesion, certain types of which are sometimes seen in young women.

- *What diagnostic tests would you order to rule out or confirm this hypothesis?*

It is also possible that the adrenal gland could be playing a part in Norma's hypertension.

- *How can the adrenal gland cause this hypertension? Describe how you would determine whether the adrenal gland is etiologic in the disease process?*

Norma is admitted to the hospital on August 27 for testing of renal function. You first order an excretory urogram. The results, available the next day, show delay in function noted on left side, with diminished visualization of left kidney at 3 minutes. Left kidney 1.5 cm smaller than right kidney in longitudinal axis. Because an excretory urogram has never been done before on Norma, you have no basis on which to compare these results.

- *What would your differential diagnosis be, including assessment and plan? Include in your plan any further diagnostic testing that you feel is indicated.*

To further confirm your diagnosis, the following tests are indicated: Radioisotope renograms, renal scans, renal angiograms, renin collection, and serum aldosterone levels.

All of the studies tend to confirm that there is a decreased blood supply to the left kidney, based on a narrowing of the left renal artery.

Results of further testing show the following:

1. Radioisotope renograms and renal scans suggest a decreased uptake in the left side.
2. Renal angiogram shows a "beading" of the proximal left renal artery.
3. Renin collections from both kidneys confirm elevated renin from the left renal vein.
4. Aldosterone levels are within normal limits.

- *Based on this data, what is your definitive diagnosis? Support it with appropriate cues. How have test results ruled out other elements of the previous differential diagnosis?*
- *What is the physiologic mechanism by which narrowing of a renal artery may produce hypertension?*
- *What management is indicated to return the patient's blood pressure to a normal level?*

You request a urologic consultation, and Norma is scheduled for surgery on September 1. A saphenous vein bypass is successfully performed, and Norma recovers without postoperative complications.

- *Should Norma continue using birth control pills for contraception? Why or why not?*

One year postoperatively, Norma's blood pressure is down to 140/90.

Author's comment. The key to establishing the diagnosis of renovascular hypertension is in thinking of it and therefore in proceeding with diagnostic studies that will ultimately lead to the diagnosis. Presence of a bruit heard anteriorly or posteriorly over either renal area is helpful but not necessarily a constant finding or even diagnostic when it is present. The rapid-sequence excretory urogram is a good screening test for this condition, particularly if there is a delay in function on one side and if that kidney is smaller than the contralateral one. Renal angiography and renin collections from each renal vein are indicated if the excretory urogram is abnormal or occasionally in the presence of a normal excretory urogram when renovascular hypertension is strongly suspected. See Chapter 9 for answers to this exercise.

EXERCISE NO. 12

In the following exercise the sex and age of the physician have been defined so as to be consistent with the dynamics of the case. A similar situation might occur regardless of the sex of either patient or physician.

You are a young male physician in the student health center of a large university. This afternoon, September 25, 1975, Kenneth Stiles has come in requesting a physical examination. You ask him why he would like to be examined. He tells you that he does not have any particular problems but has not had an examination since his precollege exam over a year ago. He just thinks it is a good idea.

Kenneth's university health chart reads as follows:

Name:	Kenneth L. Stiles
Student no.:	572684
Date of birth:	6/14/1955
Local address:	204 N. Crowley Hall
Phone:	7-2684
Class:	Sophomore
Major:	Engineering
Medical information:	1/17/75, Dr. Thompson. Chief complaint: sore throat; temperature 102 F; culture and sensitivity studies show β-hemolytic streptococcus infection; sensitivity to penicillin G. ℞: ampicillin 500 mg. q.i.d./10 days

You proceed with a general history, review of systems, and physical examination, which are unremarkable until you begin to do a genital examination. When you examine Kenneth's penis and testes, you notice that Kenneth becomes visibly tense and uncomfortable. You find no physical abnormalities.

- *Do you think it is appropriate to investigate Kenneth's discomfort? If so, how would you pursue? If not, why?*

You decide it is appropriate to gently query Kenneth on his reaction and ask him if this part of the examination is making him uncomfortable. "A little, I guess" is his tense response. You then explain to him that the next part of the examination involves examining his prostate gland rectally, and you ask him if he has any concerns about it. "You don't have to do that, do you? I mean, I'm really not old enough to worry about that stuff, and my family doctor said he did that last year."

- *What would be your response to Kenneth?*

You decide to try to discover the cause of Kenneth's anxiety and to gently explore his feelings about his sexuality. How would you approach Kenneth about his discomfort and his sexuality?

- *Given what you know about Kenneth, what might you think are possible sources of his discomfort? List no more than three possibilities and possible ways to follow up on these.*

You complete the physical examination (omitting the rectal exam) and note no physical abnormalities. CBC and urinalysis are normal. Then you have the following conversation with Kenneth.

You: You seemed to be very uncomfortable when I examined your penis and testes. Can you tell me why?

Kenneth: I don't know. I guess I just don't like to be touched.

You: Does that affect your sex life?

Kenneth: Oh, no, not with girls; I don't mind women.

You: Would you mind telling me something about your sexual history?

Kenneth: No, guess not . . . (pause). I started screwing when I was 14, and I've been screwing ever since. I usually date a lot of women. Once

	in a while I get thick with one, but I think it's better with a lot of women.
You:	How often do you have intercourse?
Kenneth:	Oh, it varies—maybe ten times a week, sometimes more.
You:	How do you feel about masturbation?
Kenneth:	OK . . . but I'd rather screw!
You:	Have you ever had a sexual experience with a man?
Kenneth:	(Tenses visibly, looks down and doesn't say anything)
You:	(After a lengthy silence) It's hard for you to talk. Would you rather not?
Kenneth:	It's . . . well . . . (looks really stressed) I've never talked about it before. Kenneth goes on to tell you that he was molested by a friend of the family when he was about 11. He never told anyone about it. You ask him if he thinks he might want to see a counselor for awhile to talk about it now. He agrees, and you refer him to a mental health service.

Index